Great Expectations

A prospective study of women's expectations and experiences of childbirth

Josephine M. Green
Vanessa A. Coupland
Jenny V. Kitzinger

Books for Midwives Press
An imprint of Hochland and Hochland Ltd

Published by Books for Midwives Press, 174a Ashley Road, Hale, Cheshire, WA15 9SF, England.

Second edition

ISBN 1 898507 58 9

British Library Cataloguing in Publication Data
A catalogue record for this book is available from the British Library

Printed in Great Britain

Contents

Volume II

Acknowledgements

We are very grateful to the Health Promotion Research Trust and the Nuffield Provincial Hospitals Trust for funding this project. We are also grateful to the grant holders: Dr M.P.M. Richards, Mr M.J. Hare and Dr D.R.R. Williams for their continued advice and support.

A very large number of people have contributed to the work reported here: midwifery staff and consultants gave us their cooperation in setting up the study, midwives and ward clerks helped us to contact participants.

The participants themselves – 825 pregnant women – were, of course, vital to the research, and we would like to thank them for their willingness to share their pregnancies and labours with us.

We could not have analysed the vast amounts of data had it not been for our dedicated data coders, particularly Jane Elliott and Jon Lawrence.

Special thanks are due to Dr Brendan Burchell, our computer consultant, whose statistical and computing expertise were tirelessly given and quite invaluable.

As ever, last but never least, we are deeply indebted to Jill Brown for her secretarial support throughout this project and to Sally Roberts for the patience and skill with which she has typed (retyped and improved!) the contents of this report through all its metamorphoses.

Preface to the Second Edition

This book represents the first commercial publication of the research study known as *Great Expectations*, previously only available as an internal publication by the Centre for Family Research (formerly Child Care and Development Group) at the University of Cambridge, UK. This volume contains all the material of the original two volumes, plus an additional chapter written especially for this book. The function of the new chapter is both to present new data and to revisit some of the original findings in the light of subsequent research. The new data include both multivariate analyses of the original data and findings from a second study which asked a number of the same questions of a larger sample of women. No substantive changes have been made to the original chapters. However, those results which are developed further in Chapter 10 are indicated in the text. The appendices, which include all the questionnaires developed for the study, have not been included in this volume. They may, however, be purchased separately from the publishers. A list of the contents of the appendices can to be found at the end of the book.

The team who carried out the original study consisted of Vanessa Coupland, Jenny Kitzinger and myself. After the funding for the study ended, Vanessa left academia in favour of social work, and is now in New Zealand. Jenny joined the Media Research Unit at Glasgow University, where her research career has flourished. Only I stayed in Cambridge, continuing to work with Martin Richards, who had been the original instigator of the *Great Expectations* project. We were awarded a further grant by the Health Promotion Research Trust, co-funder of *Great Expectations*, to examine the effects on pregnant women of routine screening for fetal abnormalities. This became the Cambridge Prenatal Screening Study. Once again, I was fortunate to have two superb co-workers, Helen Statham and Claire Snowdon. The CPSS, which is described in Chapter 10, was used as a vehicle for re-examining some of the points that had arisen in *Great Expectations*. Many of its findings have been published (see list of publications), but some are presented here for the first time. In 1994, the Health Promotion Research Trust, which had only ever been intended as a short-term venture, was being wound down. I was invited to bid for its last £20,000. I requested the opportunity to employ a research assistant with expertise in multivariate statistical techniques who could work with both the *Great Expectations* and CPSS data sets to try and help me to resolve some of the mass of information that these two studies had generated. My bid was successful and in June 1995 Kostas Kafetsios joined the team. The new results which appear in Chapter 10 are Kostas' invaluable contribution. Finally, in October 1996, I too left Cambridge to join Mary Renfrew in building up a new maternity-related research group at the University of Leeds. My new colleagues have been wonderfully supportive, and I would like particularly to acknowledge the cheerful assistance of John Berry in literature searching and obtaining hard-to-find reprints.

Josephine M Green
Leeds, July 1997

Introduction

For many years there has been a broadly held view that many women prefer to hand over responsibility for their care to the professionals who are looking after them and do not wish to take an active part in planning their care or making decisions about it. Alongside this view is a growing acceptance that other women will want to be fully informed and in control of their care. These are usually thought to be better educated, more articulate and, by definition, middle-class women.

Anecdotal evidence about the fate of this latter group tends to surface at conferences and debates about maternity care. So well-informed are these women, so keen are they to do well and for things to go according to plan that, so the story goes, disillusionment and disappointment almost inevitably await them.

In 1987 Jo Green and colleagues set out to establish whether these commonly held views reflected the way that women felt. How did they feel about the issues of choice and control? Were they important to the majority of women? Did class and educational background influence the way they felt? Did women with 'Great Expectations' feel better or worse about their experiences than women whose expectations were low or even non-existent?

The results of this study focus on women's responses to these questions and should be required reading for all involved in maternity care. This is the study to turn to if you are ever tempted to make decisions about maternity care in the genuine – but often mistaken – belief that women want decision making to be in the hands of the professionals.

The book addresses the issue of control in some detail. Teasing through its many pages an interesting and subtle picture emerges. Being in control doesn't seem to mean that women want to be asked and informed about every single test, procedure and intervention. What it does seem to mean is that women feel in control when they trust that the person caring for them will respond positively should they say that they wish their care to be arranged or altered in a particular way.

The findings of this study have already influenced policy for maternity services in this country. The Select Committee on Health (1992) received evidence from the researchers and this is evident in the Committee's final report. *Changing Childbirth* echoed many of the central messages of the study. The decision to publish this work in an extended form is extremely timely. Professionals are increasingly keen to base their practice and beliefs on firm evidence and this study gives them exactly that.

Jo Green and colleagues are to be congratulated on this gem of a study. Firstly for showing so clearly how research can be used to explore, and in this case explode, the myths that can build up around an issue as complex and emotive as maternity care. Secondly for acting as an inspiration to the many researchers who must often ask whether their work will ever really affect practice, and finally for the objectivity of their work which makes their results even more powerful.

Kate Jackson OBE
Former Director of The Changing Childbirth Implementation Team

Volume I

CHAPTER ONE

The Research in Context

Introduction

Childbirth is a means to an end, the ultimate fulfilment of a woman's role, an agony to be endured, the most dangerous journey of anyone's life, a joyous and fulfilling experience in its own right and so the list goes on. To any one woman it may be any, all or none of these things and her experiences may or may not conform to her expectations.

Those expectations are likely to have been derived from her own previous experiences, from what she has heard from other women, from television, magazines, doctors, antenatal classes and more generally from her cultural background. Women must surely have always had expectations of some sort about the experience of childbirth but advances in obstetric analgesia and subsequent pharmaceutical and technological developments have added many more parameters and choice points to the process. Thus discussion of 'expectations' of childbirth nowadays generally relates to pain or obstetric interventions, and the extent to which choices will be made by the woman herself or by her medical attendants.

A central debate revolves around the twin issues of natural childbirth and control. On one side critics have argued against the medical monopoly over childbirth and have emphasized a woman's right to a fulfilling experience of childbirth and to maintain control over her own body. In particular they have challenged any unquestioning or routine use of interventions and more generally the medical management of labour. On the other side some obstetricians have argued that childbirth today is safer than it has ever been thanks precisely to the increased medicalization of the process and the use of modern technology. According to this view all women have to do is to follow the advice of the experts.

The clash of these two perspectives has led to various disturbing cases in recent years such as the precedent of the first application for a court order in Britain to force a woman to have a caesarean section against her will (Antenna, 17th February 1988, Channel 4) and the suspension of a consultant obstetrician on the grounds of alleged incompetence (Savage, 1986).

Concern has been voiced (from both sides) that whilst increasing women's choice and control in childbirth is potentially very positive, it may also have negative effects. In particular, it is argued that women, especially primiparous women, may now have unrealistic expectations both regarding the amount of choice and control available to them in any one hospital, and about childbirth itself. The National Childbirth Trust (NCT), for example, has been singled out for criticism by many doctors, midwives and some mothers for apparently fostering just such unrealistically high expectations among its clients.

This report documents a study which explored women's expectations and experiences of childbirth and their subsequent satisfaction or dissatisfaction, mood and feelings about their babies. We have tried to consider a wide range of factors which might be important to women, in particular the many different ways in which the concepts of choice and control might be interpreted. These possibilities will be discussed later in this chapter but first we will place our research in the context of other research which has looked at women's experience of childbirth and the factors which may predict and mediate it. We will then go on to consider the relevance of our focus on choice and control, and finally we will look at certain stereotypes of women that appear in debates about childbirth.

Literature review

The general context

Since the mid 1970s there has been increasing concern on the part of organizations such as AIMS (Association for Improvements in Maternity Services) and the NCT, as well as among some professionals, about the medicalization of childbirth. The focus of the concern has mainly been the use of routine interventions in labour, the scientific validity of which remains unestablished (Lumley and Astbury, 1980). However concepts such as the active management of labour and the desirability of hospital birth for low risk women have also been questioned. Consequently, some women have become much more questioning of the necessity of intervention, and more assertive and confident in their ability to make decisions for themselves, particularly in normal labours. This has been accompanied by a popular literature on the modern experience of childbirth which has increasingly focused attention on issues of medical control and decision making, sometimes from a feminist perspective (Arms, 1975; Haire, 1978; Kitzinger, 1987a; Oakley, 1980; Riley, 1977). It has also prompted a number of studies of women's knowledge and experience of obstetric techniques. Cartwright (1977, 1979), for example, carried out a much quoted study on induction, Kitzinger has looked at epidurals (1987b), induction (1978) and Kitzinger and Walters have looked at episiotomies (1981), whilst others have examined the experience of fetal monitoring (Garcia et al., 1985; Molfese et al., 1982) and caesarean section (Affonso and Stichler, 1978; Bradley et al., 1983). There has, in addition, been a growing recognition of the importance of women's expectations as determinants of their reactions to the experience of childbirth.

We are not going to present a comprehensive review of this large body of literature, but we will describe briefly those findings which are particularly relevant to expectations and psychological outcomes. Inevitably we find that many of these expectations relate to the experience of pain. We will therefore begin by looking at some findings in this area before focusing on some of the independent variables which appear to be related to expectations of childbirth.

Pain and pain relief

Since the mid-nineteenth century when ether and chloroform were first introduced into obstetrics, the main concern for many, maybe most, women, and indeed staff, has been the alleviation or even complete removal of the pain of childbirth with pain-relieving drugs. However, the advent of natural childbirth and psychoprophylactic techniques which have appealed to some, mainly middle class, women has enabled such women to feel that they can control the pain themselves without resorting to medically prescribed drugs. Arney and Neill (1984) describe how obstetrics has responded to the challenge posed by the natural childbirth movement. They show how the medical profession now takes account of the subjective experience of pain and argue that the understanding of pain in childbirth has changed:

> 'Pain is no longer something which necessarily must be obliterated. It is now something to be appreciated, understood, worked through, and above all managed in order to ensure an optimal childbirth experience.'

However, researchers have paid relatively little attention to the subjective nature of pain. Nettelbladt et al. (1976), reviewing the field in the mid 1970s, found only a few studies which examined the importance of psychological factors in the experience of childbirth pain (although there has been more work since then). In their own prospective study, involving a sample of 78 middle class primiparous women (primips), Nettelbladt et al. (1976) found that pain was associated with the desirability of the pregnancy, as well as with ambivalence about motherhood, anxiety about childbirth pain and lower educational levels.

Also important was the inability to control behaviour during contractions and inadequate support from the midwives. They concluded that women's past experiences and present situations influence the experience of pain in childbirth.

In a study of 104 mainly working class women in Scotland, Niven and Gijsbers (1984) also found that pain was related to the desirability of the pregnancy as well as to expectations of labour and the stressfullness of birth; unfortunately they do not define what is meant by 'stressfullness'. Importantly, they found that lower levels of pain were associated with positive, but presumably realistic, expectations of labour, while women with 'unrealistically high expectations' about pain and their ability to cope with it reported strong negative reactions postnatally. Such women had apparently expected labour to be 'virtually painless' but it should be noted that this study was retrospective and did not ask about expectations until after the event. They also reported that the intensity of labour pain was related to a number of obstetric factors: parity, duration of the second stage and artificial rupture of the membranes, although other studies (Nettelbladt et al., 1976) failed to find such relationships.

Morgan looked at women's experience of the effectiveness of and satisfaction with pain relief in labour (Morgan, 1982; Morgan et al., 1982a, 1982b). A retrospective study of 1000 women who gave birth at a London teaching hospital was carried out. Epidurals were offered to everyone for whom they were not contraindicated. The assumption of the midwives seemed to be that women would choose the promise of a painless labour and the authors describe the fact that only just over half of the women chose an epidural as 'curious' (1982a). Pain relief was greatest in the epidural group, but this group also had a much higher incidence of assisted delivery and longer labours. However, the same proportion of women had 'as much pain as they expected' (70–72%) whatever method of pain relief they experienced. By contrast, Woollet et al. (1983) found that two thirds of their sample of working class women said that they had experienced more pain than expected. Morgan (1982) found little relationship between pain scores and satisfaction with childbirth. On the contrary, 16 per cent of women who had epidurals and no other medication were dissatisfied compared to 8 per cent who had no analgesia at all, despite the fact that the epidural group had the lowest pain scores and the no analgesia group the highest. Dissatisfaction related more to assisted delivery (see also McIntosh, 1986).

Although Morgan and her colleagues obtained interesting results, the work is subject to all the problems of retrospective research, as well as some confusion as to what constitutes expectation (see critique in Editorial of the *Bulletin of the Society for Reproductive and Infant Psychology*, 1983).

The effects of preparation for childbirth

Before going on to report research which has looked at the effects of childbirth preparation, it is important to point out that such research must be viewed with caution because of consistent methodological shortcomings (Clark, 1986). There is a fairly large amount of research on the effects of childbirth preparation, most of which is American and limited to small middle class, well-educated and non-random samples.

Lumley and Astbury (1980) highlight the dangers of attempting to compare the results of different studies which look at the outcome of 'antenatal preparation' and 'childbirth preparation' classes. Problems include varying definitions and types of antenatal preparation, varying definitions of the obstetric complications used as outcome measures, changes over short periods of time in the management of labour and non-comparable populations. Beck and Hall (1978), in a review and critique of studies of the effectiveness of psychoprophylaxis, conclude that methodological errors in research design compromise and in some cases invalidate research results. They stress the importance of random allocation to experimental and control groups and the desirability of a group of controls receiving an attention-placebo treatment. Very rarely have studies on childbirth preparation met such rigorous standards of research design (for exceptions, see Astbury, 1980; Timm, 1979).

Effects of preparation on pain

Several not very comparable studies report lower levels of pain in labour for women who have attended childbirth preparation classes. Brewin and Bradley (1982) in their study concluded that this was because trained women had greater perceived control over the process of labour. Charles et al. (1978) carried out a retrospective study of 95 prepared (i.e. trained) and 154 unprepared American women of mixed parity. They developed an overall pain scale reflecting the intensity and duration of pain during labour, transition and delivery, and also an equivalent enjoyment scale. The two scales were independent and not highly correlated. The prepared women in their study had significantly lower levels of pain, higher levels of enjoyment and greater effective control of pain than did the controls.

The differences between the groups were not explained by differences in parity, socio-economic status and psychological attitudinal characteristics. In a retrospective study of 104 mainly working class women, Niven and Gijsbers (1984) found an association between attendance at antenatal classes and lower levels of affective pain i.e. the qualitative, subjective aspects of how pain is experienced such as with fear or dread. Tanzer (1972), in a small study, found that controlling for parity, trained women reported less pain than did untrained women.

However, other studies do not find an association between childbirth preparation and reported pain (Davenport-Slack and Boylan, 1974; Melzack et al., 1981; Bennet et al., 1985; Clark, 1986).

Other effects of childbirth preparation

While some early studies reported shorter labours and fewer obstetrical complications, more recent work gives evidence that the length of labour and incidence of complications is unrelated to childbirth education (see summaries by Lumley and Astbury, 1980; Jones and Dougherty, 1984; Clark, 1986).

One consistent finding is that women trained in childbirth education use less analgesia and anaesthesia than untrained women (Enkin et al., 1972; Huttel et al., 1972; Doering and Entwisle, 1975; Charles et al., 1978; Timm, 1979; Bennett et al., 1985; Clark, 1986). Reported psychological benefits include lower levels of pain, increased satisfaction with birth, increased self-esteem and decreased postpartum depression (Enkin et al., 1972; Huttel, et al., 1972; Tanzer, 1972; Doering and Entwisle, 1975; Davenport-Slack and Boylan, 1974; Charles et al., 1978).

Several studies have highlighted the importance of control and active participation in childbirth and concluded that maintaining such control is indeed one of the benefits of childbirth preparation (Huttel et al., 1972; Davenport-Slack and Boylan, 1974; Willmuth, 1978; Clark, 1986). Felton and Segelman (1978) carried out a small prospective study which examined the extent to which Lamaze training brought about changes in mothers' (and fathers') perceptions of being in control. They compared three groups: one with Lamaze training, one with Red Cross training and one who had attended no classes. Red Cross classes teach the physiology of childbirth and babycare. Before birth, none of the women felt in control with regard to possible unexpected events during labour and delivery but Lamaze trained women felt confident they would be able to control their own bodies. However, after birth, Lamaze trained women were significantly more likely to see themselves as 'control agents', i.e. as having been in control. To a lesser extent women who attended Red Cross classes saw themselves in control (these classes put less emphasis on active participation in childbirth than Lamaze classes do).

In another retrospective study on the effects of childbirth preparation, Doering and Entwisle (1975) interviewed 269 middle class women of mixed parity nine weeks after delivery. Different degrees of preparation for childbirth and knowledge about childbirth were taken into consideration, from attendance at Lamaze classes down to no preparation of any kind. Each degree of preparation was associated with more awareness at delivery (in terms of the amount of medication used) and awareness in turn was significantly associated with positive attitudes to the birth and to the baby. Awareness was interpreted by the authors to mean retention of control in labour. They concluded that even minimal training (i.e. just concerning the physiology of labour and delivery) is worthwhile and produces positive results.

Other research on the benefits of preparation has focused on intervention rather than psychological factors. For example, in a large but retrospective British study Jones and Dougherty (1984) tested the hypothesis that attendance by low-risk women at hospital antenatal classes and clinics is associated with 'patterns of intervention which tend towards natural childbirth'. The aspects of natural childbirth tested for were: spontaneous onset, no augmentation, no analgesia or anaesthesia, normal delivery, high Apgar score and baby breastfed. Only breastfeeding was significantly and independently associated with antenatal class attendance.

Motivation

It may be asked whether it is the motivation to attend classes rather than the preparation itself which is important. A person who chooses childbirth preparation classes might be the same type of person who perceives childbirth positively and copes well with the pain.

Huttel et al. (1972) carried out a randomized controlled trial of 72 women in a part of West Germany where the psychoprophylactic method of childbirth preparation was unknown. Primiparous women were randomly assigned to a childbirth preparation treatment group, or to a control group which did not receive training. Women in the treatment group who did not attend at least four of the five offered classes were excluded from the study, as was anyone who gave birth by caesarean section. Prepared women used significantly less medication than the control group, were observed to have more self-control during labour and delivery, had more positive attitudes towards future pregnancies and were less depressed in the week following delivery. Although this study is more sophisticated than most others in this field, Beck and Hall (1978) point out that the much higher attrition rate in the treatment group (28% versus 7%) suggests that the two groups may have differed from each other in several important ways which could confound the results.

Enkin et al. (1972) compared three groups of women matched for age and parity. The women were not randomly assigned to groups. The first group received psychoprophylactic training, the second group were too late in their applications to receive training and the third did not request or receive training. The trained group required significantly less medication than the other two, rated the experience of labour and delivery more positively and rated themselves as less depressed following delivery. However, although this was an attempt to consider the effects of motivation, the group who applied late for training may have done so precisely because they were not as highly motivated as the group who applied earlier.

In a third study by Timm (1979), 118 low-income women were randomly assigned to one of three groups – antenatal hospital classes, an attention-placebo knitting group, and a no-treatment control group – along the lines of the three-group principle recommended by Beck and Hall (1978). Women were excluded from participation in the study if they had attended or planned to attend an antenatal class, and in this way Timm controlled for motivation to attend classes. The women who attended antenatal classes used significantly smaller amounts of medication than the other groups.

The results of these studies, whilst not conclusive, would seem to show that preparation may indeed be the key factor rather than motivation to attend classes *per se*.

Social class

Social class is a major confounding factor in studies of childbirth preparation classes. Most women who undergo training, particularly the more specific NCT or Lamaze-type training, are middle class and consequently most of the studies are of middle class women. Nelson (1982, 1983) criticizes much of the childbirth preparation literature for ignoring social class differences in what women want, expect and get out of childbirth. She attributes this to the wholesale adoption by researchers of a middle class model of childbirth which 'assumes that the outcome of preparation – knowledge, control, cooperation and an avoidance of medication – are definite, clearcut and desirable'. Her data suggest that working class women in fact do not view such outcomes as benefits and have very different ideas about childbirth. In her study, preparation for birth made little difference to the attitudes of middle class women, but a great deal of difference to those of working class women. Their attitudes converged with those of the middle class group. We will discuss this study further in a later section.

Satisfaction with childbirth

A number of factors in addition to childbirth preparation have been found to be associated with satisfaction with childbirth, or with what generally seems to be called 'a more positive birth experience'. Norr et al. (1977) and Clark (1986) found an inverse relationship between satisfaction and use of medication/anaesthesia, whilst difficult delivery or forceps delivery has been linked to dissatisfaction (Norr et al., 1977; Nordholm and Muhler, 1981) as have birth complications (Clark, 1986).

Satisfaction has been linked positively to a partner being present during labour and delivery (Davenport-Slack and Boylan, 1974; Norr et al., 1977; Bennett et al., 1985; Clark, 1986) and women's participation in and control over the process of childbirth (Davenport-Slack and Boylan, 1974; Norr et al., 1977; Clark, 1986). However, these findings have not necessarily been confirmed by other studies.

In a large retrospective English study, Jacoby (1987) found that women's views about the way their labours were managed were clearly related to the procedures they experienced. They were most likely to be dissatisfied if they experienced a procedure which they preferred not to have. However, with regard to anaesthesia, women were more likely to be dissatisfied if they wanted an anaesthetic but did not get one.

The emphasis on pain and pain control by both women and staff carries with it the assumption that the less painful birth is, the more satisfied women will be. Clark's (1986) study provides partial evidence for this. However, as we saw above, this was not what Morgan (1982) found and other studies have also failed to demonstrate such a relationship (Davenport-Slack and Boylan, 1974; Willmuth, 1978). Humenick (1981) pointed to this apparent lack of relationship between reported pain and satisfaction with the childbirth experience and argued that the 'key' to satisfaction is not pain management but control or 'mastery' in childbirth. In the mastery model, pain management is only one of several factors which can influence satisfaction. Increased mastery is hypothesized to be attainable through the assertive, self-reliant behaviour encouraged in preparation classes.

Humenick and Bugen (1981) tested this hypothesis with a group of 33 well-educated primips who attended Lamaze classes. Women's prenatal attitudes towards childbirth participation and their psychological characteristics were evaluated at the end of training and their childbirth experiences at three weeks postpartum. Some support for the mastery model was found: assertion, independence and decisiveness increased postnatally and were significantly related to women's perceived participation in birth.

They concluded that women may not want much pain relief and will want to rely on their own resources because of the importance to them of maintaining control. However, they themselves acknowledge that their study has many problems making it difficult to generalize the results; the sample was not random but a highly motivated and selected group, there was no control group and the sample was very small. Also, while the mastery model was set up as an alternative to the model of pain management as a key to satisfaction in childbirth, they did not in fact compare the two models by looking at pain itself in their sample, nor, most curiously, did they attempt any direct measure of satisfaction. Their 'Labour/Delivery Evaluation Scale', which might have been seen as an indication of satisfaction, did not in fact correlate significantly with increased assertion, independence and decisiveness.

The measurement of satisfaction

A number of authors (Oakley, 1983; Zastowny et al., 1983; Lumley, 1985) have drawn attention to the difficulties inherent in measuring satisfaction. Firstly there is the well known tendency of women to feel relieved, grateful and generally positive after the safe delivery of a healthy child (Riley, 1977), and to be 'loyal' to their own birth (Shearer, 1983). It thus requires a sensitive measure to detect any elements of dissatisfaction which co-exist with such feelings, and which will avoid problems of ceiling effects. In addition, women appear to feel the need to rationalize adverse experiences, thus making dissatisfaction still more difficult to detect.

Other difficulties include the fact that the assessment of satisfaction is often made while the woman is still in hospital. She may, therefore, perceive the person carrying out the assessment as connected to the hospital and not want to say anything that may offend or seem critical. Questions are generally closed, allowing little scope for the expression of subtle feelings. In many cases it is questionable whether it is really 'satisfaction' that is being tapped at all. A recent paper by Lomas et al. (1987) proposes a new measure, the 'Labour and Delivery Satisfaction Index' (LADSI) which attempts to avoid some of these problems. While this has not been entirely successful in overcoming the problems listed above (see Shearer 1987), the LADSI is capable of distinguishing between women with high and low mood scores. However, the evidence presented does not rule out the possibility that the LADSI is primarily a reflection of current mood. It may well be that the subtleties of satisfaction are simply not measurable or are not sufficiently stable over time to allow them to be distinguished from more transient emotional reactions. However, the goal of measuring these so-called 'soft' outcomes (as opposed to 'hard' ones such as infant mortality) and of employing a 'critical approach to studies of women's opinions about their care' (Garcia et al., 1985) is to be encouraged.

Expectations and experiences of childbirth

For multiparous women the main sources of information on which to base expectations will be their previous experience, and several studies have demonstrated this. For example, Ounstead and Simons (1979) in a retrospective study compared two groups of women, one of which had experienced induced labour, and looked at their preferences for future labours. A third of those who were induced wanted an induction if they became pregnant again, whereas 91 per cent of those who had gone into labour spontaneously hoped for the same again. Among the women who had had epidurals (93% of the induced group and 37% of the spontaneous group), half wanted one in a future pregnancy compared to only 20 per cent of those who had not had one. In Cartwright's (1977) study only 17 per cent of the women who had been induced wanted the same again, but 63 per cent of those who had had an epidural wanted one again.

Whilst multiparous women have the advantage of previous experience, for the majority of primips the main source of information is often childbirth education or preparation classes. It may therefore be expected that such classes play a unique role in shaping and formulating the expectations of women who have not given birth before. Clark (1986) looked at the relationship between childbirth education and the development of realistic expectations of birth (i.e. expectations which are matched by actual events), in a study of Australian primips and their partners.

Expectations after antenatal class attendance were no more likely to be fulfilled by the events of birth than expectations held before attendance. Clark concluded that childbirth education plays little or no role in providing women with realistic expectations. However, although expectations were generally unrealistic, women tended to 'err on the side of caution' and for most, childbirth turned out better, not worse, than expected.

As previous experience introduces complications, many studies have limited themselves to primips. It is also assumed that previous experience gives multips more realistic expectations of childbirth than primips whose information is necessarily second hand. However those studies which have compared multips and primips do not lend unequivocal support to this assumption.

Booth and Meltzoff (1984) looked retrospectively at 267 women's expectations and experiences of both psychological and emotional, as well as physical and environmental aspects of birth. They found that primips and multips did not differ greatly in their expectations but primips had significantly higher expectations than outcomes. This was due to poorer outcomes rather than particularly high expectations on the part of primiparous women, who had many unexpected obstetric interventions. However they did have overly high expectations on two psychological measures: body control and control over health care decisions.

Nelson (1983) did not find that parity made much difference in terms of prenatal attitudes, although it was important once women went into hospital. Stolte (1986) in a small, retrospective study of 70 women found that three-quarters of the women had experiences which differed in some way from their expectations, and regardless of parity, women had unrealistic expectations about the effectiveness of pain relief.

Such studies do not support the hypothesis that primips necessarily have unrealistically high expectations. However, the studies by Booth and Meltzoff (1984) and Stolte (1986) were retrospective which raises questions about the validity of their findings. Nelson's (1983) results are more reliable because the study was prospective. The study is also of interest because it is one of a number that have looked at social class attitudes and expectations towards childbirth.

Nelson argues that it tends to be assumed that all women share a view of a childbirth experience which is as natural as possible and which is in conflict with the medical model of childbirth. She maintains that this is in fact only a middle class view which is foisted upon working class women and has little relevance for them. She supports this argument with the data from a careful prospective study of 322 women giving birth in a New England teaching hospital. She found that working class and middle class women had 'different attitudes towards childbirth during pregnancy, different experiences during childbirth and different postpartum evaluations of their experiences'.

Working class women (educational level is used as the measure for social class) felt more negative about pregnancy itself. They did not feel that being pregnant was especially desirable in itself and they were more anxious about labour and delivery. They viewed intervention and pain relief favourably because the priority for them was freedom from the pain and to get labour over quickly. In contrast, middle class women sought participation in the process of birth and wanted freedom from technological intervention. Both groups were concerned with safety but defined it differently, middle class women in terms of no medical interference, and working class women in terms of having medical intervention. (McClain (1983) shows how adherents to particular birth choices play up the risks of rejected alternatives whilst discounting the risks of the chosen option.) However, despite the positive attitude of working class women towards intervention, 54 per cent of them felt that a natural childbirth would be best for their baby (compared to 69% of middle class women), something which Nelson ignores completely, although it shows that many working class women related favourably to some aspects of natural childbirth.

In the event, both groups of women had experiences approaching their hopes, middle class women giving birth more actively and working class with more medication and intervention. However, neither group had all their choices met or their hopes realized. Postnatally, working class women reported that childbirth was worthwhile in spite of the pain, and did not value the process of birth, hardly ever using the word 'experience'. Middle class women focused on the process as a rewarding and fulfilling experience and commented on the hard work involved.

The question of class and expectations has also been examined by Hubert (1974) and McIntosh (1986) in prospective studies, and in a retrospective study by Woollet et al. (1983). All of these lend support to Nelson's thesis that working class women have very different hopes and expectations from those incorporated in the middle class model. In each of these studies working class women anticipated and experienced childbirth as a time of fear and pain, and Hubert found that for some women this did affect their attitudes to their babies. In McIntosh's study in Glasgow, women had very negative expectations antenatally, especially fear of pain and of losing control. As with Nelson's working class women, they wanted to get birth over as quickly and painlessly as possible. Intervention rates were very high: less than half the women had a non-instrumental normal delivery. Over half (53%) felt birth had been better than they expected – perhaps this is not surprising, given their extremely low expectations. Intervention was seen as inevitable and pain relief was welcomed. This was also true of the London women studied by Woollet et al.

Nevertheless, satisfaction was related to lower levels of intervention. A major source of dissatisfaction was lack of information from staff. Reid et al. (1982) found that the working class women interviewed as part of a study of a Scottish community antenatal clinic were also very concerned about avoiding pain in labour as far as possible.

However, Morgan et al. (1984) asked women about their general attitudes to obstetric care in childbirth a year after delivery and found little relationship with social class or any other demographic variable, although psychological well-being did influence some opinions. Women were asked in a questionnaire to indicate the extent to which they agreed with thirteen statements on different aspects of childbirth, including pain in labour and medical attention. Morgan et al. found that women were in agreement with some aspects of both the natural childbirth and medical models but in full agreement with neither. The majority, irrespective of social class, were in favour of medical attention and fetal monitoring, whilst 45 per cent thought pain was an essential part of the emotional experience of childbirth.

Caution is required in the interpretation of these results since the methodology is dubious in several respects, e.g. several of the thirteen statements offered to women do not particularly represent either the natural childbirth or medical establishment views, and neither are the options necessarily mutually exclusive.

The studies reviewed do indicate that working class women on the whole view medical intervention positively. In addition it seems fair to conclude that working class women do not have high expectations of childbirth – on the contrary, they sometimes seem to have very negative expectations and then have their worst fears realized.

One major problem is that few studies appear to compare directly the attitudes or expectations of women from different social backgrounds. Rather they examine the views of women from a particular geographic and demographic population and look to see how far they diverge from some hypothetical position, often that of the natural childbirth 'school'. Thus we find papers beginning with a blanket comment on the activities of the natural childbirth 'movement', and the 'insistence' of women to participate in their own births. McIntosh (1986) for example, writes:

> 'The natural childbirth movement has, in various guises, been a powerful voice in the maternity arena in recent years. Many women, it is claimed, are increasingly opposed to the medicalization of labour and delivery and seek a form of childbirth that is more "natural"...'

The choice of words such as 'guises' and 'claimed' suggests a lack of neutrality bordering on hostility towards the ideology of natural childbirth.

Thus, the method adopted by some researchers seems to be first to set up 'the natural childbirth movement' as a strawperson, then to present results from particular populations which do not accept a natural childbirth philosophy, and then to conclude that natural childbirth is therefore a middle class hobbyhorse or is confined to a 'vociferous' minority. McIntosh, for example, concluded that the desire for natural childbirth is likely to be a middle class one whilst providing no evidence for such a statement, merely that it is not the goal of the working class women he interviewed. Similarly, Ounstead and Simons (1979) (whilst saying nothing at all about the social class background of their informants) concluded that a group of women exist who favour active obstetric management as well as another group 'who insist on natural childbirth at all costs'. Yet they provide no evidence at all for the existence of such a dogmatic group.

Reaction to motherhood

As we have stated, we are interested in the relationship between prenatal hopes and expectations and postnatal reactions to childbirth. The traditional measures of outcome are depression/mental health, adaptation to motherhood, satisfaction and relationship with the baby. Many women experience some degree of depression after childbirth and about 1 in 500 develop postpartum psychosis (Breen, 1975; Kendall, 1985; Leverton, 1987).

As many as 80 per cent of women (Affonso and Domino, 1984) suffer postnatal 'blues', which typically start at two to four days after birth and last up to ten days, having a short-term impact on daily mood and function. Some authors argue that the blues are incompletely understood clinically and should not be dismissed as irrelevant or unimportant (Cox et al., 1982). The term 'postnatal depression' refers to a condition of undefined onset which is more persistent than the 'blues' and which can culminate in feelings of inadequacy, inability to cope with everyday life, social withdrawal, and generally a feeling of more bad days than good. It is thought to affect 10–15 per cent of mothers, although reported incidence varies between 3 per cent and 27 per cent (Affonso and Domino, 1984; Leverton, 1987; Pitt, 1968).

In practice, postnatal depression covers a wide variety of symptoms and diagnoses whilst the transient blues and the psychoses characterized by thought disorder or severe depression are more clearly delineated.

Researchers and clinicians define and measure postnatal depression in different ways which is one reason why its reported incidence varies widely (Arizmendi and Affonso, 1984). The categories 'postnatal blues', 'postnatal depression' and 'puerperal psychosis' are, of course, medical constructs. Some researchers have challenged the emphasis of such constructs on the abnormality of childbirth (with its concomitant hormonal 'imbalances') or on the woman's inner subjectivity (and possibly flawed personality) and the implicit idea that unproblematic adaptation to motherhood is normal and difficulties are not (Oakley, 1980). It has been suggested that when the prevalence of depression in the general population of women of childbearing age is taken into account, childbirth itself does not necessarily bring an increased risk of non-psychotic depression (Bardon, 1972; Romito, 1988). Cooper et al. (1988), for instance, found the prevalence, incidence and nature of such problems within a year of childbirth were similar to that in non-puerperal women. Other researchers have challenged the psychological or biomedical focus of previous research. Instead they have chosen to focus on external factors, such as obstetric interventions, socio-economic conditions and the implications of societal expectations of motherhood (see Affonso and Domino (1984) for a review of theories and factors implicated in postnatal depression).

Here we review several studies which have particular relevance to our own. One of the most important studies in this area was that of Oakley (1980) who charted women's passage to motherhood from early pregnancy to five months postpartum. Her sample consisted of 55 middle class primips all living in the same area of London. She differentiated between four components of mental health or 'depression' which women may experience after childbirth: postnatal blues, anxiety, depressed mood and depression.

In Oakley's sample 84 per cent of the women had postnatal blues, 71 per cent were anxious, 33 per cent were categorized as depressed mood and 24 per cent were depressed (she estimates that a clinician would have found 15% to be depressed). Each component of mental health was associated with a different set of predictor and vulnerability factors:

1. Postnatal blues were related to various aspects of birth management: instrumental delivery, dissatisfaction with the management of the second stage and epidurals.

2. Depression was associated with medium to high use of technology, low degree of maternal control, dissatisfaction with the birth management and lack of previous experience with babies.

3. Depressed mood was associated with current life situations such as bad housing, a segregated marital role relationship and lack of employment outside the home (see also Brown and Harris, 1978).

4. Satisfaction with motherhood was associated with previous socialization: strength of maternal self-image and orientation towards the feminine role (see also Breen, 1975).

5. Feelings for the baby were related to feminine role orientation (see also Raphael-Leff, 1985) and current life problems.

On the basis of these results Oakley concluded that 'unproblematic adaptation to first-time motherhood is unusual', and further, 'that it is normal to experience difficulties'. Her study is important in underlining that postnatal 'depression' is associated with normal, not abnormal, patterns of stress and coping and that the factors associated with negative well-being are intrinsically linked to the everyday mundane experience of motherhood.

Breen (1975) was in many ways interested in similar processes of psychological change with the birth of the first child, although her approach was psychological and psychoanalytic, whereas Oakley's approach was sociological. Both Oakley and Breen emphasized the problems in looking at adaptation/adjustment to motherhood as an outcome measure. As Breen noted, such a focus implies that pregnancy is a hurdle to be overcome, and that healthy adaptation is a return to the pre-pregnant stage. However, adjustment was the focus of Breen's prospective study of 50 mainly middle class women. A control group consisted of 20 non-pregnant women. One third of her sample were at least mildly depressed at ten weeks postpartum ('depression' here is being used in a more general way and includes anxiety and somatic manifestations). Discrepancy between women's expectations of their child and the reality was an important factor.

One third had difficulties with their babies (defined by giving a worse rating for 'own baby' than for an 'average baby'). No measures differentiated between women who did not have any problems in early pregnancy and those who did experience difficulties postpartum. Acceptance of pregnancy did not predict adjustment to motherhood. Breen concluded that problems in postnatal adjustment were related to an over-idealization of motherhood and femininity:

> 'In sum, those women who are most adjusted to childbearing are those who are less enslaved by the experience, have more differentiated, more open appraisals of themselves and other people, do not aspire to be the perfect selfless mother but are able to call on a good mother image with which they can identify and do not experience themselves as passive, the cultural stereotype of femininity.' (ibid. p. 193)

In another psychoanalytically based longitudinal prospective study, Raphael-Leff (1985) proposed a model of two basic orientations towards mothering, each involving a different vulnerability to distress in early motherhood. The 'Facilitator' feels she is fulfilled as a woman through pregnancy and motherhood, views babies as sociable from the start and adapts herself to the baby in every way that she can. The 'Regulator', on the other hand, sees babies as pre-social and her main task as socialization which may be shared with other carers. She finds fulfilment in various ways but not motherhood, instead feeling threatened by the baby's dependence on her.

Raphael-Leff found very high rates of depression in both groups: 36 per cent of Facilitators and 44 per cent of Regulators experienced a depressive syndrome over the course of the first two years. However, she suggests that different vulnerability and precipitating factors in each group precipitated such distress. She also suggests that if depression is a result of motherhood rather than childbirth (as argued, for example, by Romito, 1988), studies which are carried out early in the postpartum period may report lower rates of postnatal distress than those which make an assessment later on.

Elliott et al. (1984) looked at the relationship between antenatal measures of psychological status, obstetric outcome and postnatal depression for 117 women of mixed parity, as part of a longitudinal study of psychological change and psychiatric status in pregnancy and the first postnatal year. The study found no relationship between antenatal psychological scores and obstetric outcome. They also found no evidence of a relationship between labour measures and postnatal depression or tension except that women with obstetric complications rated themselves as *less* depressed and happier postnatally than those with no complications (see also Paykel et al., 1980). However, the reports of labour pain, distress and fear seem rather unreliable; assessments were made during labour and were based on 'brief conversations' (sic) with the women. Elliott et al. constructed a technology score using weightings as similar as possible to those of Oakley (1980). In contrast to Oakley's results, there was no relationship between the amount of technology used and depression. (However, all 117 women studied were under the same consultant which may have reduced the variation in the amount of technology used.) Whereas Oakley argues for a causal relationship between medium to high use of obstetric technology and depression, Elliott et al. suggest that how the woman perceives the intervention rather than technology *per se* may be the critical factor. Nevertheless, they acknowledge that the measures of obstetric outcome used may have been inappropriate and do not exclude the possibility that unsatisfactory management of labour may have led to depression in some cases. In Jacoby's (1987) study carried out four months after birth, 21 per cent of the respondents said they had felt depressed some or most of the time since their baby had been born. Women who had experienced certain procedures (induction, epidural, stitches, shave and enema) were more likely to report feeling depressed. Also, women who said they had felt depressed were subjected to a higher than average number of procedures.

Concern that interfering in the physiological process of labour may have adverse effects on the mother-baby relationship has contributed to the debate over the routine use of obstetric technology. Robson and Kumar (1980) provide some limited evidence for this. They followed 112 primips through pregnancy and also two smaller groups of multips and primips were studied after birth. A relationship was found between a delay in maternal affection and experience of artificial rupture of membranes (ARM) in addition to either a painful, unpleasant labour or more than 125 mg of Pethidine. The most painful labours were those where an ARM had been done at an early stage. In fact, about 40 per cent of the primips and 25 per cent of the multips reported that their immediate reaction to their babies had been one of emotional indifference, which suggests that it is far from being an unusual response. However, most had developed strong positive feelings towards their babies within one week of delivery and there were no effects at three months postpartum. At one year, very few women expressed feelings of guilt about their initial reactions, saying they had been prepared for them by antenatal classes (which does not support the hypothesis that classes instill over-high expectations in women).

Some support for Robson and Kumar's finding of an association between ARM and initial negative feelings towards the baby is given by Oakley's (1980) more general finding of a link between high/medium use of technology and medium/poor feelings for the baby.

Ball (1987) carried out a study examining the role of postnatal care and support by midwives in women's transition to motherhood and their ability to cope with this major life change. She followed 279 women of mixed parity and varying social class from 36 weeks pregnant to six weeks after birth, interviewing them in hospital between two and three days after birth. Data were also obtained from the midwives attached to the three hospitals involved in the study. An emotional well-being score for each woman was constructed from the scores of five emotional well-being factors (depression, coping ability, anxiety, sleep disturbance associated with anxiety and self confidence). Nineteen per cent of the sample were defined as having low emotional well-being by this method, i.e. were considered to be emotionally distressed. Ball found that three interacting sets of factors were significantly associated with maternal emotional well-being six weeks after birth:

1. Maternal and family factors acting together to create a pattern of vulnerability, in the same way as Oakley's (1980) research demonstrated (anxiety, loss of identity, lack of warm confiding relationship with male partner, stressful life events).

2. The mother's feelings immediately after birth, satisfaction with motherhood and perception of the baby's progress.

3. Self-image in feeding in the days after the birth, which was adversely affected by two aspects of postnatal hospital care – conflicting advice and lack of sleep.

Ball suggested that satisfaction with motherhood acted as a 'boost' to women's emotional well-being.

In their review of postpartum depression, Affonso and Domino (1984) list the following factors (among others) as increasing vulnerability to postnatal depression: previous psychiatric history, marital problems, lack of social support, stressful life events, ambivalence and anxiety about the pregnancy, unmet expectations relating to labour and delivery, obstetric complications, unanticipated birth events, stressful labour or delivery, obstetric intervention and physical illness of the mother or baby. Additional factors shown to be important in the studies reviewed here are: lack of previous experience with babies, self-image and orientation to the feminine role, dissatisfaction with the birth management, lack of maternal control in labour/delivery, self-image in feeding (i.e. how competent a mother feels in feeding her baby) and postnatal care and support.

Although Affonso and Domino (1984) point to a relationship between depression during pregnancy and postpartum depression, Oakley (1980) highlights the general failure of researchers to establish such a connection. Depression does not appear to be related to parity, marital status or social class (Leverton, 1987).

To conclude, the review of previous work produces sometimes conflicting results on women's expectations of childbirth and the predictors of how women feel after childbirth. This probably results, at least in part, from different methods of assessment. In addition, most of the studies are small scale and many are retrospective. The samples are often not strictly comparable, the studies frequently lack control groups.

The variables analysed and the techniques used to analyse or measure them differ from study to study, and the appropriateness of the statistical analyses employed also varies. Expectations of pain, for example, may be measured differently according to the researcher's own perspectives. All these factors make it very difficult to compare results across studies in any rigorous way. Instead, we have chosen to highlight themes or results which relate to our own study and which we will explore in our own data.

Choice and control as themes in childbirth

In this section we will look at the twin concepts of choice and control in childbirth: the ways in which these interrelate and the stereotypes that have been constructed around these concepts.

Women's 'right to choose' in relation to their role as major users of the health service has been a popular theme in the last two decades. What we see here is partly an extension of a prevailing ideology that sees choice *per se* as desirable. The theory would seem to be that the act of exercising choice gives satisfaction irrespective of the inadequacy of the options. That such assumptions carry the danger of obscuring more fundamental issues has been argued elsewhere (Richards, 1982). The trouble with choice is that 'it implies that there exists a comprehensive set of options to choose from and that the chooser is in a position freely to exercise choice in an informed way' (ibid). In practice, choices are made in highly constrained contexts that preclude both of these possibilities. As a recent report by the World Health Organization (1985) observed:

> 'For most pregnant women in most countries there is little or no choice with regard to where she will receive officially sanctioned care, who will give her the care and what the care will or will not include.' (p. 76)

'Choice and control' are often spoken in the same breath as if they were synonymous, or as if choice automatically led to control. The theme of control itself emerges out of many different roots and has correspondingly different meanings. In Lamaze's (1958) theory, 'control' was about internal control i.e. women developing and maintaining control over their own behaviour. Other theories, however, emphasize that a positive childbirth experience is dependent on relinquishing internal control. The focus then is on flowing with one's body rather than trying to assert control over the childbirth event or distance oneself from it (Dick Read, 1933, 1944).

The concept of 'external' control during labour, control over your environment and what is done to you, is one that goes hand in hand with the 'right to choose' ideology and the lay challenge to medical expertise.

It is this external sense of control which is most likely to be experienced as lost immediately a woman enters the hospital institution. Hence, for some women maintaining control may mean having their babies at home.

We should also comment on the difficulty of distinguishing in practice between perceived control and real or actual control. It is possible that perceived control may in fact diverge greatly from how much control the woman 'actually' has, but that this difference is in fact unimportant. Thus, it may be the subjective feeling of being in control that is the important variable in determining a woman's reactions to her birth experience, regardless of whether by some objective measure she is seen to lack or retain control.

Relationship between 'choice' and 'control'

It will be clear that the relationship between choice and control will be a function of the particular interpretations of these concepts being used. 'External' control, for example, is achieved in part through active participation in decision making. Choice is therefore a necessary prerequisite, and an absence of choice implies an absence of control.

However, it does not follow that having choice, for example about a birth companion or attendants, the kind of obstetric care received, pain relief, position and interventions, will necessarily lead to a sense of either 'internal' or 'external' control. On the contrary, it could be argued that choice actually decreases one's sense of being in control by increasing anxiety. Other prerequisites for 'external' control are information and responsibility. Both of these are inherent in recent developments in antenatal care such as fetal movement (kick) charts and women carrying their own notes. In this sense women may be seen as having more control. For example, a woman carrying her own notes has physical control of them, is free to read them, comment on them, or even to lose or destroy them. However, she usually has no choice about whether she carries the notes or not, nor does she necessarily have any more choice over other aspects of her care. Clearly this is an example where there is no necessary relationship between choice and control.

Control and the experience of childbirth

Notwithstanding the confusions of terminology, hypotheses exist about the ways in which control may relate to women's experience of childbirth. For example, it has been argued that encouraging women to assert 'internal' control, i.e. control over their behaviour, leads to tension and inflexibility in the woman who is unable to 'listen' to what her body is telling her to do. Similarly, allowing women to be involved in decision making may serve to confuse them and increase their anxiety levels which may have several negative effects such as an inability to relax. It may lead to panicky feelings, and so to a sense of being out of control rather than in control. Related to this some people have suggested that 'giving' women control, particularly in the area of decision making, may burden them with a sense of over-responsibility which they cannot cope with. This could have severe repercussions if 'things go wrong', leading to self blame, guilt and depression for some women. Furthermore, an inherent danger in women's desire to be in control of what happens to them during childbirth is that they are set up for conflict with midwives and doctors who also want to be in control. Staff may feel threatened and put on the defensive by assertive behaviour from women which they may interpret as aggression. There may be consequent poor interactions between the staff and the women who are put in a vulnerable position in this way.

On the positive side, the literature just reviewed suggests that being in control, or perceiving that you are, leads to a more positive birth experience, increased satisfaction and less depression. A better relationship with the baby may also develop as the woman is more likely to approach motherhood with confidence (Flint, 1986b). However, it has also been argued that the concepts of choice and control are essentially middle class notions and may not in fact have any relevance to the vast majority of working class or less well educated women. As we have seen, there is evidence suggesting that working class women may indeed have different priorities.

Common stereotypes embodying assumptions about choice and control

The research that we have reviewed reflects a number of different ideas about childbearing women. Such ideas or assumptions are inevitable: we all work with internal models in order to make sense of the world and reduce its complexities to manageable proportions. Internal models frequently result in a series of stereotypes of kinds of women: what they want and do not want and how they should be treated. Examples have already been given from the research literature, for example what 'middle class' women want as opposed to 'working class' women (McIntosh, 1986; Ounstead and Simons, 1979).

Stereotypes also appear in material written for the general public, for example, Toynbee's depiction (1986) of 'lentil-eating earth goddesses' obsessively and selfishly promoting the cause of natural childbirth. These stereotypes have also been obvious to us in the writings of some obstetricians and in our own observations on labour wards in Phase I of this research (Green et al., 1986; Kitzinger et al., 1988). In this context, stereotypes of women may give particular cause for concern because the way in which a doctor or midwife categorizes a woman is likely to influence the way in which that woman is treated. As one consultant commented:

> 'I warn some women with very specific expectations that that in itself, the expression of them, can provoke an anti-reaction in the attendant. I hear it at the desk, you know, the way people are described and one knows immediately that that woman is not going to have the sort of sensitivity she hoped for.'

Such descriptions often take the form of caricatures which are not necessarily intended to be taken literally, but reflect underlying internal models and often a hostile, or belittling attitude. One example is the description of a woman who wants an 'active' birth as someone who wants to 'hang from the chandeliers' or 'squat in a corner' – two phrases which are often used in pejorative ways although they may also be used affectionately by people who are in favour of active birth. Another example is the characterization of the woman who wants a natural birth as obsessive and naive. This woman has romantic views about 'primitive societies' and believes that in other countries women 'step behind a proverbial bush for a short time and emerge with the baby in one arm and nonchalantly swinging the placenta by the cord with the other' (Francis, 1985, p. 70). Such women run the risk of being advised by hostile professionals that:

> 'There are vast stretches of wilderness... those who want a natural birth should go there.' (Consultant quoted in *Nursing Mirror*, Sept 5th, 1984)

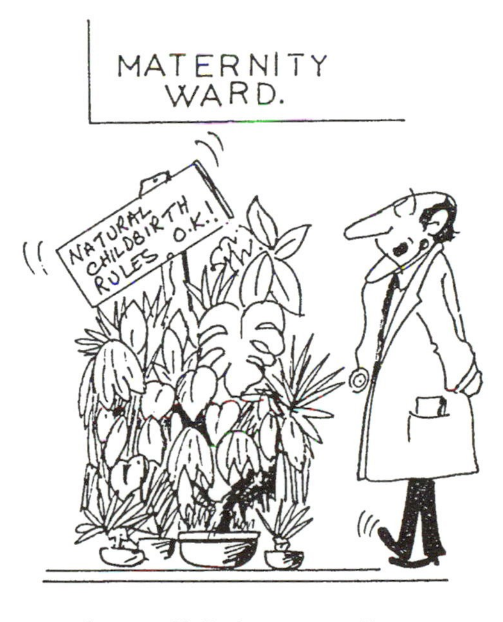

Come, come, Mrs Brookes — aren t we taking our anti-hospital delivery campaign a little too seriously?

Reproduced with kind permission of Peter Bellamy

'Women who come in with long lists' is another popular image (short lists are apparently unknown). This caricature reflects staff's negative attitudes to birth plans. As a midwife in Phase 1 of our study commented (Green et al., 1986):

> 'It's the same as if they are known to be NCT, they are just written off – "Oh Christ, here we go again!". They are labelled, it's very negative. How many midwives say "oh great! They actually know what they want"?'

The point made by this midwife is an interesting one in that it shows how the same stereotype of women can be interpreted positively or negatively according to the stance of the 'beholder'. To conclude this chapter we will present just three stereotypes of women that are commonly encountered, and show how each caricature may be viewed either positively or, more commonly, negatively.

First, there is the well-educated, middle class NCT 'type'. This woman has firm ideas about what she wants and demands choice and control in childbirth. She is seen as having overly high expectations of getting her own way and as placing a great deal of importance on childbirth as a fulfilling experience. With such unrealistically high hopes she is bound to be disappointed and feel a failure when everything does not go according to plan. Therefore she is likely to end up with severe postnatal depression. Consumer support groups representing pregnant women, such as the NCT, are held responsible for her attitude; she has been hoodwinked by a lot of natural childbirth propaganda and is naive about the pain and dangers of childbirth. It is also implicit that she is probably a primip since no-one who has actually experienced birth could be so deluded. In addition, she may have a rigid and intellectual approach to labour, and so be unable to 'let go', thus possibly inhibiting her contractions. This woman is believed to focus on childbirth as an experience in itself, for itself, almost to the exclusion of the baby at the end, and may be held to be more concerned with women's rights than with the baby's safety. As the author of a recent commentary in the *British Journal of Obstetrics and Gynaecology* asks aggressively:

> 'What of the patient who insists against advice on having the baby at home, standing up, supported by her partner and claiming that the emotional fulfilment transcends all other priorities...?' (Macdonald, 1987, p. 834)

The positive version of this 'NCT type' is somebody who, far from being inflexible, naive and unrealistic, is well-informed, reasonable and rational. She chooses to attend childbirth preparation classes, even if she has attended them in previous pregnancies, in order to be well-informed on all possible events and outcomes of birth. Her aim is to be able to communicate on an equal basis with the staff in order to work in partnership with them. Although setting her own goals for childbirth, she is able to adapt to changing circumstances due to having worked out her feelings and choices in the face of such circumstances beforehand. A birth plan might well be the tool she employs to do this. She is not naive about the pain of childbirth and neither is she anti-intervention in itself, as long as she remains in control of decision making. However she takes an intelligent and critical stance about routine interventions and is aware of the side-effects of drugs. She does place a lot of importance on childbirth as a fulfilling event, but maximizes the possibility of this by her calm and informed approach, and furthermore she is in no doubt that the safe delivery of her baby is her paramount goal.

The second image of child bearing women that we will consider tends to be the preserve of the old-style paternalistic obstetrician: woman as an emotional creature, irrational and constitutionally incapable of making sensible decisions. For example, Francis (1985, p. 72) writes:

> 'It is not widely appreciated that pregnant women are not only emotionally unstable, they are intensely egocentric.'

He goes on to say that this egotism is:

> '...probably atavistic and necessary for self preservation when we lived in caves. However, in this egocentric state, encouragement to participate can result in a fierce demand to dictate.'

The logical conclusion of such a position is to deny women active participation in the childbirth process because of the dangers inherent in their biologically determined inability to reason. Given this set of assumptions, it is clearly inappropriate and even reckless to offer pregnant women anything other than the most medically circumscribed choices for the management of pregnancy and birth, and the possibility of sharing control should be eliminated altogether for fear of abuse by unreasoning and unreasonable women. Indeed, Francis does talk about the 'illogicality of women' to invalidate requests for low-tech births and, as one would expect, he dismisses the importance of previous experience of labour as a basis for making decisions about the care in a future pregnancy.

In many ways the stereotype of pregnant women as being too unstable to make sensible choices would seem to be unfashionable and fading fast in popularity. Certainly, few obstetricians would state their beliefs as baldly as Francis does. Nevertheless, the conclusion of this position, that the views of staff are always more valid than those of the woman giving birth, still underlies the approach of many doctors and midwives together with an accompanying resentment towards women and lay people who try to maintain control of decisions during childbirth.

The positive view of 'woman, the non-rational creature' is one encountered most commonly in American writings which emphasize the spiritual nature of birth. In this portrayal the pregnant woman is at one with nature and the cosmos, she follows her instincts and flows with her body, the tides and the moon. Giving birth is about truth, godliness and beauty, it draws on psychic energy and the life force as much as on physical endurance. It is a mind-expanding and uplifting as well as a bodily experience. The proponents of this view are:

> '...concerned with the sacrament of birth – the passage of a new soul into this plane of existence. The knowledge that each and every childbirth is a spiritual experience has been forgotten by many people of this culture.' (May, 1975)

Women's experiences in childbirth join them spiritually together:

> 'The wisdom and compassion a woman can intuitively experience in childbirth can make her a source of healing and understanding for other women.' (ibid)

The natural place of spiritual birth is more in the country, in small rural communities where people are in harmony with one another and with nature than in alienating hospital environments. This image of pregnant women and birth is in its own way as much out on a limb as Francis' views, but we include it as an example of how non-rationality may be perceived in a very positive light.

The final stereotype that we will consider is that of the working class uneducated woman, a woman out of control of her fertility, often portrayed as a young unmarried mother or as already having more children than she should. She is seen as wilfully ignorant, the type who books late and may fail to turn up to antenatal clinic appointments. She is unconcerned with the possibilities of emotional fulfilment through the process of childbirth and refuses to even consider the question of pain and how to cope with it. Childlike, she abdicates all responsibility to the staff. Consequently, this woman goes into the maternity unit thoroughly unprepared for the rigours of the hours ahead. She apparently learns little in the process and next time round still firmly buries her head in the sand, like the proverbial ostrich.

To some midwives and doctors, on the other hand, she is the ideal patient. She lays no claim to special knowledge so she accepts that the staff know best and she does what she is told. Being more down to earth she just gets on with the job without any airy-fairy notions of fulfilment and satisfaction, recognizing that it is the end product that matters rather than the process.

Professional reactions

The stereotypes that we have described and staff's reactions to them revolve around the issues of how much information women should have and how much choice and control they can retain. If women want to maintain control over childbirth, they can be seen as challenging the staff's professional autonomy. As a midwife said to us:

> 'If I go to the dentist I don't expect him to say to me "Now what kind of filling would you like to have?" I mean what are we all trained for?' (Phase 1, Midwife interview)

Professionals can feel very threatened by women competing with them for control in their area of expertise. This is most eloquently demonstrated by this quotation from the President of the American College of Obstetrics and Gynaecology:

> 'We are under siege from consumerists, environmentalists, Women's Liberationists, civil rightists and other special interest activists yet to be organized... we must take the offensive against the faddists who would supplant proven excellence within the medical profession with popular mediocrity.' (Stone, 1979)

Or, as one of the midwives we interviewed said:

> 'If I disagree with a patient I don't mince my words... don't forget she is lying there and if she was capable she wouldn't come in, she wouldn't come in if she felt in control.'

Professionals like the ones quoted here are challenging the idea that they should have to put up with women who assert their right to make choices and maintain control.

On the other hand, some staff do welcome well-informed women and see their own role as facilitators rather than directors of childbirth. They are committed to supporting women in making their own choices, and to acting according to the woman's wishes:

> 'It's her decision, if it's unsafe, if she's adamant then I go along with her.' (midwife interview)

There is yet a further question to pose: what about the effect on women themselves of having choice? The rationale behind a lot of women-centred obstetric care is that choice and control are good for us in a number of ways. For example, it is argued that if women maintain control during labour they are more likely to become confident, competent and happy mothers. As the obstetrician Wendy Savage wrote:

> 'Over the years I have been practising, I have learnt that women need to be able to talk as equals with doctors, to be informed of the choices available to them and encouraged to make up their own minds... I have realized how important it is for a woman to feel in control of the birth process if she is going to emerge as a confident parent.' (Savage, 1986)

Similarly, midwife Caroline Flint has argued that allowing women choice and control in labour is important because:

> 'The mother has to be all powerful, all knowing, a total deity really, a goddess. And to be a godlike person you need confidence above all else, and to be a mother happily and confidently we need confidence in our ability to mother. We need self respect and we need acknowledgement that this baby is the mother's baby, her responsibility.' (Flint, 1986a)

It has also been suggested that women in labour should not only be 'allowed' choice and control but indeed have a moral obligation to take it. Women are urged to take responsibility for decision making during pregnancy and labour and are advised to use libraries in order to research into obstetric care:

> 'If all this seems a lot of extra work, remember that you owe it to yourself and your unborn baby to be well informed and accurately informed...' (Brackbill et al., 1984)

The woman who abdicates this responsibility may be viewed very negatively. One midwife disparagingly commented:

> 'Some people are quite happy to hand over responsibility for their lives – you know, they live off the dole and they hand over their care...' (Phase I, Midwife interview)

It is clear that people hold many different beliefs about how important, and how appropriate, it is for pregnant and labouring women to make choices and to be 'in control'. It is also clear that 'control' is a commodity which professionals view very much as their own preserve: the more liberal may 'allow' or 'give' women control but for women to 'take' control is, to use another popular phrase, 'going too far'. Clearly, beliefs about choice and control are inextricably bound up with issues of information and assertiveness. It is these themes that are explored in our study and we will refer back to the images discussed here when we document our findings.

CHAPTER TWO

Methodology

Our research has come to focus on two central questions:

1. In what way, if any, are women's expectations and experiences of childbirth associated with postnatal psychological outcomes?

2. What is the importance of having choice and control to pregnant and labouring women, and what do they understand by having control in childbirth?

Hypotheses

Earlier studies in this area, as described in the previous chapter, led us to formulate the following hypotheses in order to address these questions. These hypotheses, unlike much of the research referred to, distinguish between 'preferences', i.e. what women would *like* to happen, and 'expectations', i.e. what they expect *will* actually happen. Hypothesis one concerns only expectations.

Hypothesis one

i) Women with high expectations who get what they expect will have positive outcomes, those that do not will have negative outcomes.

ii) Women with low expectations who have better experiences than expected also have positive outcomes but if their low expectations are realized they will have neither particularly positive nor particularly negative outcomes.

iii) Women with no expectations will have positive outcomes irrespective of events in labour (as long as the baby is alright).

This hypothesis assumes that if you do not have high expectations you cannot be disappointed. It further assumes that if you have no expectations at all then events will be relatively unimportant – so long as the baby is healthy these women will be happy. Hypothesis one, however, takes no account of what women actually want to happen. This aspect is incorporated into hypothesis two.

Hypothesis 1

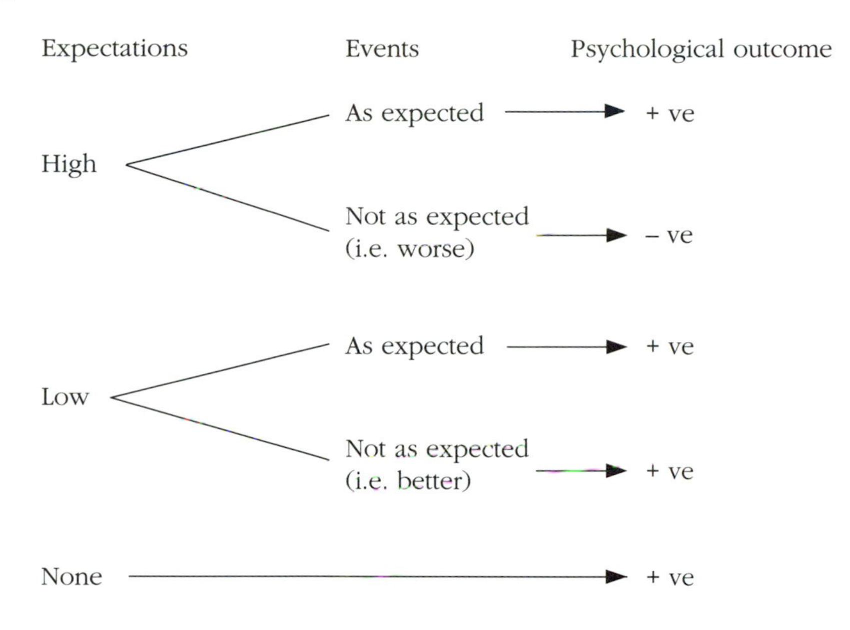

Hypothesis two

In hypothesis two, expectations do not matter as long as preferences are met. If, however, they are not met then women with high expectations have worse outcomes than women with low expectations. Women with no preferences, as those with no expectations, will be happy whatever happens.

Hypothesis 2

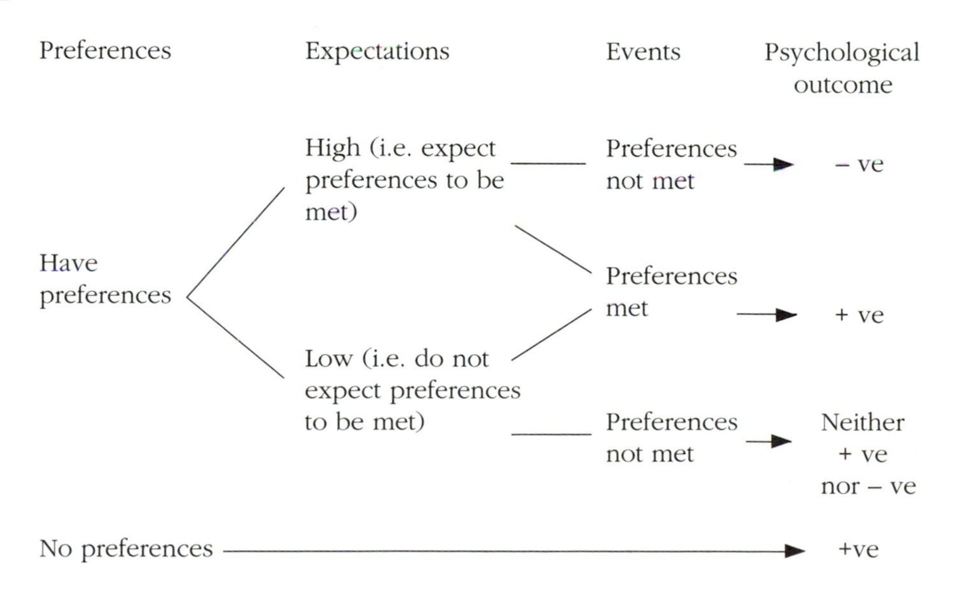

Hypothesis three

This hypothesis places more emphasis on what women *want* rather than what they *expect*. Contrary to hypothesis two, not having preferences met will lead to a negative outcome for women with low expectations as well as those who expected their preferences to be met.

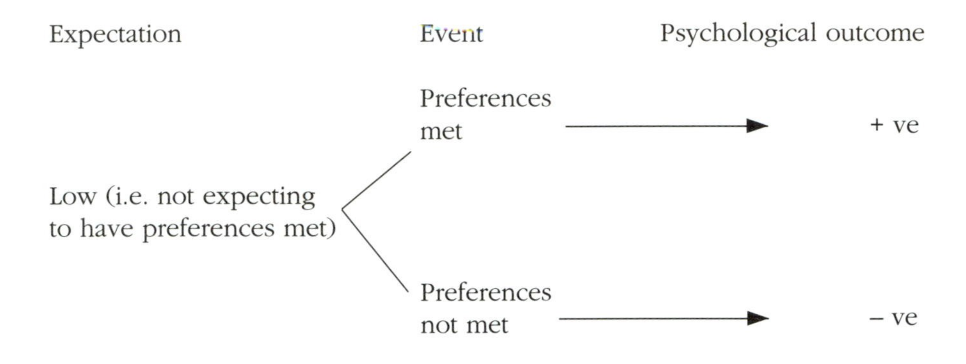

The fourth hypothesis addresses the question of parity, expectations and psychological outcome.

Hypothesis four: Primips are more likely to have negative outcomes

This is based on the sub-hypotheses that i) not having expectations met tends to lead to negative outcomes, ii) primips have no previous experience, therefore their expectations will be less realistic, therefore their expectations are less likely to be met.

Hypotheses five and six are alternative hypotheses about control.

Hypothesis five

Women who want control and get it will have positive outcomes, those who want it and do not get it will have negative outcomes. Women who are not concerned about control will have positive outcomes because they cannot be disappointed. Therefore, overall, women who want control are less likely to have positive outcomes.

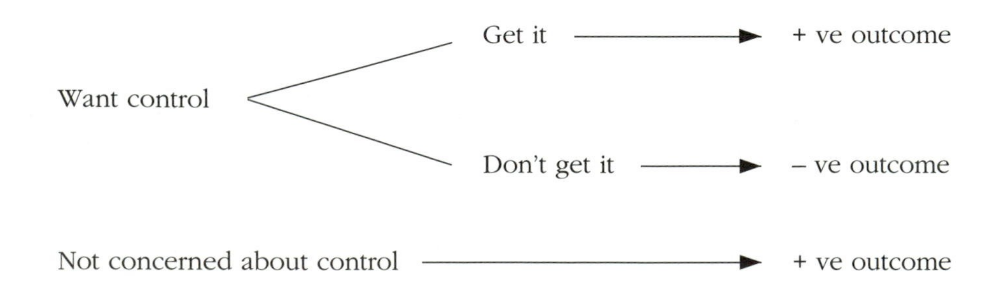

Hypothesis six

Experiencing control leads to positive outcomes irrespective of wants and expectations, i.e. 'control is good for you'.

In control ⟶ + ve outcome
Not in control ⟶ – ve outcome

Hypotheses seven and eight introduce the factor of social class/education.

Hypothesis seven

Middle class or highly educated women are likely to express a greater *desire* for control in the areas of decision making and what staff do to them in childbirth than are working class or less educated women.

Hypothesis eight

Middle class or highly educated women are likely to express greater *expectations* of having control in the areas of decision making and what staff do to them in childbirth than are working class or less educated women.

The corollaries to hypotheses seven and eight are that middle class educated women have more scope for negative outcomes.

The final two hypotheses are concerned with the relationship between obstetric interventions carried out on women in childbirth and their subsequent psychological outcome.

Hypothesis nine

Major interventions, for example, caesarean section, forceps delivery and induction, are more likely to be associated with poor psychological outcome than are minor interventions such as enemas and shaves.

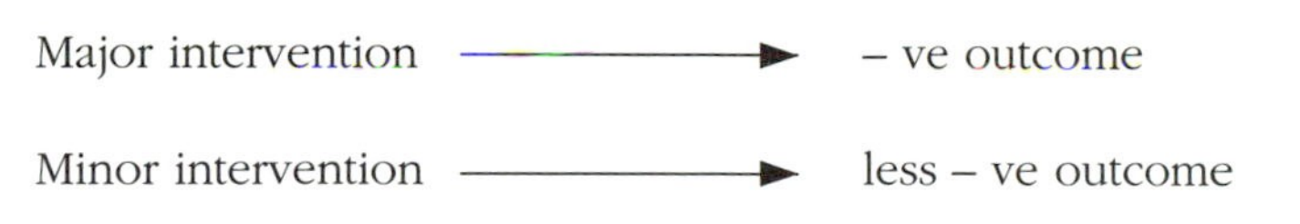

Hypothesis ten

Women experiencing a greater total number of interventions are more likely to have negative psychological outcomes than women experiencing a smaller total number of interventions.

Many interventions (major or minor) ⟶ – ve outcome

Fewer interventions ⟶ less – ve outcome

Research design

In designing this research we wished to remedy some of the gaps in the existing knowledge that have already been described. The study therefore started from the following fixed points:

1. Design: The study should be *prospective*, i.e. women should be identified and questioned before the birth of their baby, and then followed up postnatally.

2. Topics to be covered: Antenatally women would be asked about their hopes and expectations of childbirth. This would include their expectations of pain and attitudes towards methods of pain relief; knowledge about and attitudes towards various common obstetric interventions; and feelings about choice and control in childbirth. Postnatally they would be asked about their actual experiences in all these areas. The postnatal questions would also cover how the woman had been feeling since the birth, her satisfaction with the birth and her perceptions of her baby.

3. Parity: Many previous studies of women's expectations have restricted themselves to women having their first babies (primips). Clearly the expectations of women who have already had children (multips) might be expected to be different given their previous experience. It was decided that this study should include both primips and multips.

4. Hospitals: The study should include more than one hospital. In particular it was intended that women booked for delivery at hospitals involved in our earlier study of medical staffing structures (Green et al., 1986) should participate, since we had the advantage of considerable knowledge about practice in these hospitals. Furthermore, some assessment of the relationship between staffing structure (and other variables identified in the earlier study) and women's satisfaction could then be made. We would also attempt to include GP and home deliveries within the same Health Districts, although we realized that there would be very few home deliveries.

Given these fixed points, various other decisions about the research design and methodology followed:

5. In order to be able to make statistically valid comparisons between hospitals, and of sub-groups (e.g. multips and primips) within hospitals, it was evident that a large sample would be needed. This, coupled with the geographical spread of the sample, meant that data would be collected via postal questionnaires. This method of data collection has been shown to yield reliable information on women's childbirth experiences (Cartwright, 1986) and has been developed by the Office of Population Censuses and Surveys (OPCS) for widespread use by individual Health Districts (DHSS, 1987).

6. Timing of questionnaires: Women's knowledge, attitudes and expectations change as pregnancy progresses. We therefore wished to collect antenatal views as late as possible, although obviously not so late that there was a significant chance of

the baby arriving before the questionnaire. The main antenatal questionnaire was therefore timed to arrive four weeks before the expected date of delivery (EDD). However, we felt that a bulky questionnaire arriving without preamble so close to the birth would be rather intimidating and would probably not get a good response. We therefore decided to make an initial approach earlier in pregnancy which would explain the research and invite participation. This seemed preferable not only for the women but also because it would save us the expense of sending lengthy questionnaires to women who did not wish to receive them. Since basic information (name, address and EDD) would be needed from respondents at this earlier stage it seemed convenient to collect other basic information (e.g. age, occupation, number of previous children) at the same time. A short questionnaire would therefore accompany the letter of invitation which would gather information unlikely to change during the rest of the pregnancy. This would have the advantage of enabling us to reduce the length of the main questionnaire, and also of giving the women a taste of what was to come.

The initial approach would be made at approximately 30 weeks of pregnancy in order to allow time for the first questionnaire to be returned to us and the main one sent to reach women by 36 weeks. Women would receive the postnatal questionnaire six weeks after the expected date of delivery, which would allow comparability with many previous studies.

Pilot study

A pilot study was carried out within the Cambridge Health District involving women booked for delivery between mid-January and mid-March 1987. The sole purpose of the pilot study was to test the questionnaires and no data analysis was carried out. Women were recruited via two GP practices, one urban and one semi-rural. The first 13 women were approached in person by one of the researchers who talked them through the questions. This allowed us instant feedback on any ambiguities or other difficulties. Thereafter, each GP practice undertook to address and post questionnaires to appropriate women so that their names would not be known to us if they chose not to participate. A total of 46 women agreed to take part in the pilot study: the original 13 who were approached in person, a further 27 out of 34 (79%) approached by post and an additional six women who were personal contacts. All were sent a second questionnaire at 36 weeks of pregnancy and 40 (87%) returned them. The final questionnaire was sent six weeks after the expected date of delivery. We were also able to pilot the postnatal questionnaire on an additional seven women who volunteered for the main study but gave birth before they could complete the antenatal questionnaires.

On the basis of the pilot responses the phrasing or positioning of some questions was altered, and a small number of questions were inserted or deleted.

Ethical approval

We also sent copies of the pilot questionnaires to local health district ethics committees. Their comments resulted in a small number of additional modifications. Most notably we added two questions to the end of the main antenatal questionnaire to discover whether women were being at all alarmed by the issues we had raised, and urging them, if so, to discuss their worries with their doctor or midwife.

Questionnaire contents

The questionnaires themselves are reproduced in the appendix.

First antenatal questionnaire (AN1)

The first questionnaire that women received along with their invitation to join the study covered mainly basic biographical and administrative information:

- expected date of delivery
- number and ages of any previous children
- place of booking
- consultant's name
- age
- marital status
- age of finishing full-time education
- current employment (if any)
- employment history
- partner's occupation and employment status.

We did not ask direct questions about ethnic origin because we did not feel that the potential use to which we could put the information justified the intrusion. However, we were aware that two of the Districts had substantial Italian and Asian populations and we hoped that it might be possible to collect enough women who belonged to these communities to be able to say something about any particular needs that they might have. We were also conscious of the fact that all the hospitals are close to Army, Air Force or Naval bases, and that Service wives might prove to be a subgroup with special problems. Accordingly, at the end of the first antenatal questionnaire, women were asked:

> 'Finally, we are interested to know about certain groups of people who we feel might have slightly different needs in terms of their maternity care. We would therefore be grateful if you could indicate by ticking the appropriate box(es) whether you belong to any of the following groups'.
>
> A. The Italian community
> B. The Asian community
> C. Women whose husbands are in the British Army, Navy or Air Force
> D. Any other group which you feel has particular needs (please specify)
> E. None of these

In addition to these relatively routine pieces of information, we also broached some more specific areas. The first of these was choice over place of delivery and consultant: did women feel that they had had a choice and would they have preferred some other arrangement? We also touched on emotional issues by asking women about their current mood and their feelings when they had first known that they were pregnant. Finally, we asked women about their smoking and drinking both before and during pregnancy. These were seen as questions of interest, firstly, as correlates of obstetric outcome and, secondly, as areas where women are expected to exercise control (i.e. self control) in order to promote their baby's health.

Second (main) antenatal questionnaire (AN2)

As a very large number of questions were being asked at this stage, we split the questions up into a 16 page A4 questionnaire and a 20 page A5 booklet. Questions in the booklet were primarily about hopes and expectations for events in labour e.g. having a partner present, having the same midwife throughout, not making a lot of noise, being in control of decisions. For each of these, 12 items in all, women rated a) how important the issue was to them, and b) their expectations of what would actually happen. These questions were followed by items on induction, acceleration, forceps and caesarean section which asked how much women felt they knew about each intervention, their expectations of experiencing them, reasons for those expectations and preferences given certain scenarios. The final question in the booklet was an open-ended invitation to describe the ways in which they felt that their hopes and expectations were influenced by previous experience.

The A4 questionnaire covered broader topics and was divided into five sections. Section A covered childbirth preparation classes, including reasons for non-attendance, and Section B dealt with information: interaction with professionals and how much information women actually wanted. We also asked women whether they felt that they knew enough to make choices about many common interventions, and, if so, what their preferences were. In Section C we asked women about their view of birth plans. We chose this as an area of focus because birth plans are a particularly high profile way of expressing one's wishes and are usually associated with highly educated women who wish to retain a high degree of control in childbirth.

Section D dealt with pain: women's expectations of pain in labour, their attitude towards coping with it and their knowledge about and preferences for different methods of pain relief.

The final section was concerned with the third stage of labour: what women knew and whether they had any preferences for its management. Our expectation was that we would find a low level of both knowledge and preference, in contrast to the topic of pain relief which has received much more publicity and on which women are expected to have some sort of opinion. Both of these last two sections asked women the extent to which they wished to be in control of relevant decision making.

Postnatal questionnaire (PN3)

The postnatal questionnaire, like AN2, was divided into an A5 booklet and an A4 questionnaire. The first part of the booklet asked about obstetric interventions: had they occurred or been discussed and how did the women feel about what had happened. There was then a series of questions matched to those on hopes and expectations in the antenatal booklet: did you have your chosen birth companion with you, did you make much noise during labour etc. and more general questions on feelings during labour. The booklet also had questions which linked up with the antenatal questions on birth plans and information and how decisions were made. The remainder of the booklet focused on the staff and women's perception of them.

The A4 questionnaire was again divided into sections. The first section collected information about the baby, both specific to the birth and subsequently, including information on feeding. The second section dealt with pain relief and the third with the third stage and stitching, asking both about what had happened and how the woman felt about it. The fourth section asked about general health and well-being since the birth and included a modified version of The Edinburgh Postnatal Depression Scale (Cox et al., 1987).

The questionnaire ended with a series of questions which assessed fulfilment and satisfaction with the birth.

Style of questions

Nearly all questions were multiple choice with women being required to tick the option which applied to them. In addition, there were open-ended questions, typically at the end of sections, which gave them the opportunity to tell us things which were not covered by the multiple choice options. Three of the postnatal questions took the form of adjective check lists: 15 or more adjectives were presented and women were required to circle all of those which they felt described their situation. This technique has been found to be very useful in other contexts (Green et al., 1983), although it is not commonly used. It has the advantage of minimizing the biases of open-ended questions while not limiting respondents to uni-dimensional positions as tends to happen with multiple choice questions. Questions of this form can also be analysed in a variety of ways which maximize the value of the data.

Psychological outcome variables

Four major variables were selected to assess the psychological outcomes or, as Oakley put it, 'how mothers feel after birth' (1980, p. 114). Three of these tapped how women felt about themselves and about the birth experience: fulfilment by the birth, satisfaction with the birth and emotional well-being. The fourth, which we have called 'Description of Baby' related more to women's relationship with their baby.

1. Fulfilment

One of the stereotypes outlined in Chapter 1 described a woman who, among other things, was overly concerned that birth should be a fulfilling experience and who ran the risk of severe postnatal depression in the event of this wish not being met. We included the question 'Was the birth a fulfilling experience' in order that this stereotype could be further explored and also because we hypothesized that wanting birth to be fulfilling was not something confined to a small, rather 'wacky' minority group but instead was of importance to the majority of women.

2. Satisfaction with birth

Chapter 1 reviewed some of the research which has suggested that satisfaction or dissatisfaction with birth is linked to a number of different factors, including difficult delivery, interventions, use of pain relief and women's participation in and control over the process of birth. The question selected as a major outcome variable was a question about overall satisfaction with birth. Women were asked to give a mark ranging from 0 to 10, indicating how satisfactory the experience of birth had been. Satisfaction with birth was treated as a continuous variable in the data analysis, with the mean score out of ten being employed as the outcome measure. We also included a series of questions in the postnatal questionnaire on how satisfied women were with having had or not having had certain interventions, about receiving pain-relieving drugs and how they felt they coped with the pain of labour. These questions were included as components in a factor analysis which aimed to explore what women were and were not satisfied with.

The factor analysis and the four factors produced by it are discussed in Chapter 8 (psychological outcome).

3. Description of baby

Researchers have been concerned with predictors of mothers' relationship with and feelings towards their babies, and with understanding the factors that contribute to a poor relationship.

Our questionnaire included a series of questions designed to tap into the mother-infant relationship at six weeks after birth. In particular, women were offered 16 adjectives which could describe their babies and were asked to circle all that applied to their own baby. To control for the different number of adjectives circled by different women, the measure used was the number of negative words expressed as a percentage of the total number circled. The variable 'Description of Baby' was treated in three categories: no negative adjectives circled at all, up to 30 per cent negative, and more than 30 per cent negative. This is discussed further in Chapter 8.

4. Emotional well-being

The final psychological outcome variable selected was a measure of mood, which we have called 'Emotional Well-Being' (EWB) since the term 'depression' is often used as a clinician's diagnostic label and we were unable to ascertain if any of our sample were clinically depressed.

A modified version of the Edinburgh Postnatal Depression Scale, a screening tool which selects potentially clinically depressed subjects, was used in our questionnaire. The six items we included were:

1. During the last week I have looked forward with enjoyment to things.
2. During the last week I have been anxious or worried for no good reason.
3. During the last week I have felt scared or panicky for no very good reason.
4. During the last week things have been getting on top of me.
5. During the last week I have been so unhappy that I have had difficulty sleeping.
6. During the last week I have felt sad or miserable.

(For an unmodified version of the Scale, with all the response categories, see Appendix.)

The answers to these six items along with those to an additional two questions 'Have you been feeling at all depressed?' and 'On the whole are there more good days than bad?' were entered into a factor analysis. (For a discussion and explanation of this statistical technique see Oppenheim, 1966.) One factor, 'Emotional Well-Being', was extracted from the analysis, accounting for 45.5 per cent of the variance, and made up from all eight variables entered into the factor analysis. (For details of factor loadings and eigenvalues, see Appendix.)

The health districts

The main sample was drawn from women expecting babies in April and May 1987 in four of the NHS Health Districts that had been involved in our earlier study of medical staffing structures. All were semi-rural, centred on towns where the major employment is light industry, service industries, agriculture-related or the Armed Forces. None of the Districts had a teaching hospital, and none were in inner city areas with their attendant special circumstances. Two of the towns had sizeable ethnic minority groups, mainly Asian and Italian.

We shall refer to the Districts by the pseudonyms of Willowford, Exington, Wychester and Zedbury. Each District has a consultant unit. In addition, in Wychester and Zedbury it is also possible to have a GP delivery within the consultant unit. Exington, however, has a separate GP unit although it is in the same hospital and also a small satellite unit for low risk women (Little Exington) approximately 15 miles away which is run essentially by midwives with just one resident SHO. Willowford, Wychester and Zedbury each deliver between 2,000 and 2,500 babies per annum. Exington is a larger District with a total of approximately 3,500 deliveries per annum. In 1985, approximately 2,800 of these were at the consultant unit, with 430 at the GP unit and 290 at Little Exington. However, the number of deliveries at these two smaller units has been increasing. Projected numbers for 1987 were over 50 per cent up on the 1985 figures for both units.

Procedure

We aimed to recruit approximately 800 women. On the basis of the pilot study we made the conservative assumption of a 70 per cent response rate and therefore calculated that we needed to send out approximately 1,150 letters of invitation. The intention was to recruit approximately equal numbers from the four Health Districts, i.e. to target approximately 280 women from each District. This number of births would take place over a shorter or longer time period for different Districts depending on the annual number of deliveries. Thus, at Zedbury, letters were sent to all women due for delivery during a six week period, while at Willowford, letters needed to be sent over a seven and a half week period to target the same number of women. At Exington, with its three different units, it was necessary to use a slightly different procedure, since 75–80 per cent of the District's deliveries take place in the consultant unit. Had we just targeted, say, a five week period for the whole District the number of women in our sample who were booked at the GP unit and the satellite units would have been too small to be statistically useful. We therefore wrote to every woman due for delivery at these two smaller units during April and May: 116 at the GP unit and 76 at Little Exington, and decreased the number of women targeted at the consultant unit accordingly.

Women were identified from hospital booking lists. This was done either by the researchers or by hospital staff, according to the preferences of local ethics committees and senior doctors and midwives. These lists also included all bookings for home deliveries in the Health District.

In all cases, the only information made available was name, address and expected date of delivery, and the only use to which this was put was to invite the women to participate in the study. The letter of invitation, the first questionnaire and a prepaid reply envelope were sent to women eight to ten weeks before their expected date of delivery. Initially we sent reminder letters to women who had not responded within four weeks, but we discontinued this practice when it became apparent that it was relatively ineffective (see below).

Women who returned the first questionnaire were sent the second one four weeks before their expected date of delivery, and the third approximately six weeks after the birth. Reminder letters were sent to non-respondents at both stages. These women had already indicated their willingness to participate by returning the initial questionnaire and their response to reminder letters consequently was much better than to those used at the earlier stage.

In addition to the three questionnaires there was an optional 'Labour Ward Record' which women and their partners could volunteer to keep (see Appendix). This was a brief summary of events on the labour ward, concentrating particularly on aspects to do with the staff. The record was completed as soon as possible after delivery, nominally by the woman's labour companion, but, in practice, often by the woman herself. It was hoped that such a record would yield detailed information, such as the number of midwives encountered, which would probably be forgotten by the time the postnatal questionnaire arrived at six weeks. We were also interested in looking at the consistency of reports immediately after the birth and six weeks later. Unfortunately it has not yet proved possible to analyse this data although we hope to be able to do so in the future.

Response rates

There were some slightly worrying inaccuracies in the hospital lists of names and addresses, specifically 16 envelopes returned by the Post Office marked 'Not known at this address'. This represents 1.4 per cent of the target population and there may well have been other inappropriately addressed envelopes which were simply thrown away. In addition, 17 replies were received from women who were not eligible for inclusion because their babies had already been born or because they had miscarried. Here again, it is likely that these 17 are only a subgroup and that others in the same position simply ignored the letter. We particularly regret any pain that our intrusion may have caused to women who had miscarried.

Detailed response figures are given in the Appendix. Overall, 842 out of 1162 initial questionnaires were returned, 810 without reminder letters, and a further 32 after reminders. This represents a response rate of 73.5 per cent after inappropriately addressed envelopes have been subtracted. However, as we have said, 17 of the women who replied were ineligible for the study, so the final sample consisted of 825 women. Of these, 18 were no longer booked at the hospital from which their name had been obtained. Five of these were transfers to the Exington consultant unit from Little Exington or the GP unit and one woman was a cross-boundary transfer from Zedbury to Willowford. The remaining 12 women had all moved house and were booked into hospitals which were not included in the study. We decided, however, that these women's experiences were still valid and they are included in the analyses except where these refer to specific units.

There was some variation in response rates between units, with the extremes both coming from within the Exington Health District: 79 per cent at the GP unit compared to 67 per cent at the consultant unit.

Response rates to the main antenatal questionnaire were, of course, much higher since these were only sent to women who had indicated a willingness to take part. Three women failed to fill in their names and addresses on the first questionnaire and therefore could not be followed up. Of the 822 questionnaires sent, 758 were returned (92%) although seven women had to be withdrawn because their babies were premature. All were sent postnatal questionnaires but the results were used only for piloting. Of the 64 questionnaires which were not returned a further small percentage are likely to have been women whose babies were born before the questionnaire arrived.

Postnatally, there was a 96 per cent response rate (n = 722). Unfortunately, one of the researchers had her car broken into, and a case containing 25 of the completed postnatal questionnaires was stolen. Happily, our system of coding the questionnaires guaranteed the women's anonymity. The women concerned were all contacted and 13 of them were good enough to complete a duplicate questionnaire. The data from the other 12 is, however, unfortunately lost. Postnatal results are therefore based on only 710 cases.

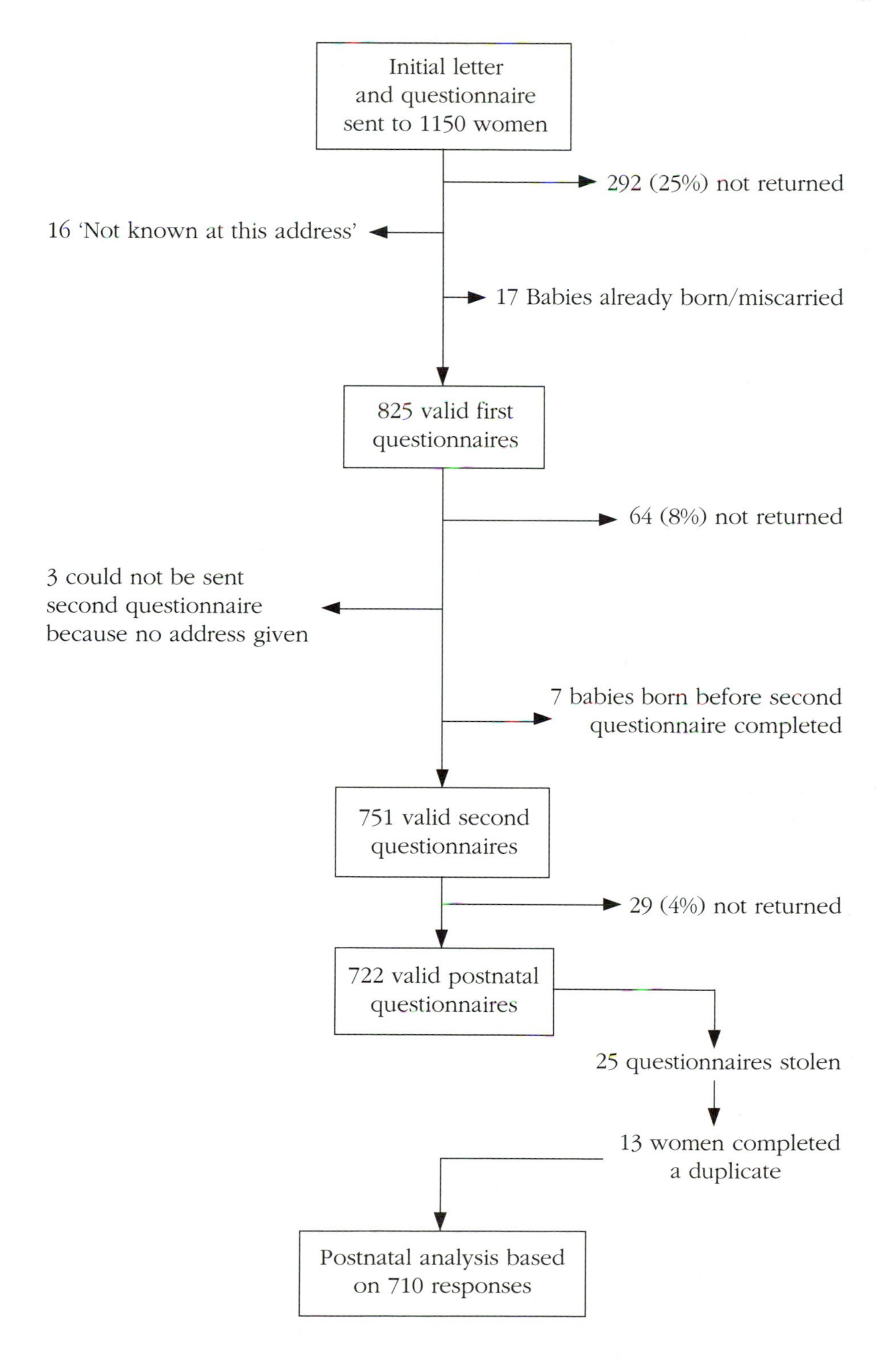

Flow diagram showing responses at each stage of the study

Data analysis and presentation

All information given on the questionnaires, with the exception of names and addresses, was coded and entered onto the computer. This amounted to approximately 700 units of information per subject, i.e. in excess of half a million characters in total. It is clearly neither desirable nor feasible to report on every aspect of this data in this report. However all the basic data has been analysed and all major cross-tabulations (by parity, education and social class and hospital unit) carried out. Chi-square analysis was used unless otherwise stated, although we shall not quote statistical details in the text. Our emphasis in the chapters that follow will be on statistically significant differences: all differences quoted are statistically significant (two-tailed) unless otherwise specified. Conversely we will only refer to a lack of significant differences between groups where this might be counter to expectations.

Percentages are always based on the number of valid responses. Since, inevitably, a small number of women may fail to answer individual questions or give invalid responses, there may be small variations in the numbers quoted in different contexts.

Quotations

Direct quotations from the women participating in the study are used throughout when they illustrate a particular point. We have always attempted to make clear the original context in which women's comments were made. Spelling has been corrected where necessary, but otherwise quotes have not been tampered with.

Organization of this report

The organization of a report of this complexity is something of a challenge. We are conscious that different readers will have different priorities and that what is of interest to one person may seem trivial to another. We are also conscious of the fact that our analysis has often led down byways of considerable interest which do not have direct bearing on the research questions. This has notably been the case for data on birth plans, third stage management, women's views on different forms of pain relief and infant feeding. Our desire to present a coherent thread of results which answer the original research questions has therefore led us to divide our results into two volumes. The areas mentioned above, as well as some smaller areas of interest, are covered in depth in Volume 2. All the main results which pertain to control or expectations are to be found in this volume (Volume 1) in Chapters 3 to 9.

An additional organizational problem is whether to present data chronologically, i.e. all antenatal data before postnatal data, or whether to organize chapters around particular topics, e.g. pain. Our solution has been a mixture of these approaches which we hope will take the best of each. Chapter 3 presents the basic antenatal data: sample characteristics, choice over place of booking, antenatal class attendance and feelings about pregnancy. Chapter 4 also presents only antenatal data: wants and expectations concerning social/behavioural aspects of labour including control, and issues to do with communication and information during pregnancy.

In Chapters 5 and 6 we tackle two of the main areas of concern in labour: pain (and ways of coping with it) and obstetric interventions. Both chapters start with women's antenatal preferences and expectations and follow through to link up with the postnatal results. Chapter 7 returns to the issues covered in Chapter 4 and looks at the extent to which social/behavioural wants and expectations were met and at the importance of issues to do with staff in labour.

Having presented our main findings, we then, in Chapter 8, describe the relationship between all of these and our four psychological outcome measures. Finally, Chapter 9 re-examines the hypotheses presented here in Chapter 2 and draws together some of the threads that have emerged. Chapter 9 is now followed by Chapter 10 which presents an update and new material.

CHAPTER THREE

Basic Antenatal Data

Sample characteristics

Parity

Questionnaires were sent to all eligible women irrespective of parity. However, there is a parity bias in the sample, as the table overleaf shows, because most of the women booked at Little Exington and Exington GP unit were multips, and these two units are disproportionately represented. Nevertheless, overall, our sample is close to the national ratio of 40 per cent primips to 60 per cent multips (OPCS, 1986 Birth Statistics for England and Wales, legitimate livebirths). It should, however, be remembered that the OPCS figures, by excluding births outside marriage, may under-represent primips.

Unit	Total		Primips		Multips	
	n	%	n	%	n	%
Exington:						
Consultant unit	87	(11)	44	(51)	43	(49)
GP unit	85	(10)	7	(8)	78	(92)
Little Exington	50	(6)	13	(26)	37	(74)
Willowford	196	(24)	79	(40)	117	(60)
Wychester	206	(25)	96	(47)	110	(53)
Zedbury	189	(23)	76	(40)	113	(60)
Other	12	(1)	5	(42)	7	(58)
Total	25	(100)	320	(39)	505	(61)

These figures include three booked home deliveries: one at Wychester, one at Willowford and one at Zedbury. All were multips. In the event there were two further (unplanned) home births: one in Willowford and one in Wychester.

Table 3.1: District booked for delivery by parity

The majority of multips already had either one (66%) or two (26%) children, as Table 3.2 shows. This compares to national figures, from the same source as above, of 60 per cent and 26 per cent respectively.

	n	%	National figures*
One	331	(66)	60%
Two	131	(26)	26%
Three	26	(5)	9%
Four	9	(2)	
Five	3	(1)	5%
Six	2	(1)	
Not given	1	(1)	
Total	503	(100)	

*Legitimate Livebirths, 1986, in England and Wales. Source: OPCS, Series FM1, No.15.

Table 3.2: Number of previous children (multips only)

Four multips in fact had no living children. One primip had a stepchild.

Virtually all multips (93%) had at least one pre-school child and 13 of them (3%) had a child under one year old. Eleven per cent of multips had two or more pre-school children.

Comparison with available national figures suggests that our sample is reasonably representative of the population although our family sizes are slightly smaller.

Marital status

The majority of the sample were married or living as married (95%). We did not distinguish between these two states. Thirty one women were single, five divorced, three widowed and two separated.

Age

The sample ranged in age from 15 to 45 years. The mean age for primips was 25.7 years and for multips, 28.4 years. The distribution of ages of the sample as a whole is shown below.

Age (years)	n	%	National figures*
16 or under	8	(1)	3%
17–19	29	(4)	
20–24	187	(23)	27%
25–29	347	(42)	39%
30–34	191	(23)	22%
35–39	55	(7)	8%
40–45	6	(1)	1%

n = 823

*Legitimate Livebirths, 1986, in England and Wales. Source: OPCS, Series FM1, No. 15.

Table 3.3: Age distribution of the sample

Our sample would seem to be broadly comparable with the population. Discrepancies are probably due to the exclusion of illegitimate births from the national figures.

Social class/education

The majority of studies of this kind classify women's social class on the basis of their partner's occupation using the Registrar General's Social Class (RGSC) Categories. However, the Registrar General's classifications have certain limitations. In an attempt to minimize these we chose to use occupational codes developed by Stewart et al. (1980) at the University of Cambridge, Department of Applied Economics. Individual codes are allocated to each of 4000 occupations. These can then be regrouped by computer either into RGSC's, socio-economic groupings, or along any of a number of other dimensions (e.g. medically related occupations) as desired.

A more serious problem is that partner's occupation is not a good indicator of the woman's own social class (see Graham, 1984; Macfarlane and Mugford, 1984). We therefore chose to maximize the available information by taking three indicators: i) age of finishing full-time education, ii) woman's own best ever job, iii) partner's current or usual occupation. 'Best ever' job means the highest status job that the woman has had since finishing full-time education. We used this, rather than current or most recent job, since the constraints of motherhood frequently lead to women undertaking lower status jobs than those for which they are qualified.

The distribution of the sample on all three of these variables is shown in Tables 3.4 and 3.5. Occupation is shown in terms of RGSC categories.

RGSC	Woman's job		Partner's job		National figures (partner's job)
	n	%	n	%	
I	23	(3)	101	(14)	32%
I	262	(33)	183	(26)	
III (non-manual)	360	(46)	81	(11)	11%
III (manual)	44	(6)	219	(31)	36%
IV	58	(7)	95	(13)	20%
V	37	(5)	37	(5)	
Total	784	(100)	716	(100)	(100%)

Table 3.4: Registrar General's Social Class of women's own best ever job and partner's occupation

An additional disadvantage of using partner's occupation as an indicator of woman's social class is that it excludes 13 per cent of the sample who either do not have partners or whose partner's jobs are unclassifiable (see Table 3.5). Even using woman's own occupation excludes the five per cent of women who had never had a paid job.

It will be seen that women's jobs cluster in classes II and III (non-manual) (79% combined) making the RGSC a poor discriminatory tool for our purposes. Comparison of RGSC's of partners' occupations with the proportions for England and Wales as a whole (OPCS Birth Statistics, 1986, Legitimate Livebirths) show our sample to be of somewhat higher social class than the population. However, given that our sampling districts are all in the South East of England where there are relatively fewer people who fall into classes IV and V, the disparity is not too great. The over-representation of classes I and II is a standard finding in studies of this kind particularly when postal questionnaires are used, and also in interview studies (Cartwright, 1987).

Fifty two women (6.3%) had partners who were unemployed at the time of the survey. This is substantially lower than the overall national figure for 1987 of 11.7 per cent (Department of Employment Gazette), but is only slightly lower than the local rates that we have been able to ascertain. Zedbury, for example, had an unemployment rate of 8.1 per cent in 1987. As might be expected, unemployment was strongly related to partner's social class ($p < 0.0001$).

Age (years)	n	%
16 and under*	418	(51)
17–18	232	(28)
19 and over	170	(21)

n = 820

* Includes three women (all of Asian origin) who never went to school.

Table 3.5: Age of finishing full-time education

This distribution shows that our sample is probably better educated than the general population. The Government Statistical Services Education Statistics for the UK (1987) show that since 1965 the proportion of girls leaving school at 16 or earlier has been approximately 80 per cent. However, some of these 80 per cent will have continued their education, for example, at secretarial colleges and colleges of further education after leaving school so the figure is not truly comparable with ours.

Relationship between parity, education and social class

Parity was not significantly related to either education or social class. However, as one would expect, education and social class were strongly related to each other ($p < 0.0001$ for both woman's own and partner's social class). Eighty three per cent of highly educated women had best ever jobs in social classes I or II compared to 17 per cent of the least educated, while 18 per cent of the least educated women had jobs in classes IV and V compared to just four per cent of the most educated. Over 50 per cent of women who had left education aged 16 or less or aged 17 to 18 years had best ever jobs in class III (non-manual), compared to only 11 per cent of the most educated women. These figures reiterate the point made above about the clustering of women's occupations into classes II and III (non-manual).

The relationship between education and partner's social class shows a similar pattern, with the majority of highly educated women (79%) having partners with jobs in classes I and II (compared to 24% of the least educated).

The relatively small numbers falling into classes IV and V mean that we will usually present findings on social class in just three categories, combining I and II, IIIN and IIIM, and IV and V. This gives more satisfactory cell sizes for statistical analysis but does mask differences within these groupings, particularly between classes IV and V. For all the reasons raised in this section we will mainly use level of education as our indicator of social advantage/disadvantage. Data relating to partner's or woman's own RGSC will only be presented where results diverge from those based on level of education, or when it is relevant to look at social class, e.g. in exploring the stereotypes presented in Chapter 1.

Minority groups

In answer to the question about minority group membership, 58 women indicated that they were members of an Italian or Asian community or were married to a member of the British Forces. A further 34 specified some other reason why they felt they had particular needs. These included: being a single parent, being unemployed, having special obstetric problems and having a partner in the American Forces. The results, broken down by Health District, are shown below.

Minority group	District*				Total	
	W	X	Y	Z	No.	%
A. Italian	–	2	–	5	7	(1)
B. Asian	3	5	2	14	24	(3)
C. British Forces	11	11	3	–	27	(3)
D. Other	13	9	10	2	34	(4)
Total	27	27	15	21	92	
% within Districts	(14)	(12)	(7)	(11)	(17)	

*W = Willowford
X = Exington
Y = Wychester
Z = Zedbury

Table 3.6: Minority group membership by Health District

It will be seen that the minority groups we specified are indeed small minorities within our sample, the largest single group being women from the Asian community in Zedbury who account for seven per cent of the Zedbury sample.

The number of women identifying with the Italian community is lower than expected given the size of the communities in Exington and Zedbury. Since both communities are well established with women of childbearing age being second or third generation, it is unlikely that language difficulties prevented women from responding, as may have been the case with some women of Asian origin. Rather, it seems more likely that these second and third generation women of Italian descent do not identify themselves sufficiently with the Italian community to indicate this on our questionnaire. An attempt has been made to investigate this issue further (Lindsay, 1987). However, because of the small numbers involved we have attempted no separate analyses of these subgroups.

Differences between Health Districts

As we have already seen, the Exington sample contains a disproportionate number of multips because the GP unit and the satellite unit are over-represented. However, the sample from Exington is also atypical in terms of a number of other independent variables which are not necessarily related to this bias. For example, there is a much higher percentage of women who are neither married nor living as married booked at the Exington consultant unit (12%) than at any of the other units (range 0–5%). The Exington women (both at the consultant unit and at the GP unit, but not at Little Exington) are also more likely to have unemployed partners: 14 per cent compared to 4–6 per cent at the other units. Consistent with these findings, the Exington sample tends to be of lower social class than those in the other districts, although differences are not statistically significant (see Appendix).

Changes over time

As we have reported in Chapter 2, the postnatal sample contained 710 women, 115 being lost from the original antenatal sample for reasons already described. There were no differences at all between women who stayed in the sample and those who did not in terms of parity. There were, however, highly significant differences in terms of all three indicators of social class/education. The effect of these is to increase the bias towards well educated women in our sample, but this is not a major shift.

	Stayed in		Dropped out	
Educational level	n	%	n	%
16 or under	342	(82)	73	(18)
17–18	207	(89)	25	(11)
19 or over	157	(92)	13	(8)
$p < 0.01$				

Table 3.7: Women who dropped out the original sample by education level

Educational level	Original sample	Final sample
16 or under	51%	48%
17–18	28%	29%
19 or over	21%	22%
Total	100%	100%

Table 3.8: Proportion of women educated to each level in a) the original sample, b) the final sample

Choice in place of booking for delivery

It is generally taken for granted that women will be delivered in the hospital nearest to where they live; if the question of choice does arise it is usually with respect to those few women who are interested in the option (or the non-option as it usually transpires) of a home delivery. For those women who do wish to choose between hospitals, information about the intervention rates and obstetric policies is difficult to come by (and interpret) and obstetricians quite frequently view attempts to acquire and disseminate such information with hostility. The publication of *The Good Birth Guide* (Kitzinger, 1979, 1983), a book of information and advice about different obstetric units, was met with outrage by some doctors. As one obstetrician complained:

> 'No other discipline in medicine has this problem. Neurosurgeons do not have to contend with the *Good Neurosurgery Guide.*' (Francis, 1985)

Yet, if a woman lives within travelling distance of two hospitals, as in Exington district, it is precisely this kind of detailed information on policy and practice which is necessary in order for her to make an informed choice. Women were asked whether they felt that they had had a choice about where to have their babies, and how they felt about this. Just under half the sample felt they did have a choice in where they were booked.

	n of women	% of women
Yes	390	(48)
No	375	(46)
Other (e.g. inappropriate answer such as 'no choice needed' or 'fine')	48	(6)
Don't know/unsure	6	(<1)
n = 819		

Table 3.9: Choice over place of booking

It is important to ask what women who answered 'yes' mean by this. Only a small proportion qualified their answers, but where they did it is possible to discern a range of meanings, or degrees of choice experienced by women. The following quotations show that some women indeed made 'real' choices, but later we look at more ambiguous responses.

Forty eight women (6% of the sample) explained that they had made an active choice between different hospitals or between Exington GP unit and Exington Consultant unit:

> 'Living [here] allows you the choice between Exington and Willowford.'

> 'I chose to go to Exington consultant unit rather than Little Exington as I feel there is more equipment available.'

Women with previous experience could more easily make decisions between hospitals. One woman pregnant with her third child explained:

> 'The staff and relaxed atmosphere at Wychester Hospital made my second labour so much easier and enjoyable that it made my first [at another hospital in the area], although 9 years ago, seem horrendous and out of my control. Therefore I've booked into Wychester for this labour and I am hoping for the same easy and relaxed labour I had last time, where I felt informed and involved totally in what was going on.'

Another 13 women stressed that they had been very assertive in order to get what they wanted (tracking down information, for example), or even had to actively fight for it:

> 'I approached them even though it is out of my area.'

> 'This time, yes [I had choice], as I had my first baby at the above hospital after a big fight with my GP and local health authority.'

Just under half the sample (46%) said that they had not experienced any choice in where to have their babies. The usual procedure is for the GP to allocate each woman to a consultant and hospital and many GPs do not discuss different options with their patients or allow them to choose. As many women do not ask about different options, booking is often left entirely to the GP. Fifteen women in our sample specifically said that there had been no question of choice and that they had been automatically booked into their particular hospital. This was probably true for many more women who did not spontaneously say so:

> 'It was just assumed I would go there by my GP.'

> 'I am automatically booked – but I was not told about it until I asked.'

A few women (7) explained that current obstetric complications, past problems or age precluded any other option than the hospital they were booked into:

> 'My feelings did not really matter, as after my first delivery I had a retained placenta. Consequently it was only common sense to book into hospital in case this situation recurred…'

This reason was generally given by women who distinguished booking between home and hospital or a small low tech unit (such as the GP unit or satellite unit) and a consultant unit, e.g.

> '[I would have liked] to be delivered at Little Exington but facilities are not good for difficult births. I've had one Caesarean section, one forceps delivery.'

(In the event the baby was born at the satellite unit. It seems that exceptions may be made.)

Perceived choice by place of booking and educational level

Perceived choice in place of booking varied between districts and hospitals.

Unit	Choice		No Choice		Other	
	n	%	n	%	n	%
Exington Consultant	28	(33)	54	(64)	3	(4)
Exington GP	49	(59)	31	(37)	3	(4)
Little Exington	34	(71)	11	(23)	3	(6)
Willowford Consultant	101	(52)	83	(43)	9	(5)
Wychester Consultant	102	(50)	86	(42)	17	(8)
Zedbury Consultant	68	(37)	104	(56)	13	(7)
n = 799						
p < 0.0001						

Table 3.10: Perceived choice by place of booking

The figures for Wychester and Zedbury include the small percentage of women booked for GP deliveries within these units. Home births have been excluded.

Both the highest and lowest degrees of perceived choice were found in the district in which women theoretically had the choice of three different units. The low risk women in this area, i.e. women booked at Little Exington and Exington GP unit, were the most likely to say they had choice, while those booked for Exington consultant unit were the least likely. This is as one would expect given the reality of women assessed as high risk automatically being booked into the consultant unit, whereas the others had the choice of the GP unit and Little Exington. This variety of alternatives did not exist in our other areas.

In practice, the greater degree of choice apparent at Exington GP unit and Little Exington was restricted to multiparous women, i.e. those most likely to be assessed as low risk: only 8 per cent of women booked for Exington GP unit and 26 per cent at Little Exington were primips, compared to 40–50 per cent at all the other hospitals. However, in general, there was no relationship between parity and choice.

Age on leaving full-time education was significantly related to whether women felt that had had a choice over where they were booked, with more of the highly educated women feeling that they had had a choice. However, there is no relationship between women's educational level and the unit at which they are booked.

Educational level	Choice		No choice		Other	
	n	%	n	%	n	%
16 or under	181	(44)	212	(52)	15	(4)
17 or 18	117	(51)	98	(42)	16	(7)
19 or over	90	(54)	61	(37)	16	(10)

n = 806

$p < 0.01$

Table 3.11: Perceived choice of place of booking by educational level

We next tried to get at some measure of satisfaction with the hospital women were booked into. Women were asked 'Would you have preferred to be booked somewhere else?' (begging the question of an alternative of course). Nearly everyone (93%) was happy with where they were booked or at least did not express any dissatisfaction with this. Of the 58 women who did expressed dissatisfaction, the proportion was highest among women in Exington consultant unit (13%) which is also the unit where women felt they had least choice. It may well be relevant that this hospital has the highest rates of intervention in our study (see Green et al., 1986), and a reputation locally of being reactionary (obstetrically speaking).

Of all the women who would have preferred to be delivered elsewhere, half (30) would have liked to have had their baby at home. However, opposition from the hospital, GP or family prevented them from pursuing this. (Only three women in our sample were in fact booked for home deliveries.) The other women who would have preferred to be delivered elsewhere explained they would have liked to go to a particular hospital which was too far away. This was usually a hospital where they had had an earlier baby and had since moved away. A few foreign women wanted to be delivered in their home country, back in less alien surroundings:

> 'Because I'm Italian and don't speak English and I would of found given birth would be better if I was back home with family.'

Discussion

The fact that so many women (93%) did not express a preference to be booked anywhere else warrants more consideration. It is a clear illustration of the difficulty of thinking in terms of 'choice', when all such considerations are made within a framework of constraints. The end result is many different understandings of choice which vary according to women's social and cultural background, their past experiences and present expectations. Some of these different understandings are illustrated in the ways in which women spontaneously qualified their answers on whether they had had a choice in the place of booking. Some pointed out the importance of the hospital's physical proximity to where they lived:

> 'I don't think choice comes into it. Willowford is my nearest hospital.'

> 'No [choice] however it would be inconvenient to myself to travel any further.'

Information about different options is vital. It was clear that some women would have chosen differently had they known about the alternatives available if they were prepared to travel:

> '... it would have been nice to have been told what place would have been available as I now understand that I could have gone to Willowford.'

Other women who did not feel they had a choice in where they were booked nevertheless believed that if they had wanted to go elsewhere it would have been possible:

> 'I could have changed if I had asked.'

It was not at all clear on what they based such certainty. Sixty nine women (8% of the sample) qualified their responses by saying that they found the hospital they were booked into was acceptable to them:

> 'Other options were not discussed and I did not ask as I am happy to go to Wychester General.'

> 'No [choice] but this would have been my choice anyway, being close and from earlier experience offering a good service and pleasant environment.'

Although most of the women who qualified their responses in these terms had previously said they did not have any choice in the place of booking, some of them in fact felt they did have a choice.

Several women interpreted the question of choice in terms of choosing between different kinds of maternity care within the same hospital:

> 'Yes, as this was my second child and there were no complications with the first, my doctor gave me the choice of the maternity unit or the... [GP unit].'

> 'No choice of hospital – but had choice of GP or consultant unit.'

The idea of having a choice seemed quite unrealistic or unfamiliar to several women:

> '...You don't expect to be asked where you want the baby as too many women have babies and everyone would not be able to have their choice.'

The final point we would make is to stress that whether choice is a relevant question or not may depend largely on how happy a woman is with whatever she ends up with. The great majority of the sample, as we have seen, were satisfied with where they were booked for delivery despite the fact that nearly half of them felt that they had not had any choice in the matter. If the outcome (regardless of whether it is actively chosen or not) is acceptable to the woman, choice of other units becomes irrelevant except in purely theoretical terms. Choice only tends to become a burning issue when women are unhappy with where they have been allocated.

Choice of consultant

The alternatives of being booked for delivery in a high tech consultant unit, a low tech GP unit or at home, clearly have very different implications for the kind of obstetric care provided during labour. Likewise, *who* a woman is booked with may be at least as important as *where* she is booked in determining how labour is managed. Consultants often have different policies on induction, acceleration, drug dosages, monitoring and so on, right through to the kind of suturing material which is used. However, few women are aware of this fact and consequently assume that the question of who they are booked with is an irrelevant one:

> 'It doesn't matter to me as long as I am getting the treatment I need.'

> 'All the consultants names were given (I know most) and I was asked who I would prefer. I didn't mind as they all do the same job.'

For the most part, women who have given birth at a particular hospital before are booked with the same consultant again (unless they raise an objection):

> 'I was under [this consultant] for my first pregnancy and was happy to do so again. I was not offered a choice in my first pregnancy but saw no reason to question it.'

Women expecting their first baby explained to us that even if they were offered a choice of consultants (rather than being automatically allocated by the GP) they would not have the information required to make a decision:

> 'The doctor asked if I had a preference but since this is a first baby I wasn't able to give a preference, therefore he selected the consultant.'

> 'I would like to have been able to choose both my consultant and midwife. However, as I do not know the hospital staff, I have just accepted my allocated consultant.'

In the event, most women are not offered a choice in the matter anyway (see Table 3.12):

> 'No choice. I was sent a letter with 3 names as signatories, I feel whoever is at the top of the list has the next mum, so to speak...'

When asked if she would have preferred another consultant, one woman answered with brevity:

> 'Did not matter. Was not asked.'

However, just over a third of the sample did feel that they had had some measure of choice about their consultant.

	n of women	% of women
Yes, had choice	271	(37)
No, did not have choice	440	(59)
Other (e.g. 'probably')	25	(3)
Don't know/unsure	6	(<1)
n = 742 (GP bookings excluded)		

Table 3.12: Choice of consultant

There were significant differences between hospital units in the answer to the question about choice of consultant.

Unit	Did have choice		Did not have choice		Other	
	n	%	n	%	n	%
Exington consultant	32	(40)	46	(57)	3	(4)
Little Exington	14	(29)	34	(69)	1	(2)
Willowford	67	(36)	111	(60)	8	(4)
Wychester	92	(48)	91	(48)	8	(4)
Zedbury	28	(17)	135	(81)	4	(2)
n = 650						
(NB: Figures exclude GP unit bookings and home births)						

Table 3.13: Choice of consultant by place of booking

Over a quarter of the women booked at the satellite unit (29%) felt they had chosen their consultant, which we find rather surprising given that only one of the Exington consultants works at Little Exington and therefore everyone is booked with him. By choosing in the first place to be delivered there other choices (such as having a woman consultant) are automatically excluded. Although it is possible that some women wish to be booked with this consultant and so opt for Little Exington, it is far more likely that they wish to give birth in the local unit and therefore end up with him automatically. Women at Zedbury experienced the least choice. They were distributed almost equally between the three consultants there.

Education was significantly related to choice over consultant ($p < 0.05$) (as it was to choice over unit). A third of those who left school at 16 or earlier said they had a choice of consultant as against 41 per cent of those who had stayed in further education beyond 18 years. However, the differences between groups were not very great (see Appendix). There was no significant relationship between woman's social class and choice of consultant, although more women in classes I and II said that they had choice.

Despite the fact that two thirds of the women said they had no choice in who their consultant was, only five per cent (36 women) said they would have preferred someone else. Reasons for preferring someone else were: want a woman doctor (4 woman), prefer own GP to the consultant (4 women), do not like the consultant (13 women), want someone else in particular, i.e. named another doctor (4 women). A couple of women stated that although they had no definite preferences they wanted a choice on principle.

However, most women did not express any sort of strong feelings on the subject. One Italian woman did describe being treated very poorly. She spoke very little English and no interpreter had been available at the hospital. (She had however received help at home filling in our questionnaire):

> 'I would of preferred somebody with more feelings, and could of explained what was going on. As I felt like a non-existing human, just number and book (next please) sort of feeling.'

Fortunately, this seemed an uncommon experience in our study hospitals, although other women, especially Asian and Italian women may occasionally have been treated shabbily and be unwilling to complain. A more common response to the question 'Would you have preferred somebody else?' was:

> 'Having met the consultant I'm a bit uncertain but wouldn't know who to change to even if I was given the chance.'

Antenatal emotional well-being

Feelings when first pregnant

We were interested in which factors may influence maternal outcome as measured by fulfilment, satisfaction with the birth, postnatal mood and relationship with the baby. It has been shown that prenatal attitudes towards the pregnancy and the fetus may be linked to the development of a good postnatal relationship between mother and child (Breen, 1975; Peterson and Mehl, 1978). A positive attitude towards the pregnancy may also be related to better birth experiences e.g. in coping with the pain (Niven and Gisbers, 1984). Consequently, we decided to look at prenatal attitudes as a potential indicator of both obstetric outcome and maternal outcome.

We felt that to ask women if they had wanted the baby would put undue pressure on them to say yes. Asking whether the pregnancy was planned is misleading since many pregnancies may be unplanned but nevertheless much wanted. Instead we asked women how they felt when they discovered that they were pregnant, offering them six options. Their answers are shown overleaf.

Feelings when first pregnant	n	%
Overjoyed	336	(41)
Pleased	266	(32)
Mixed feelings	180	(22)
Not very happy	19	(2)
Very unhappy	13	(2)
No particular feelings	11	(1)
n = 825		

Table 3.14: Reaction on discovering pregnancy

As we can see from Table 3.14, three quarters of the sample were pleased or overjoyed on discovering that they were pregnant. Only a small number of women (32) were actually unhappy, and 11 women rather sadly seemed indifferent saying that they had no particular feelings either way. However, nearly a quarter of the women said that they had had mixed feelings on finding that they were pregnant.

The parity breakdown for feelings when first pregnant shows little difference between multips and primips, except that women pregnant for the first time were more likely to say they were 'overjoyed' rather than just pleased. Clearly, the experience of being pregnant for the first time with a wanted baby can be extra special and is reflected in these responses.

Parity	Overjoyed	Pleased	Mixed	Not v. happy	Very unhappy	No particular feelings
Primips	162 (50%)	68 (21%)	73 (23%)	5 (2%)	6 (2%)	8 (3%)
Multips	174 (35%)	198 (39%)	107 (21%)	14 (3%)	7 (1%)	3 (1%)
n = 825						
p < 0.0001						

Table 3.15: Feelings on discovering pregnancy by parity

We then asked women how they had felt overall during pregnancy. This is not necessarily a straightforward question to answer because it is possible to feel very differently across the whole range of emotions in different periods during the pregnancy. However, we believed that we would pick up anyone who felt that depression or low mood dominated their pregnancy, for whatever reason.

Feeling	n	%
Reasonably cheerful most of the time	565	(68)
Depressed/low spirited/worried/anxious	56	(7)
Mood swings	189	(23)
Other	14	(2)
n = 824		

Table 3.16: Overall feeling during pregnancy

As Table 3.16 above shows, 68 per cent of women felt they had been reasonably cheerful throughout pregnancy, slightly less than the proportion who had felt overjoyed or pleased on first discovering they were pregnant. The same proportion who had mixed feelings initially had mood swings throughout pregnancy (though they are not necessarily the same women). Seven per cent of women felt depressed, low-spirited or generally anxious.

Finally, we compared women's overall feeling during pregnancy with their initial feeling on discovering they were pregnant. Here a clear pattern is evident with women who were initially unhappy (or who had no particular feeling) more likely to feel depressed or have mood swings during pregnancy: 16 per cent of these women felt depressed compared to only 5 per cent who had been overjoyed initially, and 42 per cent had mood swings compared to 20 per cent who had been overjoyed initially. Only 42 per cent of those who had been initially unhappy about the pregnancy felt reasonably cheerful during the subsequent antenatal months compared to three quarters of those who had been overjoyed. It seems then that initial reaction to pregnancy is a good indicator of mood throughout. However, it must be noted that we are comparing a small number of depressed women to a much greater number of happy women (see Appendix).

For antenatal attitudes towards pain and expectations of pain during labour, see Chapter 5 on pain and pain relief.

Childbirth preparation classes

Women in different areas were attending a wide variety of preparation classes and the type of class offered by different units also showed considerable variation. Willowford, for instance, offers 'active birth' classes closer to the National Childbirth Trust (NCT) classes than conventional hospital childbirth preparation teaching.

Type of class attended

Forty two women (6% of the sample) were attending NCT classes at 36 weeks of pregnancy and another seven per cent were attending classes run by their GPs. The majority, however, were attending classes run by midwives or the hospital. Ten per cent of the women had not yet attended or not yet decided to attend classes (this was only about four weeks before their expected date of delivery); a further 46 per cent of the sample had not so far attended classes and were definitely not intending to do so. However, almost half of the sample were attending classes during their current pregnancy.

Attending classes	Primips		Multips		Whole sample	
	n	%	n	%	n	%
Am/have attended	236	(81)	96	(21)	332	(44)
Will attend	12	(4)	13	(3)	25	(3)
Undecided	18	(6)	34	(7)	52	(7)
Won't attend	27	(9)	316	(69)	342	(46)

Table 3.17: Attendance at childbirth preparation classes during current pregnancy

Number of classes attended at 36 weeks of pregnancy

Taking into account only the 332 women who were attending classes, women had, at this point, attended (on average) between four and five classes each. However, the attendance for individual women ranged from just one class (29 women) to nine classes or more (22 women). Some women attended two sets of classes. On the whole they described the classes as 'good' or 'very good' (80%) with just 19 per cent describing the classes as 'mixed' and only one woman saying her classes were poor.

Reasons why women did not attend classes

The following question was answered only by the 342 women who had no intention of attending classes:

'Why are you not planning to attend any childbirth preparation classes? Please tick whichever apply (you may tick more than one).'

I know all I need to know from any previous birth(s)	40%
I know all I need to know from things I've read and/or talking to other women who have had babies	10%
It is not convenient for me to attend classes (distance, time, childcare problems etc.)	52%
There's no point, you can't learn how to give birth	9%
I get the information I need from the antenatal clinic	6%
I have attended classes for my previous birth(s) and I feel I can remember all I need from them.	52%

Percentages are of non-attenders who ticked each option

The reason given most frequently for not attending classes was that it was not convenient. This was ticked by 52 per cent of the women who answered the question. Some women mentioned having no childcare for younger children and not having any way of getting to classes. Half of the women (52%) said that they had attended classes for previous births and felt they could remember all that they needed. Forty per cent ticked the option 'I know all I need to know from any previous birth'. Ten per cent of the women felt they knew enough from reading and/or talking to other women and nine per cent felt that there was no point going to classes as 'you can't learn to give birth'. Only a few felt that they did not need classes because they received the information they needed from the clinic (6%). (These last two options were, in any case, rarely ticked in isolation.) On average women ticked 1.8 reasons each.

Women's feelings that previous experiences of childbirth (and/or of antenatal classes) made going to antenatal classes this time around unnecessary are reflected in the fact that primips were much more likely to attend antenatal classes than multips. By the time they had received our second questionnaire 81 per cent of primips had attended classes as opposed to just 21 per cent of multips.

Relationship between education and attending antenatal classes

As expected, the more educated women were more likely to attend classes than the less educated women. Only 36 per cent of the women who left school at 16 or earlier were attending classes as opposed to 63 per cent of those who had stayed in full-time education until 19 or later. (A similar relationships exists for social class.)

Education did not appear to be associated with women's assessment of how good classes were, but it did relate to the reasons they gave for not attending classes. The less educated women were more likely to say they did not attend classes because 'you can't learn to give birth' ($p < 0.01$). The highly educated women, on the other hand, were more likely to say that they could remember enough from classes attended during a previous pregnancy ($p < 0.001$) – a fact that probably reflects the tendency of more educated women to attend classes in the first place.

Educational level	You can't learn to give birth		Know enough from previous class attendance	
	n	%	n	%
16 or under	25	(13)	76	(39)
17–18	5	(5)	68	(67)
19 and over	0	(0)	34	(71)

Percentages are of women of a given educational level.

Table 3.18: Reasons for not attending classes by education

Relationship between antenatal classes and parity

As we have already mentioned, women approaching their first birth were four times as likely as multips to have attended antenatal classes. Only 21 per cent of multips were attending classes and, interestingly, 25 per cent of these were attending NCT classes. By contrast 81 per cent of the primips were attending classes and only 8 per cent of these were going to NCT classes.

Parity, like education, was not associated with women's views on how good or informative their classes were but it was related to the reasons given by non-attenders for not going to classes. Obviously, it was the multips who ticked the options 'I know all I need to know from any previous birth(s)' (ticked by 43% of the multips not attending classes), and 'I have attended classes for my previous birth(s) and feel I can remember all I need from them' (ticked by 56% of the multips not attending classes). No primips ticked these options much to our relief! Primips, however, were more likely to tick the option 'I know all I need to know from things I've read and/or talking to other women who have had babies'. This was ticked by a third of the primips who were not attending classes. Second hand knowledge was substituted for knowledge gained from personal experience. Interestingly, primips were also more likely to say that 'you can't learn to give birth'.

Relationship between class attendance and unit booked for delivery

Women booked for delivery at Little Exington and the Exington GP unit were less likely to attend classes than women booked at the consultant units – a fact which probably simply reflects the predominance of multips at these units. Women who were booked at each of the four consultant units were equally likely to attend classes. Not surprisingly, women booked at the GP unit were more likely to attend antenatal classes run by GPs than the other women.

It is worth noting the one striking relationship between where women were booked for delivery and their reasons for not attending classes. Seventy five per cent of the non-attenders booked at Little Exington said that it was too inconvenient to attend classes as opposed to, at the other end of the spectrum, only 33 per cent of women booked at Exington consultant unit. It seems unlikely that women were just saying it was inconvenient to attend classes as an easy 'excuse' but rather they were responding to particular situations – women booked at Little Exington have to go into Exington consultant unit for NHS antenatal classes. Numbers were too small to carry out analysis of women's perceptions of the classes they attended by unit booked for delivery.

CHAPTER FOUR

Social/Behavioural Aspects Of Labour: Antenatal Data

Wants and expectations

One of our concerns was to investigate the relationship between antenatal wants and expectations and maternal outcome, especially where wants or expectations are not fulfilled. Women's expectations about pain and their preferences concerning pain relief are considered in the appropriate section in this report (Chapter 5), as are feelings about obstetric interventions (Chapter 6). This chapter is concerned with social/behavioural aspects of labour, e.g. who will be there and how decisions will be made.

Twelve questions were asked with the same format. Part a) asked how important it was that some particular thing happened and part b) asked what they actually expected would happen. We will report here briefly the answers to each of the twelve questions. Tables of results are given in the Appendix.

1. **Do you want a birth companion (husband/partner/mother/friend) with you at all times throughout your labour?**
   Ninety four per cent of the sample wanted this, 85 per cent wanting it 'very much'. Four per cent did not mind. Only 66 per cent were sure that it would actually happen, with a further 26 per cent thinking that it probably would.

2. **Do you want to be delivered by a midwife or a doctor?**
   This question was included because many staff in the first phase of our research believed that women had a preference. In fact, half said that they did not mind while 46 per cent preferred a midwife. Only 4 per cent preferred a doctor (probably those booked for elective caesarean sections). Seventy nine per cent actually expected to be delivered by a midwife; this is a pretty good estimate of national figures (OPCS figures for 1984 show 78% of women having non-instrumental vaginal deliveries). Fourteen per cent had no expectations.

3. Do you want to be looked after during labour by a midwife that you have already met?

Our expectation was that most women would prefer this option although, in fact, only 62 per cent said 'yes' and 37 per cent said they did not mind. Perhaps their answers were tempered by their expectations: 49 per cent thought it unlikely and 27 per cent had no expectations. This still leaves 18 per cent who did think it likely and 7 per cent who were sure that they would be looked after by a familiar midwife. This figure actually disguises a massive difference between units: at the Exington GP unit 62 per cent thought that they definitely or probably would have a familiar midwife compared, at the other extreme, to only 13 per cent at the Exington consultant unit. This difference is also reflected in these women's wants: only 18 per cent at the GP unit did not mind whether or not they were looked after by a familiar midwife compared to between 35 per cent and 43 per cent at the other five units. It could be that the GP unit women chose the GP unit precisely because they cared more about this issue and saw the GP unit as their best bet for having their wishes met.

4. Do you want to have the same midwife with you throughout your labour and delivery?

Only 13 per cent of women did not mind, the remaining 87 per cent all wanted this continuity. However, only 49 per cent expected it and 23 per cent thought it unlikely. There were differences between units in both wants and expectations similar to those for the previous question.

5. How important is it to you *not* to have lots of different people coming in and out of the room while you are in labour?

Caroline Flint (1986b) and others have drawn attention to a lack of privacy in hospital labour wards, with many comings and goings which are irrelevant to the labour in progress. We were therefore interested to know women's expectations and how strongly they felt about the issue. Only 12 per cent said that they did not mind, with 55 per cent preferring not and a further 33 per cent saying that they definitely did not want lots of comings and goings. However, expectations were also high. Eleven per cent were sure that there would not be lots of different people, 51 per cent thought that there probably would not be while only 19 per cent thought that there would be. The same number (19%) had no expectations. There were no differences between units in terms of what women wanted but there were differences in expectations. In particular, expectations were notably lower at Exington consultant unit.

6. Assuming that there are no complications, who would you think should make most of the decisions about your labour?

We saw this as a key question about choice and control: are women happy to leave all decisions up to the staff and, if not, what degree of involvement do they want? We gave five possible options for women to choose from, and their responses are shown in Table 4.1.

	n	%
Staff should just get on with it, that's their job	6	(<1)
Staff should make the decisions but I'd like to be kept informed	199	(27)
Staff should discuss things with me before reaching their decision	269	(36)
Staff should give me their assessment of the situation but I should still be the one in control of the decision	260	(35)
I don't mind	6	(<1)
n = 740		

Table 4.1: Assuming that there are no complications, who would you think should make most of the decisions about your labour?

In other words, nearly three quarters of the women want an active part in decisions, not just to be 'kept informed'. Responses to this question were significantly related to level of education, with the more educated women wanting a greater involvement in decision making. However, there was still a clear majority even among the least educated women (65%) who wanted at least to have issues discussed with them.

Women's expectations were not as high as their ideals, but 55 per cent still expected either to have issues discussed or to make decisions themselves. Thirty eight per cent thought that the staff would make the decisions but keep them informed, while five per cent thought that the staff would just get on with it. Multips and less educated women had significantly lower expectations than primips and more educated women. This may explain why expectations of involvement were significantly lower for Exington where we sampled relatively more multips and where women were less well educated. At all the Exington units and at Zedbury the modal response was that staff would keep them informed. By contrast, at Willowford and Wychester the most common expectation was that staff would discuss things before making a decision.

The next question was identical except that it specified decision making in an emergency.

7. **In an emergency who do you think should make the decisions?**
   The same response options were offered as for question 6. This time a clear majority (72%) saw decision making as the staff's responsibility although the majority of these (65% of the sample) wanted to be kept informed. However, 21 per cent wanted discussion and six per cent still wanted to be in control of decisions. Unlike non-emergency decision making, these responses were not related to women's level of education, however their expectations were (perhaps with reason).

	Educational level					
Expectation	16 and under		17–18		19 and over	
	n	%	n	%	n	%
Staff alone	95	(26)	40	(19)	17	(11)
Kept informed	211	(58)	131	(64)	111	(69)
Discussion	45	(12)	27	(13)	27	(17)
My decision	10	(3)	7	(3)	6	(4)
Don't know	5	(1)	1	(<1)	0	(0)
Total	366	(100)	206	(100)	162	(100)
$p < 0.01$						

Table 4.2: Expectations of involvement in emergency decision-making by level of education

8. Do you want to be in control of what doctors and midwives do to you during labour?

This question is clearly tapping some of the same ideas as the previous two but goes beyond mere decision making. It is also the first of a series using the word 'control' in specific contexts. We were interested to know if there were women who explicitly did not want to be in control of what was done to them. Assuming that most women did want control, we also wanted to know how important an issue it was. One woman, although saying that she 'did not mind', added:

'I found these difficult to answer, as I feel no-one should be *in control* but the decisions more of a consensus.'

Once again results show a strong relationship with level of education.

	Educational level					
Want control?	16 and under		17–18		19 and over	
	n	%	n	%	n	%
Very much	120	(33)	75	(37)	79	(50)
Quite like	161	(44)	98	(48)	65	(41)
Don't mind	76	(21)	27	(13)	13	(8)
Prefer not	7	(2)	5	(2)	2	(1)
Definitely not	0	(0)	0	(0)	0	(0)
Total	364	(100)	205	(100)	159	(100)
$p < 0.001$						

Table 4.3: Do you want to be in control of what doctors and midwives do to you during labour? (by educational level)

As Table 4.3 shows, only a very tiny minority of women would prefer not to be in control of what is done to them and not a single woman in the whole sample said that she definitely did not want to be. The biggest difference between groups of different levels of education is in the 'Don't mind' category (a consistent finding throughout this study), with 21 per cent of the least educated women 'not minding' compared with only 8 per cent of the most highly educated women. The other difference lies in the strength of feeling: 50 per cent of the 19 and over group wanted it 'very much' compared to 33 per cent of the 16 and under group. There were also highly significant differences, in the expected direction, in the expectations of women with different levels of education. Overall, 61 per cent of women had positive expectations, 24 per cent had none and 15 per cent had negative expectations. Expectations were highest at Willowford and Wychester and lowest at the Exington consultant unit. There were also parity differences here: notably, 19 per cent of multips had negative expectations compared to 8 per cent of primips. Primips were, quite reasonably, more likely to have no expectations.

Other characteristics of women who did/did not want 'external' control are considered in greater depth later in this chapter.

9. How important is it to you not to lose control of the way you behave during labour?

This was the first of three questions about 'internal' control. We had thought that control of one's own behaviour might be the sense in which control was most important to women (Bing et al., 1961). In fact, only 25 per cent said that it was very important, 51 per cent said quite important and the remainder said that it was either not very (20%) or not at all (4%) important. There were no significant differences related to level of education, although there were when we came to look at expectations; the higher a woman's level of education, the greater her expectations of not losing control. Interestingly, this is one question where the 'no expectations' option is ticked by similar proportions of women of different educational levels (approximately 28%). There were also expectation differences between multips and primips with multips having higher expectations of staying in control of their behaviour. These parity differences account for such differences as exist between units. Note the interesting fact that multips have *lower* expectations of *'external'* control than primips, but *higher* expectations of *'internal'* control. In other words, they are more cynical about the staff (see also their views on Birth Plans, Vol. 2), but they have more confidence in themselves.

10. How important is it to you to feel in control during contractions?

A further aspect of 'internal' control concerns the idea of being in control during contractions. This was very important to 37 per cent of the sample and quite important to a further 54 per cent. However, there are several possible meanings to being in control during contractions. This question is not sufficiently sensitive to differentiate between them. There is the idea of not feeling overwhelmed by the intensity of contractions, of staying 'on top' of them. Closely connected to this is the technique of breathing through one's contractions, advocated and taught in some childbirth preparation classes. However, there is also the suggestion that 'being in control' means being able to let go of rigid controlled behaviour and going with the contractions. There were no differences by education or parity. In the case of expectations there were again no differences by education, but multips and primips had significantly different expectations, primarily in the 'no expectations' category (30% of primips versus 16% of multips). Overall 64 per cent of women had positive expectations and 15 per cent negative.

11. How important is it to you to be sure that you do not make a lot of noise during labour?

We had thought that making a noise might be what people had in mind when they spoke of losing control of their behaviour. However, answers to this question, while broadly associated with question 8, show that this is not something that is very important to many women. For example, one woman who had said that it was '*very* very important' not to lose control of the way she behaved, said that it was 'not at all important' not to make a lot of noise. Those women to whom it was important or very important tended to have a lower level of education (47% of the 16 and under group compared to 32% of those with higher education). Multips were twice as likely as primips to say that it was very important (14% compared to 7%). Most did not expect to make a lot of noise (55%), while 18 per cent thought they would and 28 per cent had no expectations. Multips were much more likely to think that they would not make a lot of noise (57% compared to 36% of primips), while primips were again more likely to have no expectations (45% compared to 17% of multips).

Table 4.4 summarizes women's feelings about control in each of the six contexts that we asked about. From this it will be clear that these questions are tapping different ideas and that women are differentiating between them. Evidently both 'internal' and 'external' control are important to women. Note that what women *want* is relatively unaffected by education and parity while *expectations* are nearly always related to both of these factors.

	% of women wanting control	% of women expecting control
'External' control		
Active part in non-emergency decisions	72 (E)	55 (E,P)
Active part in emergency decisions	27	17 (E)
Control of what staff do to you	82 (E)	61 (E,P)
'Internal' control		
Control of your own behaviour	77	45 (E,P)
Control during contractions	92	65 (P)
Not making a lot of noise	43 (E,P)	54 (E,P)

KEY: E means that there are significant differences between women of different educational levels.
P means that there are significant differences between multips and primips.

Table 4.4: Summary of different questions to do with 'external' and 'internal' control: percentage of women who wanted/expected control

12. How important is it to you that giving birth will be a fulfilling experience?
When the pilot version of the questionnaire had been circulated one doctor told us that most of his patients would not know what this meant. We therefore included 'Don't even know what this means' as a response option. It was ticked by only 19 women (3%) who represented all levels of education and approximately equal numbers of multips and primips. Two women, both educated beyond the minimum school leaving age, pointed out that it was the baby rather than the birth that was fulfilling:

'It is after the birth it is fulfilling – can't say I think giving birth is much fun.'

Another said baldly: 'This question sounds as if a man wrote it.'

In fact, having a 'fulfilling experience' was very important to 40 per cent of the sample and quite important to another 42 per cent, with no significant differences by education or parity. Unlike many of the other questions in this section, expectations were just as high as wants, with 41 per cent being 'sure' that the birth would be fulfilling and another 42 per cent thinking that it probably would be. Only 12 per cent had no expectations while 5 per cent thought it would not be. Interestingly, there is no difference at all between the expectations of multips and primips on this question. With regard to educational level the main difference is to be found in the caution of the more highly educated women. They were more likely to say that the experience would 'probably' be fulfilling (53%) than to be 'sure' (29%), while for the least educated women the pattern was reversed: 45 per cent were 'sure' while 39 per cent said 'probably'. The most educated women were also slightly more likely to have no expecations (13% versus 11%): an interesting reversal of the usual pattern. This data would seem to challenge that aspect of the stereotype of the middle class highly educated woman which credits her with unrealistically high hopes and expectations of fulfilment.

Relationship between wants and expectations

What women said they wanted and what they expected were significantly related for all of the above questions. Notably, women who 'did not mind' were least likely to have any expectations. Conversely, women who did mind generally had some expectations, even if these did not coincide with what they wanted. We were particularly interested in the expectations of those women who had strong feelings about the issues raised in these questions: were they actually expecting to have their ideals met? Not surprisingly, there is considerable variation depending the question. For those items where women may feel able to influence events, such as the presence of a birth companion, women with strong preferences (in either direction) usually expected to get what they wanted. Conversely, in the case of events over which there is little perceived control, such as being delivered by a midwife that you have already met or the number of people coming in and out of the room, only a minority of women felt sure that their preferences would be met. Table 4.5 looks only at those women who expressed strong feelings about particular aspects and, within them, picks out only those who were sure that their wishes would be met and those who did not think that they would be. Women with intermediate expectations, e.g. who think that they will 'probably' get what they want, are omitted from this table. The questions referred to in the table are those questions 1–12 discussed previously.

How accurate these expectations proved to be will be discussed later in this report.

		Certain that wishes will be met		Think that wishes probably will not be met		Total with* strong feelings
		n	%	n	%	n
Issue						
1.	Birth companion	473	(74)	17	(3)	635
2.	Who delivers baby	117	(64)	5	(3)	183
3.	Known midwife	39	(26)	43	(29)	149
4.	One midwife throughout	53	(22)	45	(18)	244
5.	Not lots of people	49	(20)	44	(18)	243
6.	Making 'normal' decisions	146	(56)	37	(14)	259
7.	Making 'emergency' decisions	21	(48)	11	(25)	44
8.	Control: staff	81	(29)	24	(9)	276
9.	Control: behaviour	27	(15)	38	(20)	186
10.	Control: contractions	43	(16)	14	(5)	274
11.	Not making noise	42	(49)	5	(6)	86
12.	Fulfilment	220	(75)	3	(1)	295

*Totals refer to those of the 725 women to whom issues were very important. Where appropriate women who had strong feelings in either direction (e.g. definitely did not want a birth companion) are included. Percentages are calculated on these totals, not the whole sample.

Table 4.5: Expectations of women to whom particular issues were very important

Information

Part of the second antenatal questionnaire focused on the information that women reported they had been given by health professionals during pregnancy. We were not interested in *how much* information and knowledge each women possessed, which would in any case be very difficult to assess, so much as discovering if women felt as informed as they wished to be. We thought that this was a factor likely to be of importance in determining who would feel in control during their labour. For a woman to get the information that she wants, it helps if she is able to discuss her concerns with the health professionals who provide antenatal care.

In answer to the question 'When talking to these professionals are you able to discuss the things you want to with them?', 33 per cent of the sample responded that they always could, and a further 51 per cent that they could most of the time.

	n	%
Yes, always	245	(33)
Yes, most of the time	380	(51)
Only occasionally	91	(12)
Hardly ever	24	(3)
Never	9	(1)
n = 749		

Table 4.6: Able to discuss concerns with health professionals?

As Table 4.6 shows, only a very small percentage of women felt they could hardly ever, or never, talk to health staff. As one would expect from other work in this area (e.g. Hubert, 1974) it was lower class (classes IV and V) and the least educated women who were more likely to feel that they had difficulties discussing problems with the staff (see Appendix).

Linked to the ability to discuss issues fully with professionals, was how assertive women felt. We asked:

'When talking to doctors are you as assertive as you want to be?' and offered three options for reply:

Yes, I am always as assertive as I want to be

Sometimes I am but sometimes I'm not

No, I'm hardly ever as assertive as I want to be

Over half of the sample (60%) said that only sometimes did they feel as assertive as they wanted to be, 31 per cent said they always were and 9 per cent hardly ever felt assertive enough.

Again as expected, the most educated women (those leaving further education at 19 years or older) and higher class women (those in classes I and II) were the most likely to feel that they were always as assertive as they wanted to be. Likewise, how assertive women felt was very strongly related to whether they felt able to discuss issues with the staff (see Appendix for details).

In Chapter 1 we considered the stereotype of the working class woman who preferred to remain in blissful ignorance, and refused to take up the advantages of antenatal education. To look at this, we next asked women the question:

'How much do you want to know about what might happen during labour?'. Five response options were given and women were told that they could tick more than one.

How much do you want to know about labour?	n of women giving response	% of sample
1. Not know anything	6	(<1)
2. Just the basics	55	(7)
3. Most things but don't want to be worried	118	(16)
4. Happy to let the staff decide	91	(12)
5. As much as possible	577	(77)

n = 747

Percentages add to more than 100 because 100 women gave two answers.

Table 4.7: Desired information about what might happen in labour

As Table 4.7 clearly shows, the great majority of women did in fact want to know as much as they possibly could. However, a number of them gave what appear to be contradictory answers – particularly, ticking the option 'I want to know as much as possible' in addition to one of the other options. Fifty nine women ticked this option as well as another. Reassuringly, no-one ticked it in combination with 'I'd rather not know anything'. However, women sometimes ticked it in addition to 'I'm happy to let the staff decide how much I ought to know', which seems to place a somewhat touching faith in the staff to decide that women should know as much as possible!

We examined how much women wanted to know in terms of their educational background in order to examine the stereotype of the wilfully ignorant working class woman. The categories 1, 2 and 4 have been amalgamated to remove small numbers and to differentiate three clearly identifiable groups – a group who are happy to know very little (or nothing) or who want to abdicate the responsibility to the staff, an intermediate group who do want to know most things but preferably not things likely to upset or worry them, and a group who want to know as much as they can. Analysis was carried out on the first option indicated by women only.

Educational level	Nothing/basics only staff decide		Most things		As much as possible	
	n	%	n	%	n	%
16 and under	75	(20)	72	(19)	224	(60)
17–18	34	(16)	28	(13)	150	(71)
19 and over	12	(8)	5	(3)	142	(89)

Percentages are of women of a given level of education

$p < 0.0001$

Table 4.8: Desired information by educational level

Table 4.8 shows a clear relationship between the amount women wanted to know and educational level. A massive 89 per cent of the most highly educated women wanted to know as much as possible and in fact there was nobody in this group who wanted to know nothing. However, a majority (60%) of the least educated women also wanted to know as much as they could about what would happen during labour and only nine per cent of them were content to just know 'the basics'. Breakdown by social class in terms of women's best ever occupation shows the same pattern as for education and is also statistically significant.

Finally, we concluded the information section of this questionnaire by asking women how much information they felt they had been given so far during the pregnancy. Their responses are shown below.

	n of women	%
Too much information	3	(<1)
The right amount of information	512	(68)
Too little information	138	(18)
Too much about some things, too little about others	97	(13)
n = 750		

Table 4.9: Amount of information received during the pregnancy

One third of the sample felt dissatisfied in some way with the amount of information they had been given. Nearly one in five women felt they had *not* been given enough information.

Lower class women and those with the least education were rather more likely to feel dissatisfied with the amount of information they had been given but the differences were not significant.

However, an interesting significant difference between multips and primips emerged (see Appendix). Although the same proportion (68–70%) felt they had received the right amount of information, a greater percentage of multips felt they had received too little information (22% compared to 13% of primips). Primips, conversely, were more likely to say 'Too much about some things, too little about others' (16% of primips compared to 11% of multips). These differences are likely to reflect the greater amount of general information with which primips are bombarded, and also perhaps, a difference in the kind of information that primips and multips are aware of not having. This is also evident in the antenatal responses to how informed women felt about the third stage of labour (see Chapter 6, Volume 2).

Finally, there were significant differences in the responses given by women booked at different units with regard to their ease of communicating with professionals and the amount of information that they felt they had received. Women booked at Little Exington consistently gave the lowest responses, for example, only 66 per cent felt that they could discuss things at least most of the time, while at the other units the range was from 82 per cent to 89 per cent. A similar pattern was found for the amount of information received.

We will return to the question of how much information women thought they had or wanted to have when we examine the postnatal results.

Choice and control

The concepts of choice and control are most clearly linked when we consider control over decision making. The second questionnaire included a total of five multiple choice questions designed to tap women's desire for control over decision making:

> How involved do you want the doctors and midwives to be in the decisions about the pain relief you might use in labour?
>
> Are you happy to leave matters to staff once the baby is actually born, or do you wish to make the decisions yourself about how the third stage of labour is managed?
>
> Assuming that there are no complications, who would you think should make most of the decisions about your labour?
>
> In an emergency who do you think should make the decisions?
>
> Do you want to be in control of what doctors and midwives do to you during your labour?

These questions appeared at different points in the questionnaire and the last three have already been discussed in the first part of this chapter. Broadly speaking, the majority of women wanted control of pain relief and other decisions in normal labour while only a minority wanted to be actively involved in emergency or third stage decisions.

In order to discover more about women who assert a strong desire for control we constructed a control score based on the answers to all five questions.

Construction of control score

A woman was given a score of one if she gave the most extreme answer indicating a desire for control and zero otherwise. There are five questions so she would get the maximum score of five if she gave the most extreme answer on all five of them and a score of zero if she did not assert a strong desire for control on any of them. Women could also score a half mark for saying that they would 'quite like' to be in control of what the staff did. We then looked at the two extremes: women who consistently expressed a strong desire for control (scoring 3.5 points or more) who we called the 'High Control' group, and women who scored zero, i.e. who never expressed a desire for control, the 'Low Control' group. There were 89 women who met the criteria for the 'High Control' group and 108 who scored zero ('Low Control'): combined they account for 26 per cent of the sample. We shall now look at the characteristics of these two groups and their responses to some of the other antenatal questions.

Characteristics of 'High' and 'Low Control' women

PARITY

The distribution of multips and primips within the 'Low Control' group is virtually identical to that for the sample as a whole (62% multips, 38% primips). Within the 'High Control' group there are relatively more primips (47%) but the difference is not statistically significant.

SOCIAL CLASS/EDUCATION

Referring back to the stereotypes discussed in Chapter 1, the woman who wants to retain control might be expected to be middle class. In fact, the social class data here is a very interesting demonstration of the problems of defining social class that were discussed in Chapter 2. If we take the usual basis for defining class, partner's occupation, we find that more lower class women had 'Low Control' scores, but the converse is not true. For 'High Control' women there is no consistent relationship with social class (see Table 4.10). Social class based on the woman's own best ever job is more clearly related to the desire for control but in fact the most significant determinant is the indicator that we argued for in Chapter 2: age of finishing full-time education.

Class	Partner's occupation				Woman's occupation			
	'High Control'		'Low Control'		'High Control'		'Low Control'	
	n	%	n	%	n	%	n	%
I and II	40	(15)	29	(11)	43	(16)	27	(10)
IIIN and IIIM	22	(8)	40	(14)	40	(11)	59	(16)
IV and V	16	(14)	23	(20)	4	(5)	18	(22)

Percentages are of women of a given class.

$p < 0.01$ for both woman's and partner's occupations.

Table 4.10: 'High' and 'Low Control' women: social class based on partner's occupation and woman's own highest status job

Age of finishing full-time education	'High Control'		'Low Control'	
	n	%	n	%
16 or less	32	(9)	63	(17)
17–18	23	(11)	31	(15)
19 or more	34	(21)	14	(9)

Percentages are of women of a given educational level.

$p < 0.0001$

Table 4.11: 'High' and 'Low Control' women: age of finishing full-time education

Table 4.11 shows that 21 per cent of the most highly educated women had 'High Control' scores compared to only 9 per cent of the least educated women. The pattern reverses for 'Low Control'. Before concluding, however, that the desire for control is an attribute of highly educated women, we should bear in mind two facts. Firstly, only 21 per cent of the most educated women asserted a high desire for control: nearly 80 per cent did not. Secondly, in absolute terms, within the group of 'High Control' women those with a high level of education did not predominate because there were fewer of them to start with. Only 38 per cent of 'High Control' women had had higher education, while 36 per cent had left school at 16 or earlier, and 26 per cent were educated to the age of 17 or 18. Thus, when we talk of the 'High Control' women we are not talking about an exclusively highly educated or middle class group.

Differences related to education

Notwithstanding the fact that only 38 per cent of 'High Control' women had higher education, we find that their answers to many questions follow the patterns that we have already seen for more highly educated women. Thus we find, for example, that 'High Control' women were more likely to attend antenatal classes (although not particularly NCT classes) and were more likely to have birth plans. They want to know more about obstetric procedures and, by their self-report, they were actually better informed than 'Low Control' women. Because, as we have already seen, the more women said they knew about most procedures the more they wished to avoid them, we also find that 'High Control' women said that they do not want these procedures. It is, however, interesting to note that the 'Low Control' women (like the least educated women) were not saying that they *did* want these interventions, rather they were saying that they did not mind or did not know enough to make a choice. This pattern seemed to be true for virtually all the obstetric procedures that we asked about. All these differences between 'High' and 'Low Control' women were highly significant with differences typically being greater than those previously described for education.

Different meanings of control

The division of women into 'High' and 'Low Control' in this section is made on the basis of their desire for control over decision making. How does this relate to aspects of 'internal' control? As we saw earlier, 'internal' control tended not to be significantly related to education. Similarly, we find little difference between 'High' and 'Low Control' women in their answers to the questions concerning control of behaviour and control during contractions, although where these types of control were important at all to 'High Control' women, they were more likely to be seen as 'very' important. However, like the most highly educated women, 'High Control' women were significantly more likely to say that making a lot of noise was *unimportant* ($p < 0.01$) as Table 4.12 shows.

	'High Control'		'Low Control'	
	n	%	n	%
Very or quite important	22	(25)	50	(49)
Not very or not at all important	67	(75)	53	(51)
Total	89	(100)	103*	(100)

$p < 0.01$

*Five 'Low Control' women failed to answer this question.

Table 4.12: 'High' and 'Low Control' women: importance of not making a lot of noise during labour

It is interesting to note that *expectations* of these various interpretations of control show a different pattern. 'High Control' women had significantly higher expectations of remaining in control of their behaviour; for once there is no difference in the proportions with no expectations. Similarly, a greater proportion of 'High Control' women expected to be in control during contractions. However, there are no differences in their expectations of making of lot of noise although this was the one question where 'Low Control' women cared more.

To summarize, a high desire for control over decision making is not significantly related to feelings about control of one's own behaviour or control during contractions and is negatively related to concern over making a lot of noise during labour. This latter finding may be because making a noise is seen as the freedom to behave as you wish in the face of social pressures to the contrary. The negative relationship should not therefore surprise us since feeling inhibited about making a noise is obviously a function of *'external'* control.

Attitudes of 'High' and 'Low Control' women to pain

'High Control' women were significantly more likely than 'Low Control' to see labour pain as different from other types of pain, the most striking difference being that 40 per cent of the 'Low Control' women answered 'Don't know'.

	'High Control'		'Low Control'	
	n	%	n	%
Yes	56	(64)	42	(39)
No	16	(18)	23	(21)
Don't know	16	(18)	44	(40)
Total	88	(100)	109	(100)

$p < 0.0001$

Table 4.13: 'High' and 'Low Control' women: is labour pain different from other kinds of pain?

In particular, 'High Control' women were likely to describe labour pain as productive while 'Low Control' women, if they did see it as different, were more likely to say that it is indescribable. There was no significant difference between the two groups in being worried about forthcoming labour pain nor in their propensity to worry about pain in general.

Pain is an area where women who want control are said to hold ideas that will be shattered by reality. There were indeed significant differences between the expectations of pain held by 'High' and 'Low Control' women, as Table 4.14 shows. However, the most notable differences were in the 'unbearably painful' and 'don't know' categories, with 'High Control' women being much less likely to give these responses (5% and 6% respectively compared to 15% and 14% of 'Low Control' women).

	'High Control'		'Low Control'	
	n	%	n	%
Not at all painful	0	(0)	0	(0)
Moderately uncomfortable	7	(8)	5	(5)
Quite painful	31	(35)	31	(28)
Very painful	40	(45)	40	(37)
Unbearable	4	(5)	16	(15)
Don't know	5	(6)	15	(14)
Total	88*	(100)	109	(100)

$p < 0.05$

* One 'High Control' woman did not answer this question.

Table 4.14: 'High' and 'Low Control' women: expectations of pain without drugs

How realistic one considers these women's expectations to be is necessarily subjective, but clearly it is not the case that 'High Control' women were expecting painless labours. The fact that so few of them expected labour *without drugs* to be 'unbearably painful' is likely to relate to their own preferences for avoiding drugs in labour. There were, in fact, highly significant differences in responses to that question as Table 4.15 shows. Note that we did not find such differences for women of different levels of education.

	'High Control'		'Low Control'	
	n	%	n	%
The most pain-free labour that drugs can give me	3	(3)	22	(21)
The minimum quantity of drugs to keep the pain manageable	45	(51)	69	(65)
To put up with quite a lot of pain in order to have a completely drug-free labour	37	(42)	14	(13)
Other	3	(3)	2	(2)
Total	88	(100)	107	(100)

Table 4.15: 'High' and 'low control' women: 'which of these options would you prefer ideally?'

The antipathy to pain-relieving drugs among 'High Control' women was particularly marked for Pethidine (76%) and epidurals (89%). Their opposition to epidurals is interesting because it has been argued that epidurals allow a woman to remain in control (Kitzinger, 1987b). However, only three per cent of 'High Control' women thought that they might 'quite like' an epidural compared with 12 per cent of the 'Low Control' women. This serves to re-emphasize the different meanings of the word 'control'.

'High Control' women were better informed about the advantages and disadvantages of the main pain-relieving drugs. Given that one of the stereotypical characteristics of 'High Control' women is that they are more interested in fulfilment than in their baby's well-being, we were particularly interested in seeing whether 'High Control' women were more or less likely to refer to the ill-effects of Pethidine on the baby. In fact, this aspect of Pethidine was mentioned by 11 of the 'Low Control'women (10%) and 41 of the 'High Control' women (46%). Even if we allow for the fact that fewer 'Low Control' women answered the question at all and calculate percentages only on responders, the difference is still striking: 57 per cent of 'High Control' versus only 19 per cent of 'Low Control'. This particular aspect of the stereotype is clearly not supported.

If 'High Control' women are not keen on using pain-relieving drugs we might expect to find them more committed to using breathing and relaxation as a method of pain relief. This is indeed the case: 58 per cent of 'High Control' women were definitely going to use breathing and relaxation compared to only 25 per cent of the 'Low Control' women. Consistent with this were generally higher expectations about the helpfulness of breathing and relaxation although none of the 'High Control' women were expecting complete pain control from using breathing and relaxation exercises (compared to three of the 'Low Control' women). 'High Control' women were also more likely than 'Low Control' women to say that they were going to use alternative methods of pain relief: 35 per cent compared to eight per cent.

One final interesting difference between 'High' and 'Low Control' women was in their preference for type of anaesthesia in the event of a Caesarean section.

	'High Control'		'Low Control'	
	n	%	n	%
General anaesthesia	27	(30)	55	(51)
Epidural	43	(48)	28	(26)
Don't know	19	(21)	25	(23)
Total	89	(100)	108	(100)

Table 4.16: 'High' and 'Low Control' women: preference for type of anaesthesia for Caesarean section

Unusually, there is little difference between the groups in the percentages saying 'Don't know'. We have already noted the disinclination of 'High Control' women towards epidurals for vaginal deliveries. The relatively high proportion of 'Don't know' replies is likely to be a reflection of the dilemma that this question poses: they do not want epidurals but they do want to be in a position to influence events. We would imagine that the 'High Control' women would have a stronger inclination to avoid a caesarean section altogether. This is supported by the answers to the question which hypothesized the near certainty of a section: 55 per cent of 'High Control' women would choose a trial of labour as opposed to 27 per cent of 'Low Control'. There was no difference between the two groups in having been told that their births might not be straightforward.

Expectations of 'high' and 'low control' women

'High Control' women are defined in terms of a consistently expressed desire for control over decision making. Do they actually expect to have their wishes met? For three of the control questions: decision making in normal labour, decision making in an emergency and being in control of what staff do to you, we asked about expectations as well as wants. For all three questions 'High Control' women had significantly higher expectations of involvement in decision making; 'Low Control' women were more likely to have no expectations. Since we have already observed a strong correspondence between what women want and what they expect, this finding should not surprise us. There were hardly any women who were expecting to experience a greater degree of involvement in decision making than they actually wanted, so it is to be expected that a low desire for this type of control will be accompanied by low expectations.

		More important to 'High Control' women?	'High Control' have higher expectations?
1.	Birth companion throughout	YES	YES
2.	Midwife delivery	YES	YES
3.	Known midwife	YES	NS
4.	One midwife throughout	YES	NS
5.	Not lots of people	YES	NS
6.	'Normal' decisions	YES	YES
7.	Emergency decisions	YES	YES
8.	Control of staff	YES	YES
9	Control of behaviour	NS	YES
10.	Control during contractions	NS	YES
11.	Not making a noise	LESS important	NS
12.	Fulfilment	YES	NS

Table 4.17: Summary of preferences and expectations of 'High' and 'Low Control' women for certain social/behavioural aspects of labour

Expectations of other aspects of labour were not, however, always higher for 'High Control' women. They were, for example, no more likely than 'Low Control' women to expect to be delivered by a midwife that they had already met or to have the same midwife with them throughout labour. However, they did care about both of these aspects significantly more than 'Low Control' women. Similarly, their expectations that birth would be a fulfilling experience were no higher than the 'Low Control' women's, although it was significantly more important to them that it should be so. Their expectations of a normal labour were, however, higher in that 'Low Control' women were significantly more likely to say that they had 'no expectations' in answer to the questions on induction, acceleration and caesarean section (see Chapter 6). This is despite the fact, already mentioned, that 'Low Control' women were no more likely to have been told that their deliveries might not be straightforward.

	'High Control'		'Low Control'	
	n	%	n	%
Definitely or probably yes	2	(2)	10	(10)
No expectations	18	(20)	46	(44)
Definitely or probably not	69	(78)	48	(46)
Total	89	(100)	104	(100)

Table 4.18: 'High' and 'Low Control' women: expectations of induction

These expectations, or lack of them, were reflected in the reasons women gave: 'Low Control' women were more likely than 'High' to say that 'every labour is different'. Similarly, as regards birth plans, they were more likely to say that 'there's no point in writing things down because you can't tell the future'.

The impression of 'High Control' women that emerges from this is that they are women who are fairly well informed and who know what they do and do not want to happen to them during labour. As such they have expectations that accord with objective probabilities (most of them will not experience major interventions), while 'Low Control' women, who have perhaps given less thought to any of these issues, are more likely to have no expectations. 'High Control' women seem more inclined to see themselves as active participants in the birth rather than as passive recipients of whatever comes their way. The desire for control over decision making can thus be seen in this context as part of a package and not necessarily as a desire to dictate *per se*.

As support for this interpretation, it is interesting to note that 'High Control' women were no more likely than 'Low Control' women to say that they were always as assertive as they wanted to be when talking to doctors.

CHAPTER FIVE

Pain and Pain Relief

Pain: antenatal data

In the second antenatal questionnaire we asked women how painful they would expect labour to be *without drugs*. They were given a set of seven options ranging from 'not at all painful' to 'unbearably painful', including the options 'I have no idea' and 'other'. This question was followed by a request to indicate whether they saw labour pain as different from other kinds of pain, and if so in what ways did they see it as different. By this approach we hoped to allow women to express both the quality and the degree of pain that they expected during labour.

How painful will it be?

Only one woman said labour without drugs would be 'not at all painful' and 29 thought it would be 'moderately uncomfortable' but the vast majority (77%) expected to to be 'quite' or 'very' painful.

Is labour pain different from other kinds of pain?

Four hundred and fifty four women said 'Yes', they did see labour pain as different, 120 said 'No' and 174 said 'Don't know'. Some women found the question itself a little odd – one woman wrote, 'Of course it is different, your teeth do not contract when they need filling'.

Those 454 women who said 'yes, it was different' were then asked to describe in what ways it was different. This was an open question and we coded up to three responses for each woman, using post-hoc coding categories.

The most popular response (given by half the women who answered this question) was to indicate that labour pain, unlike other pain, was 'productive':

> 'It's different in that one can cope better with it knowing that it will bring forth something beautiful at the end of it.'
>
> 'There is a very good natural reason for the pain – the joy of the baby hopefully will be a kind of painkiller.'

Or, as one woman succinctly commented:

> 'It's for a good cause!'

This perception of birth pangs as a 'Pain with a purpose' helped women to approach it positively:

> 'It is pain worth bearing for the results and therefore can be dealt with using mind over matter better than senseless pain.'

The second most common response was to say that the pain of labour, unlike other pains, had a definite end:

> 'I suffer migraine badly – I prefer labour, at least I know there's an end in sight.'

> 'You know it's only temporary – seeing light at the end of the tunnel helps you to cope.'

Almost a quarter of the women who answered this question emphasized this 'light at the end of the tunnel' approach to labour pain and this was closely tied in with the idea of the patterns and progress of painful contractions. As one woman commented:

> 'They come in a form of pattern so you get to know when to expect them and can prepare yourself for them. Also knowing that they will gradually build up to a climax and then subside makes them easier to cope with.'

Another woman (who had previously had a caesarean section for 'failure to progress') described the pain of labour as:

> 'Waves of pain getting closer together, becomes very difficult to cope with especially when not getting any further on with the birth.'

Eight per cent of the women who described labour pain commented positively on the gradual build up of pain:

> 'Unlike other pain, labour pain builds up gradually allowing adjustment to and acceptance of increasing intensity; unless the process is accelerated or interfered with.'

> '… there is a gradual build up of pain as your contractions get stronger so it is not so noticeable, and by the time you're in the second stage of labour they are talking you through it step by step… making you feel that it won't be long before everything will have been worthwhile.'

However, sixteen women described the opposite sensation (sometimes explicitly linking this to a previously induced labour):

> '… this pain is the most intense I have ever experienced. It is all consuming and as I was induced appears to never let go.'

Just over 12 per cent of the respondents also made comments to the effect that the pain of labour was indescribable:

> 'This is very difficult to put down in writing. I don't feel I can explain the pain but it is completely different from other kinds of pain – sorry if this isn't good enough!'

> 'With other kinds of pain you can always describe it, but people never seem to know how to describe labour pains.'

Even some women who had written at length about other areas were rendered inarticulate when asked to describe labour pain.

Forty nine women (11%) said labour pain was worse than other kinds of pain. These tended to be the women who had ticked the statement 'unbearably painful' to describe the pain they would expect in a drug-free labour. As one woman wrote:

> 'No words could describe the pain and agony that I went through when my daughter was born. I felt as though I was being torn in two, I never thought that it would be so painful.'

Or as another wrote:

> 'From my experience it's like being tortured slowly and repeatedly.'

This emphasis on the extreme pain of labour was tied in with the feeling that it was inescapable:

> 'Put it this way, 2 Panadol take away a headache. It takes an injection of Pethidine to dull the pain of labour even slightly. I don't mean to be rude but that is the only way I can explain it.'

> 'You can't just stop it when you want (with pills, injections etc.)'

Ten per cent of the respondents commented that labour pain was 'soon forgotten' and another 10 per cent said that it was a natural and healthy pain that did not indicate that anything was wrong. A few added that pain was an inherent part of natural childbirth:

> 'You need to experience it, to be completely in touch with your baby, and its birth naturally.'

Some women explicitly stated that bearing the pain was an active choice made for the good of the baby, or which allowed full involvement in the birth and that this 'self-inflicted' (as one woman put it) nature of the pain made it more bearable:

> 'Labour pain is something we choose to have – other types of pain we have no choice.'

The 'Other' category is an amalgamation of various different responses. These include, for example, a few women who found comfort from the fact that the pains of labour were experienced by many other women:

> 'It is universal – experienced the world over by women through generations.'

Others emphasized that it was a pain they expected and could prepare for:

> 'You know its going to happen, and if you want babies, its something you have to put up with!'

Some women complained that with labour pain you just had to 'grin and bear it' rather than languishing in a sick role:

> 'Very painful but at the same time one has to work hard at doing the right things at the right time – any other pain one just suffers without any other demands being made upon one.'

> '... if you hurt yourself your immediate reaction is to pull the hurt part towards you but in labour you have to push past this even though part of you is saying stop (e.g. you don't run on a broken leg!)'

As one woman put it:

> 'You are not ill so you get no sympathy.'

Women's expectations and understanding of pain are intertwined with their view of the quality, as well as the degree, of pain and how it can, or should, be relieved. Feeling that the pain was something they were choosing to go through, knowing that their labour was progressing, feeling the gradual build up of contractions and looking forward to seeing their baby were all seen as helping women to deal with the pain.

Although we did not ask women directly about their source of information about pain this was often hinted at. As expected, most women referred to previous experiences about labour or what other women had told them. A few explained that their expectations of pain reflected what they had read or heard in antenatal classes and some gave very specific references such as the Jehovah's Witness who referred us to Genesis 3:16, and 4:1-2:

> 'Unto the woman he said, I will greatly multiply thy sorrow and thy conception; in sorrow thou shalt bring forth children; and thy desire shall be to thy husband, and he shall rule over thee.'

The effect of previous experience

One of the questions we were interested in was how previous experiences of labour might affect women's expectations and perceptions of pain. We found that multips were more likely than primips to emphasize that labour without drugs would be painful: 16 per cent of the multips thought that a drug-free labour would be 'unbearably' painful as opposed to just 7 per cent of the women having their first child. However, there was also a tendency for multips to be *more* likely to say that labour without drugs would be 'not at all painful' or just 'moderately uncomfortable'.

It would seem that while multips are more likely to tick the extreme options in response to this question, the primips tended to stick to describing the expected pain of a drug-free labour as 'quite' or 'very' painful (77%) and a substantial proportion (13%) said they had 'no idea' about how painful it would be.

There was also a difference between the responses of multips and primips to the question 'Do you see labour pain as different from other kinds of pain?'. Forty two per cent of primips said 'don't know' as opposed to just 11 per cent of the multips. However, of the women who felt they *did* know, the majority of both multips and primips said 'yes' it was different.

Women's expectations of pain and their education

Women who had left full-time education at 16 or younger were more likely than the more educated woman to describe the expected pain of labour (without drugs) as 'unbearably painful'. Sixteen per cent of the least educated women ticked this option as opposed to just three per cent of the most highly educated women. However, the most educated women were more likely to describe drug-free labour as 'very' painful and when the category 'very painful' is amalgamated with the category 'unbearably painful', there is no significant difference between the educational groups. It would seem therefore that there is something specific about the phrase 'unbearably painful' which seems to make this description less acceptable to the more educated woman. One woman (a teacher), for instance, had originally ticked 'unbearably painful' but then crossed that out, commenting:

> 'Extremely painful, but I would not say "unbearable" because it would have to be "borne" and if drugs were not available, I would not expect it to be likely that the pain would be such that the woman died instead of bearing the pain. (Sorry if this sounds pedantic – I do not mean it to be!)'

Women's expectations of pain and unit booked for delivery

There was some idea among staff at other units that women who booked for delivery at Willowford were expecting a) drug-free labours, and b) that such labours would not be too painful (Phase 1).

There was no relationship between women's views of the pain of a drug-free labour and where they were booked for delivery. The apparent differences were related to parity variations in the populations sampled. However, there were differences in whether or not they ideally hoped to avoid drugs: 32 per cent of those at Willowford ideally wished for a drug-free labour as opposed to 13–28 per cent at other units ($p < 0.01$).

Do women worry about pain in labour?

Seven hundred and thirty nine women answered the question 'Are you worried about the thought of pain in labour?'. The option 'very worried' was ticked by 12 per cent, 'a bit worried' by 67 per cent and 'not at all worried' by 22 per cent. There was no significant relationship between concern about the pain and level of education. There was, however, a relationship with parity. Of women who had previous experience of childbirth, 26 per cent were 'not at all worried' as opposed to just 15 per cent of the women pregnant for the first time. The responses of the women who had not experienced childbirth clustered in the 'a bit worried' category (75%). Only 9 per cent of primips were 'very worried' by the thought of labour pain as compared to 14 per cent of multips. There was a strong overall relationship between being worried about labour pain and being worried about pain in everyday life. However only 15 per cent of those who were 'very' worried about labour pain said that that was their normal response to pain, and indeed 30 per cent of them said that they were not normally at all worried by the thought of pain. These subgroups would be worthy of further investigation.

Pain: postnatal data

Was the pain of labour as expected?

Twenty per cent of the sample found that the pain of labour was not at all as they had expected and 38 per cent said that it was as they had expected in some ways but not in others. The primary way in which the pain of labour differed from their expectations was that for 143 women (21% of the total number of respondents), it was more painful than they had expected:

> 'They don't call it labour for nothing! The pain was more intense that I ever thought imaginable.'

However, 87 women (13%) found it less painful than expected:

> 'There was hardly any pain at all.'

> 'It wasn't a pain that I had felt before, it was, in a strange way, pleasurable, the intensity of it gave me the incentive to persevere with the labour.'

Eight per cent of women described the sensations of labour pain as more 'powerful' or 'overwhelming' than expected:

> 'It was far more enveloping than I'd expected – I couldn't seem to get outside it.'

Seven per cent said the specific sensations were of a different kind from what they had expected (more of an ache than a pain or a dragging sensation rather than a stabbing sensation):

> 'I didn't expect the contractions to be like period pains. I thought it would be a muscular feeling like when you get an involuntary twitch.'

Six per cent found the pain was in a different place from that expected, e.g. in the back or legs rather than in the stomach:

'Because the pain was unexpectedly in my back it seemed a lot worse.'

	n	% of all women who experienced labour
More painful	143	(21)
Less painful	87	(13)
Harder work/more powerful	57	(8)
Different sensations	52	(7)
Pain in unexpected part of body	39	(6)
Continuous pain	22	(3)
Painful at unexpected time during labour	21	(3)
Pain did not last as long as I expected	19	(3)
Pain went on longer than expected	13	(2)
I coped better than expected	13	(2)
I coped less well than expected	12	(2)
Hard to explain	9	(1)
Other	20	(3)

(Up to three descriptions were coded for each woman)

Table 5.1: Ways in which labour pains differed from expectations

Expectation/experience of pain and parity, class and education

Primips were much more likely than multips to be surprised by some aspect of the pain.

	No, not at all		Yes, in some ways, No in others		Yes, exactly	
	n	%	n	%	n	%
Primips	91	(36)	126	(50)	37	(15)
Multips	42	(10)	129	(32)	230	(57)

Percentages are of women of a given parity.

$p < 0.00001$

Table 5.2: Was the pain of labour as expected (by parity)

Also, higher class women were less likely than lower class women to find the pain 'exactly' as expected.

	No, not at all		Yes, in some ways, No in others		Yes, exactly	
	n	%	n	%	n	%
I and II	37	(15)	124	(50)	86	(35)
IIIN and IIIM	77	(24)	107	(34)	135	(42)
IV and V	16	(22)	18	(25)	37	(52)

Percentages are of women in a given social class grouping.

$p < 0.001$

Table 5.3: Was the pain of labour as expected (by social class)

A similar pattern exists with respect to education – the most educated women were least likely to state without qualification that the pain was exactly as they had expected.

Women's antenatal expectations of pain and their actual experience of pain

It has been argued that women who go into labour expecting it not to be very painful are unprepared for the realities of childbirth and therefore will suffer more. Deutsch (1945), for example, believed that anxiety about childbirth is a form of psychological preparation which acts as a major defence against the stressful events of labour and which is psychologically beneficial to women. Others, however, have argued that women who go into labour expecting it to be very painful will be tense and frightened and will therefore experience *more* pain than a more relaxed woman (Dick Read, 1933). When we compare women's responses to the antenatal question, 'Without drugs how painful would you expect labour to be' with their postnatal descriptions of their labour pains (with and without drugs) we can begin to explore these issues. If anything our findings would tend to support the second hypothesis, i.e. that women who expect natural childbirth to be fairly pain-free find labour relatively easy. Only 14 per cent of the women who expected labour (without drugs) to be not at all painful or only moderately uncomfortable found, in the event, that labour was more painful than they expected, whereas 19–21 per cent of those who expected labour (without drugs) to be more painful found their labour pains worse than expected (perhaps they had over-inflated ideas about the degree of relief drugs could provide).

	Expectation of pain in labour without drugs							
	Not at all painful/ Moderately uncomfortable		Quite painful		Very painful		Unbearably painful	
	n	%	n	%	n	%	n	%
Found labour more painful than expected	4	(15)	42	(21)	72	(23)	17	(20)
Found labour less painful than expected	2	(7)	24	(12)	45	(14)	6	(7)
Labour was neither more or less painful than expected	21	(78)	134	(67)	196	(63)	61	(73)
Total number of women	27	(100)	200	(100)	313	(100)	84	(100)

Table 5.4: Antenatal expectation of pain by experience of pain

Desires for a drug-free labour and postnatal descriptions of the pain

Women who had wanted a drug-free labour were more likely than other women to find labour unexpectedly painful (25% versus 15% of those who wanted the most pain-free labour drugs could provide).

It may be these women that staff are referring to when they talk of women with high expectations 'setting themselves up' for failure. However, that generalization does not take into account the fact that most (75%) of those who ideally would prefer to cope without drugs did not find their labours unexpectedly painful or that of the women who expected the pain of labour to be only moderately or quite uncomfortable, 85 per cent did *not* find their labour unexpectedly painful. (The women who saw natural childbirth as more painful were in fact slightly *more* likely to be surprised by the pain they experienced during labour.)

In the majority of cases, it would seem that women who expect moderate pain and hope to cope without drugs were more likely to experience moderate pain than other women and to use fewer drugs. Most women with low expectations (i.e. expected a drug-free labour to be very or unbearably painful) also got what they expected – they may be less often disappointed, but they were more likely to find, as expected, that labour is very painful.

As we will see in the next section, women who expected a drug-free labour to be only moderately or 'quite' painful or who ideally preferred to cope without drugs were more likely to be both dissatisfied and satisfied with the way they coped with the pain. They saw dealing with the pain as their responsibility, something they could be satisfied or dissatisfied with whereas the other women were more likely to say they had no feelings either way.

Pain relief: antenatal data

General attitude towards drugs in labour

'Which of these options would you prefer ideally?'

The most pain-free labour that drugs can give me

The minimum quantity of drugs to keep the pain manageable

To put up with quite a lot of pain in order to have a completely drug-free labour

Other (please say what)

Only nine per cent of respondents wanted 'the most pain-free labour that drugs can give me'. The majority of women (67%) wanted the minimum quantity of drugs to keep the pain manageable and the remaining 22 per cent said that they would prefer 'to put up with quite a lot of pain in order to have a completely drug-free labour'. Forty per cent of the 'pain free' group were 'very worried' about the pain of labour compared with only five per cent of the 'drug free' women ($p < 0.0001$).

Relationships between general attitude to drugs in labour and education

Women's general attitudes towards drugs in labour were not significantly related to their level of education. There was no relationship between women's attitudes and their partner's occupation or their own 'best ever' job. It seems that it is no longer (if it ever was) just a 'middle class minority' who are concerned about the use of drugs in labour.

Multips were just as likely as primips to say that they would prefer 'to put up with quite a lot of pain in order to have a completely drug-free labour'. However, multips were slightly more likely ($p < 0.05$) to want 'the most pain-free labour that drugs can give'.

Preferences regarding specific drugs

We also asked women about their preferences regarding specific drugs: epidurals, Pethidine (or alternative such as Meptid), and Entonox which we called 'gas and air' because, although this is inaccurate, it was the term most familiar to women themselves.

GAS AND AIR

Almost half the women were predisposed to use gas and air and over a quarter 'didn't mind'. Only four per cent did not feel they knew enough about it to make a choice. This is an interestingly small number given that 22 per cent did not feel they could list any advantages or disadvantages of gas and air. Women evidently have feelings about what they want and do not want even if they feel unable to answer a formal question about the advantages and disadvantages of a particular method.

	n	%
Definitely do not want	47	(6)
Prefer not to have	106	(14)
Don't mind	201	(27)
Would quite like	195	(26)
Definitely do want	167	(22)
Don't know enough to make a choice	30	(4)

Table 5.5: Preferences regarding gas and air

PETHIDINE
There was much less enthusiasm for Pethidine, with only a fifth of the sample being predisposed to use it. A quarter did not mind either way, but almost half (48%) wanted to avoid Pethidine.

	n	%
Definitely do not want	95	(13)
Prefer not to have	264	(35)
Don't mind	185	(25)
Would quite like	104	(14)
Definitely do want	47	(6)
Don't know enough to make a choice	50	(7)

Table 5.6: Preferences regarding Pethidine

EPIDURAL
Epidurals elicited the strongest negative reaction. Almost half the sample definitely rejected the use epidurals in labour. This was quite striking given the general pattern of response to the questionnaire as a whole. Overall, 79 per cent of the sample did not want an epidural, six per cent did not mind and nearly nine per cent were in favour.

	n	%
Definitely do not want	344	(46)
Prefer not to have	248	(33)
Don't mind	41	(6)
Would quite like	40	(5)
Definitely do want	24	(3)
Don't know enough to make a choice	49	(7)

Table 5.7: Preferences regarding epidural

There is no clear association between women's educational level and their wishes about epidurals during labour. However, more women would prefer an epidural for a caesarean section and there were class and education differences on this (for further discussion see Volume 2).

Pain relief and control

Women's knowledge and feelings about each specific type of pain relief are discussed in Volume 2. Here we will just note the frequency with which women mention 'control' as a positive aspect or 'loss of control' as a negative aspect of drugs. Between them, 583 women made 287 references to the positive or negative relationship of gas and air with control e.g. 'gas and air is good because you're in total control of it yourself' or 'gas and air is bad because it makes you too woozy to be in control at your own delivery'. (This is 287 references, not 287 women, as some made references to both positive and negative effects of gas and air on control.) There were 166 references to control by the 578 women who wrote about Pethidine, and 180 among the 577 women who wrote about epidurals. The actual word 'control' was used a total of 377 times in the answers to these questions about pain-relieving drugs.

Women's wishes concerning staff involvement in decisions about pain relief

We asked women: 'How involved do you want the doctors and midwives to be in the decisions about the pain relief you might use in labour?'.

> I will leave it totally up to the staff to make the right decision
>
> I would like the staff to advise me and I will probably take their advice
>
> I would like the staff to advise me but I will still make up my own mind even if my decision is different from their advice
>
> I do not want any staff involvement in the decision
>
> Other – please say what

Only four per cent of women wanted to leave decisions about pain relief totally up to the staff and, at the other extreme, only 0.7 per cent wanted no staff involvement. The vast majority (95%) wanted staff advice but were equally divided between saying they would probably follow the staff's advice (48%) and wanting to still make up their own minds even if their decisions were different from what the staff advised (48%). Practically everyone appeared to want some involvement in decisions about pain relief (in contrast, as we shall show later, to decisions about third stage management).

The most highly educated women were more likely than the less educated to want to make their own decision even if it was different from the advice of the staff.

A similar trend is evident in relation to class as defined by woman's best ever job, though not in relation to class as defined by partner's occupation. There was no relationship with parity.

Education level	Leave it totally up to staff		Probably follow staff advice		Listen to staff but make own decisions		No staff involvement		Other	
	n	%	n	%	n	%	n	%	n	%
16 or under	18	(5)	192	(52)	159	(43)	1	(<1)	2	(<1)
17–18	6	(3)	104	(49)	100	(47)	1	(<1)	0	(0)
19 or over	0	(0)	59	(37)	96	(60)	3	(2)	2	(1)

Percentages are of women of a given educational level

$p < 0.001$

Table 5.8: Wishes about staff involvement in decisions about pain relief by education

Pain relief: postnatal data

Drug use

GAS AND AIR

Just over two thirds of the women (69%) used gas and air and most of them found it 'very' effective (42%) or at least 'partly' effective (48%). It is interesting to note that some women, as we had also noticed antenatally, saw gas and air as somehow 'natural', and not really a drug at all. 'The drugs were no use at all [but] the gas and air relieved everything'.

Most women did not feel under any pressure to use (or not to use) gas and air, but 64 women (10% of those who answered this question) did feel pressurized to use it: 'Gas and air made me feel sick but the midwife kept giving it to me but I didn't want it'. Most women (87%) were pleased about their use/non-use of gas and air, or else had no particular feelings either way. Nine per cent had mixed feelings or were unhappy:

> 'I don't think I would have it again as it seemed to make me feel as if I were not in control, amd made me feel helpless and alone. I couldn't make sense of what people were saying to me at one point and had a tendency to fight it rather than relax. I found it frightening so stopped taking it.'

Women who felt pressurized into having gas and air were more likely to express unhappiness or mixed feelings about what happened than women who felt pressurized *not* to use it.

	n	%
Yes, a lot	6	(1)
Yes, a bit	58	(9)
No, not at all	544	(87)
On the contrary, I felt encouraged not to have it	15	(2)
Quite the opposite, I felt under a lot of pressure not to have it	3	(<1)

n = 626

(53 women failed to answer this question)

Table 5.9: Did you feel under pressure to use gas and air?

	n	%
I am pleased about it	404	(61)
I have mixed feelings	44	(7)
I am quite unhappy about it	16	(2)
I have no particular feelings either way	170	(26)
Other	30	(5)

n = 664

Table 5.10: How do you feel now about having had, or not had, gas and air?

PETHIDINE (OR ALTERNATIVE SUCH AS MEPTID)

Over half the sample (53%) used Pethidine (although ten women were unsure whether or not they had had it). Only 21 per cent of those who used Pethidine found it 'very' effective while 29 per cent found it not at all effective. Most women had not felt under any pressure to use Pethidine although ten per cent had:

> 'I was given Pethidine and was not asked. I was prepared to have the baby without it but was just given it as *they* thought I was in too much pain.'

A further two per cent had felt under a lot of pressure *not* to use it. Only 57 per cent were pleased about their use (or non-use) of Pethidine. Fifteen per cent had mixed feelings about it or were quite unhappy about what happened. It was overwhelmingly women who *had* Pethidine who expressed dissatisfaction with what happened rather than those who did not have it. Only ten women who did not have Pethidine (4%) said they had mixed feelings about this, whereas 61 women who *did* have it (17%) expressed mixed feelings in addition to a further 28 women who said they were 'very unhappy' about having it. Those who did not use Pethidine (or Meptid) were more pleased about what happened than those who did (see Appendix B9).

	n	%
Yes, a lot	18	(3)
Yes, a bit	44	(7)
No, not at all	522	(83)
On the contrary, I felt encouraged not to have it	34	(5)
Quite the opposite, I felt under a lot of pressure not to have it	10	(2)

n = 628

(48 women failed to answer this question)

Table 5.11: Did you feel under any pressure to have the injection?

	n	%
I am pleased about it	371	(57)
I have mixed feelings	72	(11)
I am quite unhappy about it	29	(4)
I have no particular feelings either way	149	(23)
Other	35	(5)

n = 656

Table 5.12: How do you feel now about having had, or not had, the injection of Pethidine or alternative such as Meptid?

EPIDURAL

Sixty six women (excluding those who had elective caesarean sections) had epidurals. Most women did not feel under pressure to have an epidural but four per cent did and two per cent felt under a lot of pressure not to have one. Most (80%) were pleased with what happened, nine per cent had mixed feelings or were unhappy. It was the women who *had* epidurals who accounted for the majority of the sample who expressed any unhappiness about what happened rather than those who did not have one. Twenty five per cent of the women who had epidurals found that they were not completely effective. Women who chose epidurals and then did not obtain complete pain relief expressed surprise, anger and disappointment:

> 'Requested an epidural, but the attempt failed, resulting in a dural tap. This meant I was bed bound for 48 hours after birth. I was very disappointed.'

This disappointment is not surprising given that a large proportion of women volunteered antenatally that they thought epidurals guaranteed complete pain relief.

	n	%
Very effective	49	(75)
Quite effective	11	(17)
Not at all effective	5	(8)

n = 65

Figures exclude epidurals for elective caesarean sections.

Table 5.13: How effective was the epidural in relieving the pain?

	n	%
Yes, a lot	15	(2)
Yes, a bit	13	(2)
No, not at all	544	(89)
On the contrary, I felt encouraged not to have it	30	(5)
Quite the opposite, I felt under a lot of pressure not to have it	12	(2)

n = 614

(57 women failed to answer this question)

Table 5.14: Did you feel under any pressure to have an epidural?

	n	%
I am pleased about it	503	(80)
I have mixed feelings	36	(7)
I am quite unhappy about it	14	(2)
I have no particular feelings either way	64	(10)
Other	16	(3)

n = 633

Table 5.15: How do you feel now about having had, or not had, an epidural?

OVERALL USE OF PAIN-RELIEVING DRUGS

In the sample as a whole 102 women (16%) used no drugs at all and a further 176 (27%) used only gas and air. Of the women who had epidurals, nearly two thirds used Pethidine as well. We do not, however, know whether they chose to have epidurals because the Pethidine was ineffective or vice versa.

Relationship between use of pain-relieving drugs and education

There were no differences by education regarding use of, or postnatal feelings about, gas and air or epidurals but the more educated women were less likely to use Pethidine and were more likely to say they were pleased about what happened (see Appendix B10). A similar relationship exists with social class as defined by the woman's best ever job. Overall the more highly educated women were more likely to have drug free labours (23% compared to 13% of other women), or to use only gas and air (33% compared to 25%) ($p < 0.001$).

Relationship between use of pain-relieving drugs and parity

Primips and multips were equally likely to use gas and air but primips were more likely to say it was 'not at all effective' (16% as against 5%, $p < 0.001$).

Primips were much more likely to use Pethidine (70% compared to 43%, $p < 0.0001$) and more likely to feel under pressure to use it (15% compared to 7%, $p < 0.05$). Primips were also more likely to now have mixed feelings about what happened (see Appendix B11). They were equally likely to find it effective.

Primips were more likely than multips to have an epidural (19% compared to 4%, $p < 0.0001$) and to feel under pressure to have one (10% comparedd to 1%, $p < 0.001$). They were also more likely to have mixed feelings about what happened (see appendix B11). They were equally likely to find it effective.

Relationship between use of pain-relieving drugs and unit

There was wide variation between units in the use of pain-relieving drugs. Women at Willowford were much less likely to use drugs. In part, this may reflect different staff attitudes (see Appendix B12 and Green et al., 1986).

	n	%
Willowford	78	(48)
Exington consultant unit	61	(68)
Exington GP unit	32	(63)
Little Exington	30	(68)
Wychester	139	(84)
Zedbury	115	(79)
$p < 0.00001$		

Table 5.16: Use of gas and air by unit

	n	%
Willowford	62	(38)
Exington consultant unit	66	(73)
Exington GP unit	30	(59)
Little Exington	19	(43)
Wychester	98	(59)
Zedbury	80	(56)
$p < 0.00001$		

Table 5.17: Use of Pethidine by unit

	n	%
Willowford	12	(7)
Exington consultant unit	11	(12)
Exington GP unit	0	(0)
Little Exington	1	(2)
Wychester	13	(8)
Zedbury	24	(17)
$p < 0.05$		

Table 5.18: Use of epidurals by unit

Relationship between women's use of drugs and satisfaction with how they dealt with the pain

The more drugs women used the less satisfied they were with how they dealt with the pain (or vice versa). Ninety per cent of those who used no drugs at all were satisfied with how they dealt with the pain as opposed to 45 per cent of those who had Pethidine and an epidural.

	Satisfied		Neither satisfied/ dissatisfied		Dissatisfied	
	n	%	n	%	n	%
No drug	92	(90)	9	(9)	1	(1)
Only gas and air	136	(77)	30	(17)	10	(6)
Epidural (with/without gas and air)	15	(63)	7	(29)	2	(8)
Pethidine (with/without gas and air)	195	(63)	81	(26)	35	(11)
Pethidine and epidural (with or without gas and air)	18	(45)	14	(35)	8	(20)

Percentages are of women in a given row.

Table 5.19: Satisfaction with how women dealt with pain by drug use

The open-ended question about pain relief and how women dealt with the pain is further discussed in Volume 2.

Relationship between antenatal and postnatal data

Did antenatal wishes about drugs affect what women had?

Women who wanted a particular type of pain relief were more likely to get it than those who did not want it. However, the effect of women's positive wishes was least effective for epidurals – less than half of the women who stated antenatally that they definitely wanted an epidural in fact had one. On the other hand, women who wanted to avoid an epidural were most likely to achieve this even though 14 per cent of those who antenatally resisted the idea of an epidural did in fact have one.

Antenatal wishes	n	%
Don't want	15	(37)
Prefer not	48	(52)
Don't mind	122	(68)
Don't know enough to make a choice	18	(67)
Quite like	131	(75)
Definitely want	131	(83)
$p < 0.0001$		

Table 5.20: Women who used gas and air by antenatal wishes

Antenatal wishes	n	%
Don't want	30	(35)
Prefer not	111	(48)
Don't mind	106	(63)
Don't know enough to make a choice	27	(63)
Quite like	54	(56)
Definitely want	31	(74)
$p < 0.0001$		

Table 5.21: Women who used pethidine by antenatal wishes

Antenatal wishes	n	%
Don't want	25	(8)
Prefer not	13	(6)
Don't mind	7	(22)
Don't know enough to make a choice	5	(12)
Quite like	9	(24)
Definitely want	7	(41)
$p < 0.0001$		

Table 5.22: Women who had an epidural by antenatal wishes

There were also some other interesting associations that could be further explored e.g. women who antenatally said they did not want gas and air but in fact did use it, were more likely to say that gas and air was not at all effective than other women were (18% compared to 9%). However, this was not true for Pethidine or epidural analgesia.

Women who used the pain relief they said they wanted and those who did not: exploring the mismatch between antenatal wishes and actual events

For ease of reference we will describe women who antenatally expressed a desire for a drug but in practice did not use it as the 'Wanted but did not get' group, and the women who antenatally said they wanted to avoid a drug but used it in practice, as the 'Didn't want but got' group.

The other women 'Got what they wanted' i.e. either had a drug and expressed indifference or a predisposition towards that drug antenatally or, alternatively, did not have a drug and expressed indifference or the wish to avoid the drug antenatally.

GAS AND AIR

Women who had gas and air, in spite of wanting to avoid it, were more likely to have felt pressurized and to have mixed feelings about what happened than either those who got what they wanted or those who antenatally said they wanted gas and air but in practice did not get it (see Appendix).

PETHIDINE

The group who 'Didn't want Pethidine but got it' and those who 'Wanted Pethidine but didn't get it' felt equally under pressure. However, the former group, those who did use Pethidine in spite of their antenatal wishes to avoid it, were much more likely to be unhappy about this than those who did not use Pethidine in spite of their antenatal wishes to do so. It is notable that although 19 per cent of the women in this latter group felt encouraged/pressurized not to use Pethidine, only 6 per cent expressed any mixed (or negative) feelings about what happened (see Appendix).

EPIDURAL

Twenty six per cent of the women who wanted but did not get an epidural felt encouraged/pressurized to avoid it, while 51 per cent of those who did not want an epidural but were given one felt pressurized in some way. The women who 'didn't want but got' an epidural were also more than twice as likely to express mixed feelings or unhappiness about what happened. In the case of both gas and air and epidural, the group of women who got what they wanted felt under least pressure and were most satisfied with events (see Appendix).

SUCCUMBING TO PRESSURE

We also looked at women who had succumbed to pressure to have a drug, women who had succumbed to pressure not to have a drug and women who either did not succumb to pressure or did not experience any either way. Succumbing to pressure was measured by answering 'Yes' to having the drug and indicating they felt under pressure to have it or 'No' to having the drug and indicating they felt under pressure not to have it.

We found that women who had succumbed to pressure to have drugs expressed much more dissatisfaction than either of the other two groups. However, succumbing to pressure *not* to have drugs does not necessarily mean that women look back on the event with dissatisfaction (see Appendix).

DRUG USE, ANTENATAL INTENTIONS AND SATISFACTION IN DEALING WITH THE PAIN

Women who wanted gas and air but did not use it were more likely to be satisfied even than women who got what they wanted. Women who said antenatally that they wanted Pethidine, but did not in fact receive it were just as satisfied as those women who had it. However, where epidurals are concerned, the most satisfied group were those who got what they said they wanted antenatally (although those who had wanted an epidural but did not get one were still more satisfied with the way they dealt with the pain than those who had not wanted one but ended up having one). These results should, however, be interpreted with caution. It could be that those who did not intend to use drugs but did in fact use them may have had unexpectedly difficult labours and consequently felt dissatisfied, rather than the dissatisfaction resulting directly from the drug use itself.

	Satisfied		Neither satisfied nor dissatisfied		Dissatisfied	
	n	%	n	%	n	%
Wanted but did not get	59	(86)	9	(13)	1	(1)
Did not want but got	40	(65)	14	(25)	8	(13)
Got what they wanted	361	(68)	123	(23)	48	(9)

Percentages refer to the proportion of women in each row.

$p < 0.05$

Table 5.23: Gas and air: antenatal wishes and what happened by satisfaction with dealing with the pain

	Satisfied		Neither satisfied nor dissatisfied		Dissatisfied	
	n	%	n	%	n	%
Wanted but did not get	38	(75)	12	(24)	1	(2)
Did not want but got	76	(54)	37	(26)	27	(19)
Got what they wanted	346	(73)	97	(21)	29	(6)

$p < 0.05$

Table 5.24: Pethidine: antenatal wishes and what happened by satisfaction with dealing with the pain

	Satisfied		Neither satisfied nor dissatisfied		Dissatisfied	
	n	%	n	%	n	%
Wanted but did not get	21	(57)	13	(35)	3	(8)
Did not want but got	17	(46)	13	(35)	7	(19)
Got what they wanted	421	(72)	120	(20)	47	(8)

$p < 0.05$

Table 5.25: Epidural: antenatal wishes and what happened by satisfaction with dealing with the pain

Antenatal expectations of how painful a drug-free labour would be and actual drug use during labour

The more painful women expected a drug-free labour to be the more likely they were to use drugs during labour. This was particularly striking for Pethidine.

Antenatal expectation of a drug-free labour	Used Pethidine	
	n	%
Moderately uncomfortable	7	(26)
Quite painful	98	(49)
Very painful	172	(55)
Unbearable	51	(61)
Have no idea	29	(69)

Percentages are of women with a given antenatal expectation.

$p < 0.0001$

Table 5.26: Expectation of pain in a drug-free labour by use of Pethidine

It is also interesting to note that the women who said they had no idea how painful a drug-free labour would be were consistently the most likely to have gas and air, Pethidine or an epidural, more likely even than women who expected it would be very or unbearably painful.

Similarly, women who said they would ideally prefer to have a drug-free labour were least likely to use drugs. Responses to the antenatal questions 'Do you worry about labour pain' and 'Do you worry about pain in everyday life' were, however, not associated with drug use during labour.

Summary

Most women (regardless of educational level) prefer to keep the drugs they use during labour to a minimum and would like to be involved in decisions about pain relief. In practice, most women used gas and air and at least ten per cent of women felt under some pressure to use drugs. Women's own expectations and staff support affected drug use – women who ideally preferred to cope with only minimum drug use were more likely to do so than other women.

In general, women were happier if they had not used a drug than if they had used it, over and above their antenatal wishes. As we shall show in Chapter 8, women who used Pethidine or epidurals were less fulfilled and satisfied than other women. Using Pethidine was also associated with low postnatal emotional well-being.

CHAPTER SIX

Obstetric Interventions

Antenatal views of interventions

The term 'intervention' covers a very wide range of procedures and the word itself, with its negative overtones, was not used at all in our questionnaires. We were interested in gauging how strongly women felt about having, or not having, each of a number of procedures and how well-informed they felt themselves to be about these. We divided interventions into two groups: i) relatively commonplace procedures which many women could expect to experience which we will call 'minor' interventions, and ii) procedures which were only likely to occur following the identification of serious obstetric problems: 'major' interventions.

Clearly, some procedures (e.g. glucose drip, continuous electronic fetal monitoring) might be seen as borderline between these categories but they have been placed in the first group for our purposes. The management of the third stage of labour, which is probably the most common intervention but about which we expected women to be fairly uninformed, is treated separately (see Volume 2, Chapter 6).

'Minor' interventions

We asked women about a total of six procedures in this group: enemas, shaving, fetal heart monitoring at intervals, continuous monitoring, glucose drip and episiotomy. For each procedure women were asked to tick one of five preference responses (from 'definitely don't want' to 'definitely do want') or a sixth option 'Don't know enough to make a choice'. Results are given in Table 6.1.

We found that the attitude towards electronic fetal monitoring differed sharply from attitudes towards the other interventions listed. Over half the women had an active preference for monitoring and over a third of these (i.e. 20% of the whole sample) indicated that they wanted *continuous* monitoring.

By contrast, the majority of women were against having all of the other four interventions listed with between 15 per cent and 28 per cent saying that they did not mind and only a handful actively wanting the procedures specified. The proportion saying that they did not know enough to make a choice ranged from one per cent for shaving (the most unpopular intervention) to 13 per cent for glucose drips.

	Definitely don't want	Prefer not	Don't mind	Quite like	Definitely do want	Don't know enough
Enema	129 (17%)	314 (42%)	206 (28%)	33 (4%)	24 (3%)	38 (5%)
Shave	264 (35%)	303 (41%)	159 (21%)	3 (1%)	8 (1%)	9 (1%)
Intermittent monitoring	5 (1%)	35 (5%)	284 (38%)	202 (27%)	203 (27%)	14 (2%)
Continuous monitoring	78 (11%)	265 (36%)	231 (31%)	92 (12%)	57 (8%)	21 (3%)
Glucose drip	93 (13%)	338 (45%)	206 (28%)	5 (1%)	4 (1%)	99 (13%)
Episiotomy	115 (15%)	407 (55%)	112 (15%)	4 (1%)	11 (2%)	91 (12%)

n = 744

Table 6.1: Preferences with respect to six 'minor' interventions

For nearly every one of these six procedures there were significant differences by both parity and level of education. The parity differences were not as wide as one might have expected, but where they did occur the pattern was that multips were less likely to say that they did not know enough to make a choice and more likely to be against having the procedures listed. The differences by educational level were, in general, also as one might expect. The least educated women were most likely to say that they did not know enough or that they did not mind, while more educated women were more likely to reject the procedures. The biggest differences were in the 'Don't mind' category, as Table 6.2 shows. There was a similar pattern for woman's own social class.

	Educational level					
	16 and under		17–18		19 and over	
	n	%	n	%	n	%
Enema	114	(31)	55	(26)	35	(17)
Shave	91	(25)	41	(20)	24	(15)
Intermittent monitoring	161	(44)	69	(33)	52	(33)
Continuous monitoring	135	(37)	65	(31)	30	(19)
Drip	103	(28)	62	(30)	38	(24)
Episiotomy	50	(14)	38	(18)	23	(14)

Table 6.2: Number of women who 'don't mind' whether or not they have each of six 'minor' interventions by age of finishing full-time education

This data would seem to support the stereotype of the middle class educated woman with her long list of 'do's and don'ts'. However, there is a lot of difference to the midwife on the receiving end between 'I definitely don't want' and 'I would prefer not to have'. As Mavis Kirkham has illustrated so graphically (1987) midwives (like the rest of us) respond much better to the conciliatory 'Well, of course, you know best but...' approach than to a bald 'I'm not having that!'. It therefore seemed of interest to look at the educational level of those women who specified 'definitely don't want' compared to those who said 'would prefer not to have'. In the table we have omitted intermittent fetal heart monitoring since so few women were against it.

	Educational level		
	16 and under	17–18	19 and over
	%	%	%
Enema	30	29	28
Shave	41	49	55
Continuous monitoring	16	24	30
Glucose drip	23	20	21
Episiotomy	24	21	20

n's are necessarily different for each cell. Numerators range from 22 to 110 and denominators from 100 to 267.

Table 6.3: Percentage of those women who wished to avoid each of five 'minor' interventions who ticked 'Definitely don't want' as opposed to 'Prefer not to have' by age of finishing full-time education

It will be seen that of the five interventions that women wished to avoid, in only two instances (shaving and continuous monitoring) were highly educated women stating their aversion more strongly than the least educated women. In all the other three cases (enema, glucose drip and episiotomy) it is the least educated women who have ticked 'Definitely don't want' proportionately more often, although for these three the differences between educational groups were not as great.

Of course, we do not know the form of words in which women actually made their wishes known to their midwives, but, if the responses to these questions can be taken as indicative, then it would seem that the stereotype of the strident uncompromising, well-educated, middle class woman is not supported. Better educated women are more likely to know what they want (or do not want) but, given that, they are not, on balance, more likely than other women to take an extreme position.

'Major' interventions

We separated this group of interventions because different questions seemed appropriate. Most people, we assumed, would prefer that there should not be any obstetric problems necessitating these interventions and we were more interested in discovering women's expectations (e.g. 'it didn't happen last time so it won't happen this time') and how keen they would be to avoid these procedures if the situation did arise. Four procedures were covered: induction, acceleration of labour, forceps delivery and caesarean section. Slightly different formats were used for the questions about each as appropriate.

INDUCTION

Women were first asked 'How much do you know about what induction involves?' (Induction was defined as 'starting labour off artificially').

Responses to the four options were:

	n	%
Nothing	42	(6)
Very little	230	(31)
Quite a bit	369	(50)
A great deal	103	(14)

We were not, of course, able to check the accuracy of these assessments, but in some cases subsequent comments suggested that women were not quite as well informed as they thought they were. For example, one woman who said that she knew 'a great deal' about induction said:

> 'I was induced at my first birth, even though my contractions were regular and everything seemed to be going OK.'

Thus indicating that she was confusing induction with acceleration. She subsequently said that she knew 'nothing' about acceleration.

Once again, as one would expect there is a very strong relationship ($p < 0.0001$) between how much women said they knew and level of education, although a majority (56%) of the least educated women still said that they knew at least 'quite a bit'. The relationship between knowledge and parity, while significant ($p < 0.001$), is not as marked as might be expected; there is, for example, no difference between the percentages of multips and of primips who said that they knew 'nothing' about induction.

The second part of the question asked women whether they expected to be induced. Responses to the five options were:

	n	%
Yes, I know that I am going to be induced	8	(1)
Yes, I think that I probably will be	47	(6)
I have no expectations either way	213	(29)
No, I don't expect to be induced	443	(60)
No, I am certain that I won't be induced	30	(4)

Differences between groups with different levels of education were not significant, although the tendency was for the better educated women to think that they would not be induced. The thirty women who were certain that they would not be induced were evenly distributed with respect to education. The majority (24) were, however, multips. Multips were, in general, more likely to think either that they would be induced or to be certain that they would not be and they were correspondingly less likely to have no expectations.

The third part of the question was open-ended and asked women if they had a particular reason for their expectations. Seventy per cent of women answered the question, although 26 per cent of these (18% of the whole sample) simply said 'No'. One woman answered 'yes' but did not elaborate.

On the whole women who *knew* that they were going to be induced gave 'medical' reasons i.e. the reasons that doctors had given them. However, women who only *thought* that they probably would be induced were more likely to cite previous experience as the reason for their expectation. We were particularly interested in the reasons given by women who did not expect to be induced. Amongst those who were certain that they would not be the most common explanations were 'medical' e.g. 'My doctor has told me that everything is going according to plan and there is no reason why I should not go into labour spontaneously'. Six women gave their personal preferences as a reason for their certainty that they would not be induced, as did a further 33 who simply 'don't expect to be induced'. For example:

> 'Yes, I have a particular reason for thinking this. 1) It's not a natural act, and I strongly believe that bearing children should be as natural a thing as the Sun shines. 2) I have set my mind on having my baby naturally and freely. 3) I have waited 23 years for this moment and no-one will spoil it for me.'

This was, however, a minority attitude. Perhaps more typical was:

> 'My pregnancy has been very straightforward with no problems whatsoever. I prefer to think my labour will follow this rather than be concerned about something which may not happen.'

This sort of 'everything is normal so far' reason was given by 23 per cent of the women who 'don't expect to be induced' and a similar number cited previous experience e.g. 'Both of my previous labours started spontaneously'. The majority of the other women in this 'don't expect' group either said that they had no reason (21%) or simply failed to answer the question (23%).

As the final part of the section on induction women were asked: 'If you were two weeks overdue and were offered an induction, what would you prefer to do?'

We felt that answers to a specific scenario of this sort would give more indicative answers than the global preference questions that we had asked about 'minor' interventions. Responses were:

	n	%
I would prefer to accept the offer of an induction immediately	287	(39)
I would prefer to wait a few more days to see if I go into labour spontaneously	313	(42)
I would prefer not to be induced under any circumstances	21	(3)
I would not mind either way	62	(8)
I don't know	55	(8)

Perhaps surprisingly, there were no significant differences between multips and primips in responses to this question. Similarly, differences between women of different levels of education were not significant.

Two women saw this as an irrelevant question but for interestingly contrasting reasons. The first (booked at Wychester) said:

> 'Nowadays women can go two weeks over due date without any concern. I'm sure it will happen quite naturally at least within these two weeks.'

The second said:

> 'At Exington you have no choice! After two weeks you are induced. This question therefore seems irrelevant.'

ACCELERATION

The pattern of questions on acceleration was the same as that for induction. We defined acceleration as 'speeding labour up artificially' and asked women first how much they knew about what it involves. Responses were:

	n	%
Nothing	171	(23)
Very little	287	(39)
Quite a bit	233	(31)
A great deal	50	(7)

It is immediately clear that women feel that they know less about acceleration than they do about induction. About a quarter of the women (23%) knew nothing about acceleration compared with only six per cent who knew nothing about induction.

Only 38 per cent felt they knew at least quite a bit about acceleration compared to 64 per cent for induction. The relationship with level of education is particularly strong; 30 per cent of those who left school at 16 or younger knew nothing compared to only 14 per cent of the group who had been educated beyond the age of 18.

The differences between multips and primips are also significant; overall, multips said that they knew significantly more than primips. However, as with induction, there was no difference between the proportion of multips and primips who said that they knew nothing.

As well as feeling relatively uninformed about acceleration, a large percentage of women (46%) had no expectations about whether or not they would be accelerated (compared with 29% for induction). Acceleration is, of course, not a procedure that is usually predictable during pregnancy, and therefore women can only respond on the basis of the perception of overall likelihood.

Do you *expect* that your labour will be accelerated?

	n	%
Yes, I know that my labour is going to be accelerated	0	(0)
Yes, I think that my labour probably will be accelerated	21	(3)
I have no expectation one way or the other	339	(46)
No, I don't expect that my labour will be accelerated	332	(45)
No, I am certain that my labour won't be accelerated	46	(6)

As with induction, primips were more likely than multips to have no expectations (55% of primips compared to 40% of multips). Multips were also more likely to be certain that they would not be accelerated (8% compared to 3%). Unlike expectations of induction, level of education was also significantly related to expectations of acceleration ($p < 0.05$). Women whose education had stopped at 16 years or younger were more likely to have no expectations, but they were also relatively more likely than other women to say that they were certain that their labours would not be accelerated. The least educated women were also least likely to give a reason for their expectations although, overall, only a third of the sample offered any reason for their expectations. These were most commonly based on previous experience or on the normality of their pregnancies to date.

Finally, we asked women how they thought that they would react in practice to the offer of acceleration:

'If the staff said that your labour probably ought to be accelerated what would you prefer to do?'

	n	%
I would prefer to have my labour accelerated immediately	242	(33)
I would prefer to wait a bit and see how it goes	310	(42)
I would prefer not to be accelerated under any circumstances	19	(3)
I would not mind either way	68	(9)
I don't know	98	(13)

These frequencies are very similar to those for induction. However, comparison of individual women's answers to the two questions shows that only 57 per cent gave the same response in the two cases. This suggests that women are not just giving blanket responses to interventions in general, but are treating each on its own merits.

One of the differences between these figures and those for induction is in the higher percentage of 'don't know' replies: 13 per cent compared to 8 per cent. For some women this was because labour is inevitably a trip into the unknown and they judged (doubtless accurately) that an appeal to their baby's safety would determine their behaviour at the time:

> 'Difficult to tell in advance, i.e. danger to baby would justify just about anything.'
>
> 'Who knows what their labour will be like? If the safety of my health and my baby's would be affected because labour is too slow, then surely it's in both our interests to speed the labour along.'

Given that this is the context in which acceleration is likely to be presented, we are struck by the fact that as many as 42 per cent of the sample said that they would prefer to wait rather than accept acceleration immediately; in practice we imagine that women would be rather more amenable to staff suggestion. We were also surprised by the lack of any difference between the responses of multips and primips since, elsewhere, multips' previous experience has tended to give them firmer views. There is, however, a highly significant difference by level of education ($p < 0.001$). Highly educated women were less likely to say that they 'Don't mind' or 'Don't know' (13% compared to 25% of the other two groups) and more likely to say that they would prefer to wait (58% compared to 38%). There were no educational differences related to the 'not under any circumstances' response.

FORCEPS

The third major intervention that we asked about was a forceps delivery. Given the variety and unpredictability of situations that might lead to the use of forceps, it did not seem useful to ask women whether they expected to have a forceps delivery. We therefore asked a single question, similar to those asked for induction and acceleration, to try to gauge the extent to which women would wish to avoid a forceps delivery: 'If you were very tired and the staff suggested a forceps delivery, what do you think you would prefer to do? (assuming that there was no immediate danger to the baby)'. Responses were:

	n	%
I would prefer to accept the suggestion of a forceps delivery immediately	128	(17)
I would prefer to wait a bit and see how it goes	278	(38)
I would prefer to avoid a forceps delivery if at all possible	294	(40)
I don't know	41	(6)

It is likely that our specification of no immediate danger to the baby is responsible for this particular pattern of results; in practice, it seems highly unlikely that 78 per cent of women would refuse to accept a forceps delivery when it was offered. It is also unlikely that forceps would be offered without at least a strong suggestion that the baby would benefit. Nonetheless, we deliberately asked the question in this way because we wanted to discover women's underlying attitudes towards forceps.

There were no significant differences related to level of education, although there was the tendency, also observed for some of the other interventions, for more educated women to 'prefer to wait a bit and see how it goes'. It was the least educated women who were proportionately more likely to want to 'avoid a forceps delivery if at all possible'. Similarly, primips were more likely to prefer to wait (45% of primips compared to 33% of multips) while multips preferred to 'avoid if at all possible' (32% primips compared to 45% of multips) ($p < 0.01$).

CAESAREAN SECTION

For caesarean sections we again asked about knowledge, expectations and preferences. 'How much do you know about what a caesarean section involves?'

	n	%
Nothing	30	(4)
Very little	230	(31)
Quite a bit	389	(52)
A great deal	96	(13)

These percentages are almost identical to those for induction, and there is similarly a strong relationship with level of education in the expected direction. Parity is also highly significant, although the actual distribution of scores is somewhat unexpected. The majority of primips (64%) said that they knew 'quite a bit' (compared to 45% of multips) while multips predominate in all the other response categories.

Expectations of having a caesarean section are as one would expect; multips were more likely to know or suspect that they would have a caesarean section, while primips were more likely to have no expectations. The majority of both multips and primips (65%) did not expect to have a caesarean section while twice as many multips as primips were *certain* that they would not have one (13% compared to 6%). There is also a significant effect of level of education ($p < 0.05$). This is not apparent among women who were expecting to have a caesarean section but, among the remainder, those with least education were more likely to have no expectations or to be sure that they would not have a section, while the most highly educated women were more likely to say simply that they 'do not expect' to have a caesarean section. Reasons for expecting a caesarean section were, predictably, medical, with a third of the 39 women who thought that they would or might have one citing previous experience. These two classes of response were also most frequently given as reasons for expecting *not* to have a caesarean section. However, a third of the women who expected not to have a section gave no reason at all and a further 18 per cent stated that they had no reason for their expectations. Some women were, however, at pains to point out to us that the interests of the baby would always predominate:

> 'I am told there is no reason as to why I should not be able to have a natural delivery. If any problems occur, then obviously in the interests of myself and my baby if a caesarean is required then I will have one.'

> 'My baby is still breech presentation. I see no reason for causing the slightest risk to her because I wish to experience labour.'

In trying to gauge how committed women were to a vaginal delivery we posited two scenarios. Firstly: 'If your consultant told you that you were *almost certain* to need a caesarean section, what would you prefer to do?'

Responses were:

	n	%
I would prefer to have an elective caesarean section (i.e. booked in advance for a particular day without waiting to go into labour)	346	(46)
I would prefer to have a trial of labour (go into labour and only if that did not work have a caesarean section)	283	(38)
I would not mind either way	32	(4)
I don't know	85	(11)

There were no significant differences between multips and primips, and the only difference by level of education was that, as with other interventions, the least educated women were more likely to say 'Don't know' (16% compared to 7% of other women). The fact that only half of the sample would prefer an elective section or would not mind seems fairly striking given the specification in the scenario of near certainty of needing a caesarean section. As with the forceps question, it seems unlikely in practice that so many women would actually resist the pressure to have an elective section. Nevertheless, it suggests a strong commitment to the idea of a vaginal delivery on the part of a substantial number of women which is unrelated to either parity or level of education. There is, however, one interesting correlate of responses to this question which runs counter to the trends reported earlier; the more women said that they knew about caesarean sections, the more likely they were to opt for an elective section. Thus 52 per cent of the women who knew 'a great deal' would choose an elective section compared to only 30 per cent of those who knew 'nothing'. These figures are at least partly explained by those women who were already committed to the idea of an elective section and who were, therefore, on the whole better informed.

To pose a situation of near certainty of needing a section allowed us to detect one particular set of attitudes. However, we were also interested in moving along this continuum and discovering how many women would still choose an elective section if the situation were less clear cut. We therefore asked 'If your consultant told you that there was *a 50:50 chance* of needing a caesarean section, what would you prefer to do?'.

The response options provided were identical to those for the previous question, and the responses were:

	n	%
I would prefer to have an elective caesarean section (i.e. booked in advance for a particular day without waiting to go into labour)	127	(17)
I would prefer to have a trial of labour (go into labour and only if that did not work have a caesarean section)	509	(68)
I would not mind either way	33	(4)
I don't know	76	(10)

For this question there were differences by both parity and education, although those for parity did not quite reach statistical significance (p = 0.06). Multips were more inclined to choose an elective section than were primips (29% compared to 13% of primips). Nevertheless, 49 primips, i.e. women who have never experienced labour, would either 'not mind' not doing so, or would actively choose an elective section. This would seem to place them at the opposite end of the continuum from the substantially larger number of women who would choose a trial of labour even if a caesarean section were almost certain. The differences by level of education were in the expected direction with 75 per cent of the most highly educated women choosing a trial of labour compared to 63 per cent of the least educated (who were more likely not to mind or not to know). Women's preferences also related to the amount that they said that they knew about caesarean sections with 43 per cent of those who knew nothing feeling unable to make a decision compared with eight per cent of those who knew a great deal. It is interesting to note that in this scenario of a 50:50 chance of needing a section, in contrast to the near-certainty scenario, the women who knew a great deal were much more likely to opt for a trial of labour while those who knew nothing were relatively more likely to choose an elective section.

Postnatal reports of interventions

We collected data postnatally on women's experiences of interventions. As in the antenatal section, we will divide these into those relatively common procedures which are unlikely to be seen as life-or-death issues, ('minor' interventions) and those likely to be associated with some perceived obstetric problem ('major' interventions). Episiotomy is considered in a separate section later in this chapter, as, again, is third stage management.

Minor interventions

Table 6.4 shows the number of women in the postnatal sample who experienced each procedure.

	n	%
Enema	147	(23)
Shave	65	(10)
Glucose drip	141	(22)
Monitoring:		
continuous	176	(26)
non-continuous	380	(56)
ARM	362	(54)

Percentages based on all valid responses (n ranges from 630 to 670). Elective caesarean sections, 'don't know' and no response are omitted.

Table 6.4: Experience of minor interventions

It will be seen that at least one 'common' procedure, shaving, was not in fact at all common among our sample (10%) which is consistent with the recent findings of Garforth and Garcia (1987) showing shaving to be on the decline as a routine practice. Similarly, enemas were experienced by only 23 per cent of the sample. The incidence of both of these procedures, and indeed of all the others in the list, varied significantly between the units, as we shall see below.

Major interventions

The number of women experiencing major interventions is shown in Table 6.5. These figures are all very close to the most recently published national figures (OPCS, 1988). The only procedure for which there is a large discrepancy is acceleration, the national figure for 1985 being only 12.1 per cent. However, those same figures show exceedingly wide regional variation, from 0.5 per cent to 31.9 per cent. Furthermore, this is an intervention which is likely to be under-recorded in hospital records, as our own data shows (work in progress).

		n	%
Induction		108	(16)
Acceleration		112	(17)
Instrumental delivery		65	(10)
Caesarean section:	elective	29	(4)
	other	32	(5)

Percentages are based on all valid responses (n ranges from 665 to 710). 'Don't know', no response, and, for the first three procedures, elective sections are omitted.

Table 6.5: Experience of 'major' interventions

Twenty nine of the 61 caesarean sections were elective (4% of all deliveries, 48% of caesarean sections). Of the remainder, four women had had a caesarean planned but went into early spontaneous labour and were operated on as emergencies. This represents 12 per cent of all planned sections. Seven women had sections following trials of labour and the remaining sections were performed as a result of unforeseen problems arising during labour.

As with the minor interventions there was considerable variation between the different units. There were also major differences between multips and primips. Both of these factors are discussed below.

Educational level and social class

There were no significant differences by level of education for any of the nine procedures listed above.

Looking at social class as defined by the woman's best ever job we find that women in classes IV and V were twice as likely to have been induced ($p < 0.05$).

Social Class	n	%
I and II	35/255	(14)
IIIN and IIIM	49/330	(15)
IV and V	20/67	(30)

Table 6.6: Induction by woman's social class

This pattern is not evident when we look at partner's occupation. There are also small class differences in the use of enemas, both by the woman's own job and by partner's occupation, with lower class women experiencing more enemas than higher class women. This is in keeping with the fact that more lower class women said antenatally that they did not know enough to choose (see below for relationship between preferences and events).

Parity

The relative incidence of the different procedures for multips and primips is given in Table 6.7.

Procedure	Primips n	Primips %	Multips n	Multips %	Significance
Enema	68	(27)	79	(20)	ns
Shave	35	(14)	30	(8)	0.05
Glucose drip	75	(30)	65	(17)	0.0001
Monitoring: continuous	83	(31)	93	(23)	0.0001
non-continuous	163	(61)	217	(54)	
ARM	139	(53)	223	(56)	ns
Induction	59	(22)	49	(12)	0.01
Acceleration	70	(26)	42	(10)	0.0001
Instrumental delivery	50	(19)	15	(4)	0.0001
Caesarean section: elective	6	(2)	23	(5)	0.05
other	17	(6)	15	(3)	

Percentages are based on all valid responses (n ranges from 630 to 670). 'Don't know', no response and, where appropriate, elective caesareans are omitted.

Table 6.7: Experience of interventions by parity

It is clear from the table that primips were significantly more likely to experience most of the procedures considered. This is consistent with other published figures (e.g. MacFarlane and Mugford, 1984). In the case of enemas the difference is not significant (p = 0.07). There is no difference in the overall proportions of multips and primips having caesarean deliveries; the difference is that multips were more than twice as likely to have an elective section. The only other procedure considered for which there is no significant difference between multips and primips is artificial rupture of membranes (ARM). In fact multips were slightly more likely to have their membranes ruptured artificially but this is because primips' membranes were more likely to rupture spontaneously at an earlier stage (see Table 6.8). When we consider only those women whose membranes did not break early on (whether naturally or artificially) we find that 72 per cent of 'at risk' primips had ARM compared to 66 per cent of 'at risk' multips. This difference is not significant but may be a reflection of the fact that primips were more likely to have electronic fetal monitoring which, if this includes a scalp electrode, requires the membranes to be ruptured. Twenty three per cent of multips (n = 93) had no electronic fetal monitoring compared to only 8 per cent of primips (n = 21).

	Primips		Multips		Total	
	n	%	n	%	n	%
Spontaneous						
Early on	70	(27)	69	(17)	139	(21)
During established labour	51	(20)	103	(26)	154	(23)
Artificial						
Pre-labour	11	(4)	21	(5)	32	(5)
During labour	128	(49)	200	(51)	328	(50)
Not specified	–	–	2	(<1)	2	(<1)
Total	260	(100)	395	(100)	655	(100)

Table 6.8: Rupturing of membranes by parity

Nine primips and nine multips who were 'not sure' have been omitted, as have women who had elective sections and those giving no response.

Differences between units

Table 6.9 shows the incidence of the various procedures at each of the six units. It will be seen that there is very considerable variation between the units. Enemas, for example, were given to 62 per cent of women at Exington consultant unit compared to only four per cent at Willowford. This presumably reflects differing unit policies rather than any differences in the populations. Similarly, the same two units represent extremes in the incidence of shaving: 31 per cent at Exington compared to just one per cent at Willowford. The substantial differences between the three Exington units are particularly noticeable for both shaving and enemas.

All the other procedures might be thought to reflect differences that we know exist in the populations served by each unit: notably the fact that the GP unit and, to a lesser extent, Little Exington cater only for low risk women. Furthermore, women showing signs of the sorts of problems that might indicate the need for these interventions would be transferred to the consultant unit. It is therefore to be expected that the GP unit has the lowest incidence of most of the procedures considered. The one exception is ARM which is actually more common at the GP unit than at any of the other units. This is despite a very low rate of electronic fetal monitoring there. It may be, however, that ARM is more frequently used at the GP unit as a method of accelerating labour: chemical augmentation is a very rare occurrence there. This is to be expected when we remember that the term 'GP unit' is a misnomer; such units are in practice run by community midwives who have limited powers to give drugs but freedom to use their discretion to hasten labour by more natural means.

Procedure	Willowford		Exington consultant		Exington GP unit		Little Exington		Wychester		Zedbury	
	n	%	n	%	n	%	n	%	n	%	n	%
Enema	6	(4)	56	(62)	27	(54)	6	(14)	9	(14)	41	(30)
Shave	2	(1)	27	(31)	6	(13)	4	(10)	9	(6)	16	(12)
Glucose drip	18	(12)	28	(33)	1	(2)	7	(17)	26	(17)	54	(38)
Monitoring:												
continuous	28	(17)	36	(40)	1	(2)	7	(16)	36	(22)	62	(43)
non-continuous	121	(75)	40	(44)	10	(20)	108	(53)	108	(53)	70	(48)
ARM	93	(57)	55	(61)	32	(67)	15	(36)	82	(51)	77	(57)
Induction	22	(14)	16	(18)	2	(4)	7	(17)	33	(20)	26	(18)
Acceleration	21	(13)	15	(17)	1	(2)	5	(12)	38	(23)	28	(20)
Instrumental delivery	12	(8)	10	(11)	–	(0)	1	(2)	24	(15)	15	(11)
Caesarean section:												
elective	9	(5)	2	(2)	–	(0)	1	(2)	7	(4)	8	(5)
other	1	(<1)	9	(10)	–	(0)	–	(0)	8	(5)	14	(9)
Non-instrumental vaginal deliveries	149	(87)	73	(78)	51	(100)	43	(98)	133	(77)	119	(76)

Unit differences are significant at $p < 0.0001$ for enema, shave, glucose drip and monitoring, $p < 0.01$ for caesarean section, and $p < 0.05$ for ARM, acceleration and instrumental delivery. Differences with regard to induction are not significant.

Table 6.9: Incidence of minor and major interventions in the six obstetric units

When the two low risk units are excluded differences between units are less marked, although still apparent. Clear differences in monitoring policies can be seen. For example, at Willowford nearly all women are monitored but only 17 per cent are actually monitored continuously. At Exington consultant unit, in contrast, one in seven women escape monitoring altogether but 40 per cent are monitored continuously. If we look separately at multips and primips within the different units nearly all the differences remain significant. Where this is not the case it is because numbers are too small. It is clear, therefore, that differences between units are not a result of different ratios of multips and primips. However, the variation between units tends to be greater for primips than for multips, perhaps because primips are more likely, in general, to experience various procedures. This is most apparent when we look at the proportion of non-instrumental vaginal deliveries (NIVD) for multips and primips at each unit:

	Willowford	Exington consultant	Wychester	Zedbury	Exington GP unit	Little Exington
Primips	84%	74%	70%	62%	100%	90%
Multips	89%	80%	83%	84%	100%	97%

Table 6.10: Percentage of non-instrumental vaginal deliveries by unit by parity

As expected, the NIVD rate is high for both multips and primips at Little Exington and Exington GP unit because problems are transferred. We will therefore focus only on the four consultant units. Amongst these the range of NIVD's for multips is only from 80–89 per cent, while for primips it is more than twice as great: 62–84 per cent. It is interesting to note that although Exington serves a higher risk multip population, the percentage of NIVD's is not dramatically lower than at Wychester and Zedbury. For primips, the very high rate at Willowford (84%) and the very low rate at Zedbury (62%) are most striking. We would, however, wish to be cautious about the reliability of our figures for caesarean and instrumental deliveries since such relatively small numbers are involved at each unit.

Episiotomies and tears

Of the 650 women who had vaginal deliveries, 474 (73%) suffered some kind of damage to the perineum: 29 per cent had episiotomies, 39 per cent had tears, 4 per cent had both.

Reason for suturing	n	% (of women who had vaginal deliveries)
Episiotomy	196	(29)
Tear	247	(39)
Episiotomy and tear	28	(4)
Don't know	3	(1)
No suturing necessary	176	(27)
n = 650		

Table 6.11: State of the perineum

Nine women had forceps deliveries under general anaesthetic and were not asked for further details. The figures discussed here therefore refer to the remaining 465 women. Of the 275 women who had tears, 38 per cent did not know what kind of tear, 35 per cent said they had first degree tears, 24 per cent had second degree tears and 3 per cent said they had third degree tears.

The actual suturing (of both tears and episiotomies) was the source of much distress. Only a third of the women found it a pain-free procedure and 19 per cent felt a lot of pain, sometimes describing it as the worst thing about the entire birth. Issues about suturing (how painful it was, postnatal problems with the stitches, who sutured, suturing material etc.) are discussed in detail in Volume 2.

Education, social class and perineal damage

There were no significant differences in what happened to women of different educational levels apart from the fact that the more educated women were more likely to know what kind of tear they had. However, there were clear class differences in terms of women's best ever job. Higher class women were more likely to need stitches. This is because they were more likely to be given episiotomies (although equally likely to tear). In all, 43 per cent of the highest class women had episiotomies as opposed to 24 per cent of the women in the lowest classes.

Social class	Intact perineum		Episiotomy		Tear		Both	
	n	%	n	%	n	%	n	%
I and II	48	(20)	81	(34)	95	(39)	17	(9)
IIIN and IIIM	92	(30)	85	(27)	122	(39)	11	(5)
IV and V	25	(35)	14	(20)	27	(38)	2	(4)

Percentages are of women within a given social class group.

$p < 0.0001$

Table 6.12: Type of perineal damage by class

Higher class women were also more likely to know what kind of tear they had and were more likely to say that they had a second degree tear.

Parity and perineal damage

Primips were more likely to need suturing than multips (90% compared to 62%, $p < 0.0001$). They were also more likely to have an episiotomy (45% compared to 19%) but slightly less likely to have a tear (35% compared to 41%). (These figures exclude women who had both tears and episiotomies which is why they do not add up to the total number of women who needed suturing.)

	Episiotomy		Tear	
	n	%	n	%
Primip	112	(45)	86	(35)
Multip	72	(19)	161	(41)

Percentages are of women of a given parity

$p < 0.05$

Table 6.13: Type of perineal damage by parity

The tears sustained by multips were less severe than those sustained by primips. Forty one per cent of the tears sustained by multips were only first degree as opposed to 27 per cent of those sustained by primips. However, in spite of this, multips were more likely to experience pain during stitching. (We could find no obvious explanation for this as they were just as likely to be anaesthetized.)

	A lot/a bit of pain		No pain at all	
	n	%	n	%
Primip	136	(61)	86	(39)
Multip	179	(74)	64	(26)

Percentages are of women of a given parity

$p < 0.05$

Table 6.14: Pain during suturing by parity

Unit and perineal damage

The most striking difference between the units was in the proportion of women who escaped the need for suturing. Forty five per cent of the women in Exington GP unit and 31 per cent of those at Little Exington did not need stitches as compared to only 11 per cent at Exington consultant unit. The fact that women in the GP and satellite units at Exington are three to four times more likely to have an intact perineum than those at the consultant unit is probably accounted for, at least in part, by the concentration of high risk and primiparous women in the consultant unit. However, significant differences still remain when parity is controlled for (see Appendix).

	Episiotomy		Tear		Both		Intact perineum	
	n	%	n	%	n	%	n	%
Exington consultant	34	(43)	30	(38)	6	(8)	9	(11)
Exington GP unit	8	(16)	20	(40)	0	(0)	23	(45)
Little Exington	12	(27)	14	(32)	3	(7)	14	(32)

Percentages refer to proportion of women in each unit.

Table 6.15: State of perineum by unit (Exington units only)

When we look at the other three consultant units – Willowford, Wychester and Zedbury – we also find differences in intact perineum rates. Thirty four per cent of women at Willowford escaped the need for any stitches as opposed to 25 per cent and 22 per cent of those at Zedbury and Wychester respectively. There are no parity differences between these units and low risk women are not being filtered away as in Exington.

Unit	Episiotomy		Tear		Both		Intact perineum	
	n	%	n	%	n	%	n	%
Willowford	25	(16)	76	(48)	4	(3)	54	(34)
Wychester	50	(32)	59	(38)	11	(7)	34	(22)
Zedbury	52	(39)	43	(32)	4	(3)	34	(25)

Percentages refer to proportion of women in each unit.

Table 6.16: State of perineum by unit (excluding Exington units)

Is the number of women with intact perineums related to the episiotomy rate?

Episiotomies are meant to be an alternative to (and an improvement on) a tear. The women in our sample were twice as likely to be given an episiotomy at Wychester and Zedbury as at Willowford. We should therefore see a proportionate increase in tears at Willowford. However, this was not the case. Women at Willowford were more likely to tear but they were also more likely to escape without any perineal damage at all. These data confirm other findings that a low episiotomy rate does not result in a proportionate increase in tears (Sleep et al., 1984).

However, it should be noted that women at Willowford, if they did tear, were slightly more likely to report having second degree tears than women at Wychester and Zedbury; they were also more likely to know what type of tear they had (see Appendix).

The low perineal damage rate at Willowford is partly accounted for by their conservative approach to episiotomies. Another possible contributing factor is that being able to get comfortable reduces the risk of perineal damage. This has been suggested by Kitzinger and Walters (1981) amongst others.

As we shall see in Chapter 7, being able to get into the most comfortable position was also something that varied between units. From our previous contacts with these hospitals (see Green et al., 1986) we knew that Willowford midwives were particularly keen to encourage women to move around to find comfortable positions, and our data confirmed that women at Willowford were more likely to say that they had always been able to get comfortable (57%) than those at Zedbury (38%). A direct cross-tabulation of these two questions (need for suturing by being able to get comfortable) confirmed that women who were always able to get comfortable were less likely to have needed stitches than those who were not.

Able to get comfortable	Needed stitches		Did not need stitches		All women	
	n	%	n	%	n	%
Always	209	(67)	101	(33)	310	(49)
Sometimes	186	(78)	54	(23)	240	(38)
Hardly ever	68	(79)	18	(21)	86	(14)

Percentages are of women in a given row.

$p < 0.05$

Table 6.17: Able to get comfortable by need for stitches

In addition, 42 per cent of the reasons for not being able to get comfortable given by the women who had stitches concerned physical constraint such as a monitor, drip or stirrups as opposed to 29 per cent of the reasons given by those who did not need stitches. Obviously, this is all interrelated with the use of/need for a variety of interventions. However, it is clear that women who are unconstrained and able to move into the positions they find most comfortable are more likely to have intact perineums than women who are unable to move freely.

Perineal damage and postnatal data

Women who had episiotomies felt less in control of what staff did to them than those with intact perineums but this was not true of women who tore (see Chapter 7).

Women who had episiotomies were also less likely to say that they found the birth fulfilling and were less satisfied with the birth (see Chapter 8).

Conclusion

Allowing the perineum to tear rather than giving an episiotomy is sometimes seen as 'bad practice' yet there is little evidence to suggest that tears are more problematic than episiotomies. Indeed, it should be noted that episiotomies (unlike tears) are associated with dissatisfaction and a sense of lack of fulfilment. There is also some evidence to suggest that prophylactic episiotomies are being carried out on women who might otherwise have escaped without any perineal damage. Staff support and encouragement to help women to move around and get comfortable might also help women to avoid both tears and episiotomies. Episiotomies and suturing are often viewed as routine procedures. However, it is clear that both are important events from the women's perspective and suturing is experienced by some women as the very worst thing about the birth.

Total number of interventions

Overall, women experienced a mean of 2.5 interventions (S.D. 1.7); median and mode were both equal to two. 'Interventions' for this count were defined as: enema, shave, electronic fetal monitoring (of any duration), glucose drip, episiotomy, ARM, induction, acceleration, instrumental delivery and non-elective caesarean section (women having elective sections were excluded from this calculation). Epidurals and other forms of pain relief were not included and neither were interventions associated with the third stage of labour (see Volume 2, Chapter 6). The distribution of the number of interventions experienced is given in Table 6.18.

No. of interventions	No. of women	%
Zero	29	(4)
1	161	(24)
2	178	(27)
3	109	(16)
4	99	(15)
5	47	(7)
6	31	(5)
7	12	(2)
8	5	(<1)
		(100)

n = 671

See text for definition of interventions.

Table 6.18: Total number of interventions experienced

Only 29 women (4%) had no interventions at all, while 95 (14%) had five or more. The total number of interventions experienced was not related to education or social class but was strongly related to parity. Primips had a mean of 3.1 interventions compared with 2.2 for multips. Only seven primips (3%) had no interventions compared to 22 multips (6%) while 64 per cent of primips had three or more compared to 32 per cent of multips. These figures are, of course, consistent with the parity differences that we have already seen for each of the interventions individually.

Experience of procedures by antenatal wants and expectations

Did women get what they wanted?

Overall, only a very small number of women with strong feelings about procedures failed to get what they wanted. However, this is partly because only a minority of women expressed strong preferences. Table 6.19 shows a very interesting relationship between antenatal wishes and experience. For three of the procedures, shave, glucose drip and any form of fetal monitoring, there is no relationship between what women wanted and what they got. In other words, women who wanted them were no more likely to get them than women who did not. This may be, in part, a statistical artefact:

	Enema	Shave	Glucose drip	Continuous monitoring	Any form of electronic monitoring	Episiotomy
Antenatal wishes						
Definitely don't want	11/115 (10%)	22/236 (9%)	15/79 (19%)	9/71 (13%)	5/5 (100%)	27/108 (25%)
Prefer not	46/271 (17%)	28/248 (11%)	68/291 (23%)	52/250 (21%)	25/34 (74%)	140/358 (39%)
Don't mind	59/170 (35%)	13/125 (10%)	34/167 (20%)	66/198 (33%)	208/252 (83%)	32/93 (34%)
Quite like	9/29 (31%)	0/3 (0%)	0/4 (0%)	21/81 (26%)	147/183 (80%)	1/3 (33%)
Definitely want	7/22 (32%)	1/7 (14%)	0/2 (0%)	22/51 (43%)	155/179 (87%)	1/6 (17%)
Don't know enough to make a choice	13/32 (41%)	1/6 (17%)	23/81 (28%)	6/18 (33%)	12/12 (100%)	18/61 (30%)
Overall percentage experiencing procedure	23%	10%	22%	26%	82%	34%
	$p < 0.0001$	NS	NS	$p < 0.001$	NS	$p < 0.0001$

Percentages are women with particular antenatal wishes re each procedure

Table 6.19: Experience of 'minor' interventions by antenatal wishes

hardly any women actually wanted either a shave or a glucose drip and only a minority got either. Nearly all women had electronic fetal monitoring and very few were against it. There is not therefore a great deal of scope for significant differences. However, in the case of *continuous* monitoring which nearly half the sample had not wanted, there was a significant relationship between antenatal preferences and what women got. Similarly, in the case of the other two procedures, enema and episiotomy, the relationship between antenatal wishes and outcome is highly significant. Broadly speaking, women who did not want these procedures were less likely to experience them than women who did.

There are, however, some additional interesting points. Firstly, we have the most noteworthy finding that women who 'don't know enough to make a choice' consistently have the highest incidence of each procedure, higher, importantly, than those women who actively wanted or preferred to have the procedure. Women who 'don't mind' also have a high incidence of each of these procedures.

There is, furthermore, the curious finding that for three of the procedures (shave, glucose drip and episiotomy) the small number of women who *wanted* them were considerably *less* likely to get them than the sample as a whole. In the same way we see that all five women who wanted no form of electronic fetal monitoring were, in fact, monitored. Again, these findings may well be artefacts arising from the tiny numbers involved and it is impossible to draw any conclusions. However, we would suggest that all these curiosities could be accounted for by the fact that the extreme views of these women were seen as irrational by staff and provoked an anti-reaction which led to their wishes (whether for or against a procedure) being denied. It would be possible to examine this hypothesis by more detailed analysis of our existing data.

It is interesting to compare these results with those of Jacoby (1987). Her data were also collected by postal questionnaire from a very large sample of women (1500). Like us, she asked women about their antenatal preferences and experiences of a range of obstetric procedures. However, her questions about antenatal preference were asked four months after the birth. This may account for the fact that a higher proportion of her women who experienced procedures said that that had been their preference. However, she also reports higher percentages than we found of women who had minor procedures that they said they would have preferred to avoid. This is partly explained by the fact that she found a much higher overall incidence of enemas, shaves and episiotomy (39%, 45% and 43% respectively compared to our figures of 23%, 10% and 34%). This discrepancy could be because of a bias in the units that we chose, but it is also likely to be a reflection of the decline in the incidence of these procedures since 1984 when Jacoby's data were collected.

Feelings about procedures

For each of the procedures considered all women were asked questions to assess their satisfaction with what had happened. The questions were in fact phrased in slightly different ways in different contexts; none actually used the word 'satisfaction' but rather asked, for example 'Do you think you *should* have had an episiotomy?'. We were thus able to detect both women who had had procedures which they thought they should not have had and women who thought that they should have had procedures which they had not in fact experienced. (A factor analysis based on all such questions is discussed in Chapter 8.)

The response options offered were 'Yes', 'No' and 'Not sure'. Our assumption is that women who say 'Not sure' probably mean that they have reservations about what happened but lack the confidence for an outright challenge to medical (or midwifery) opinion, even six weeks after the event. This is supported by the fact that relatively more women said 'Not sure' with regard to procedures such as glucose drips about which, as we saw antenatally, there was a lot of ignorance while they were more openly critical where they were more confident in their antenatal views, for example, with regard to shaving.

Minor interventions

Table 6.20 shows the numbers of women who were dissatisfied with the decision reached for each of the minor interventions considered. For the purposes of this table 'Not sure' answers have been amalgamated with more directly critical answers.

	Did have		Did not have	
	n	%	n	%
Enema	40/145	(28)	45/492	(9)
Shave	19/64	(30)	9/559	(2)
Glucose drip	35/139	(25)	25/483	(5)
Episiotomy	49/220	(22)	50/411	(12)
Continuous monitoring	30/171	(18)	see below	
Other electronic fetal monitoring	38/353	(11)	2/112	(2)

Percentages are of women who did/did not experience that procedure. Numbers do not correspond exactly with earlier tables since some women failed to answer this question.

Table 6.20: Dissatisfaction with the decision to have/not have six 'minor' interventions

It is immediately clear from the table that women who experienced procedures were more likely to query the decision than women who did not. This is, of course, exactly what one would expect, particularly since the majority of women antenatally specified a preference to avoid most of these procedures. We can, in fact, break the table down further and look at women's views in relation to their antenatal preferences. This is done in Table 6.21, omitting those women who did not express any preference in either direction. This confirms that dissatisfaction is highest among women who experienced a procedure that they had not wanted and lowest amongst those whose wishes to avoid a procedure had been met. Women who had wanted procedures that they had not received were, on the whole, less likely to query the decision than those who had not wanted them but got them anyway.

	Did have				Did not have			
Antenatal attitude:	Pro		Anti		Pro		Anti	
	n	%	n	%	n	%	n	%
Enema	2/15	(13)	22/57	(39)	8/33	(24)	24/325	(7)
Shave	1/1	(100)	17/49	(35)	1/8	(12)	2/429	(1)
Glucose drip	0/0	(0)	24/83	(29)	1/6	(17)	10/282	(3)
Episiotomy	0/2	(0)	35/166	(21)	1/7	(14)	31/297	(10)
Continuous monitoring	3/43	(10)	15/57	(26)	22/84	(26)	64/258	(25)
					Had continuous monitoring			
Non-continuous monitoring (excluding women who were pro continuous monitoring)	14/148	(9)	5/22	(23)	9/54	(17)	2/4	(50)
					Had no monitoring			
					0/36	(0)	0/9	(0)

Women who had no preferences antenatally have been omitted

Table 6.21: Dissatisfaction with the decision to have/not have 6 'minor' interventions by antenatal preference

Note that when we exclude women who had actually wanted *continuous* monitoring, dissatisfaction with not having any monitoring drops to zero. (This was true for women who had been neutral about intermittent monitoring antenatally as well.) This seems slightly surprising given the positive way in which monitoring seemed to be viewed by our sample.

In general, we can see that the most satisfied group of women were those who did not want procedures and did not get them. This was also true in Jacoby's study (ibid). This was particularly clear for those interventions which are likely to be a matter of unit (or consultant) policy rather than a direct response to need. It was evident, for example, that the trend away from routine shaving and enemas pleased many women:

> 'I was very pleased to discover that in recent times it is not compulsory to have the above. Also I was given much more choice in how I wanted things to be.'

> 'With my first baby there was no choice at Exington consultant unit about an enema. I thought it was almost as bad as having the baby and it was one of the reasons I had my baby at Little Exington as I found out it was not a matter of routine there.'

'I am very glad I didn't have any [enema/shave/glucose drip/episiotomy]; I think they make you feel degraded when they do any of these.'

Electronic fetal monitoring, as we have seen earlier, is viewed much more positively by women than other interventions. This is reflected by the fact that a smaller percentage of women expressed dissatisfaction about monitoring decisions than about the other procedures listed. Women who were monitored continuously were more likely to query the decision than those monitored intermittently. Furthermore, of the 38 women who were unhappy with the intermittent monitoring that they received, 12 actually wanted more monitoring, not less.

The final 'minor' intervention that we considered was ARM. The phrasing of this particular question allowed for the additional response option of 'Didn't mind', which gives us a slightly different pattern of responses. Of the 361 women whose waters were broken artificially, 16 per cent said that they had not minded whether they were broken or not and 11 per cent queried the decision. Among those 142 women who were 'at risk' for ARM but did not have their waters broken, 11 (8%) 'didn't mind' and eight (5%) queried the decision.

Women's objections to what had happened could be divided into objections to the actual procedures (and their side-effects) and objections to the way in which the decision was made. Most comments about enemas fell into the first category:

'Having an enema was more upsetting for me, than having the baby. Because you are uncomfortable, in pain and sweat (I hate them).'

'Enema done at last minute was not very effective in Labour Ward!! and caused a great deal of embarrassment.'

Very little was said about any discussion or decision making with regard to either enemas or shaving.

However, comments about ARM, monitoring and episiotomy were more likely to describe situations in which women's wishes had been disregarded or procedures carried out without prior discussion or warning:

'I was never asked (re ARM) – they just came in and did it.'

'I suppose I needed an episiotomy although feel that a small tear might have been preferable. The trouble is that I don't remember being consulted – it was, I think, presented as a "fait accompli" and I suppose I must have gone along with it. I wish I had really asked why and whether it was really necessary.'

'My episiotomy was not very agreeable they just said stop pushing or they would cut me. I said I was not pushing, the baby was making its own way out, and I said if they wanted to cut me they would have to freeze me first. They just said there's no time and cut me. Luckily I didn't feel a thing.'

Similar comments were also made by women who had *wanted* interventions:

> 'Midwife refused repeated requests on my part for an episiotomy rather than be left to tear. Result was second degree lacerations.'

> 'I requested that my waters be broken as I was having a strong desire to push and I had to persuade the midwife to do it.'

Major interventions

Table 6.22 shows the numbers of women querying the decision made for each of the four major interventions. The comparability of these figures is somewhat confounded by the fact that 'Didn't mind' was a response option for induction, acceleration and instrumental delivery but not for caesarean section. Note, however, that none of the women who had instrumental deliveries ticked the 'Didn't mind' option. It seems unlikely that any of those having caesarean sections would have done so either.

	Did have				Did not have			
	Queried decision		Didn't mind		Queried decision		Didn't mind	
	n	%	n	%	n	%	n	%
Induction	22/108	(20)	15/108	(14)	15/551	(3)	9/551	(2)
Acceleration	18/111	(16)	15/111	(14)	28/543	(5)	14/543	(3)
Instrumental delivery	8/44	(19)	0/44	(0)	5/600	(<1)	4/600	(<1)
Caesarean section	9/60	(15)	N/A		25/591	(4)	N/A	

Table 6.22: Dissatisfaction with the decision to have/not have each of four major interventions

Once again we see, as expected, much greater dissatisfaction with decisions among women who experienced procedures than among those who did not. However, the proportions querying decisions were generally much lower than they were for minor interventions discussed above. This is precisely what one would expect. Firstly, even though the experience of these more major procedures may actually be a lot more unpleasant than the minor ones, women are much more likely to have been given a plausible obstetric reason for carrying them out. They may indeed have been experiencing protracted and distressing labours prior to the intervention or they may see the intervention as having saved their baby from danger. They are, therefore, much more likely to have been actively welcoming of these interventions than, for example, women who had shaves and enemas. Secondly, cognitive dissonance theory (Festinger, 1957) would predict that the more major the intervention, the more women would feel the need to believe that it had been necessary. Thus, we find that only 15 per cent of women who had caesarean sections queried the decision compared to 30 per cent of the women who were shaved. This was also reflected in the qualitative data; these more major interventions tended to be treated with pragmatic acceptance as medical necessities, even when it was clear that no explanation had been given:

> 'The fetal heart monitor of the baby is getting distress so the doctor said we have to use forceps. At that time the doctor had no chance to ask me, they just got on with it. I suppose there was no time to be lost, the baby must be delivered at once.'

> 'I was very impressed with the care I received. The decision to have a forceps delivery is very vague, now and at the time, but there must have been anxiety about the baby.'

There were more objections to inductions, primarily about the effects of the procedure:

> 'I wish I hadn't been started so fast then I think I would have coped better. I was really rather upset about the whole affair. It all happened far too quickly and then before it could all sink in about being in labour I was in too much pain to think about it.'

> 'I started small contractions three weeks early. So I was given a drip to get me properly started. I then had contractions every two mins for 10 and a half hours. Then when I was starting to push I didn't have the energy so the baby had to be a forceps delivery so I had to have an episiotomy. Thinking back I wish they had let me start on my own.'

It was noticeable that elective caesarean sections were seen as much more satisfactory than emergency ones. This is consistent with previous research (see Garel et al., 1988; Oakley and Richards, 1988), and probably relates also to the fact that most elective sections were carried out under epidural rather than general anaesthesia. For example, one woman, who had had an elective section under epidural, in answer to 'What would you say was the worst thing about the birth', answered, 'Nothing, I loved every minute of it'.

Even those who felt that the situation had been coped with as well as possible could see the desirability of an elective:

> 'The emergency section was dealt with in an impressive and professional way and I received very attentive postnatal care. I do feel though that better antenatal care could have pin-pointed problems and an elected caesarean section would have avoided an otherwise traumatic experience for myself and my husband.'

We will not be going into detail here about women's experience of caesarean section although further analysis of this data would be possible. Due to the fact that giving birth by caesarean section is so qualitatively different from a vaginal delivery these women have been excluded from a number of subsequent analyses:

'When I got home I did feel as though I hadn't given birth as I had no sensation from my birth canal that the child has passed through as with my other two children. It was rather an odd experience as though I had a baby without giving birth to it.'

Third stage management

The original report included a condensed version of Volume 2, Chapter 6 in this chapter. We have removed the duplicated material apart from the conclusion.

Conclusion

Our hypothesis that a significant proportion of women do not realize that the third stage of labour is routinely managed by the staff was confirmed. A large minority of women knew very little or nothing about the third stage of labour, including many women who had given birth previously. Furthermore, the majority of the women had had no opportunity to discuss the third stage with health professionals during the antenatal period or in any previous pregnancy. These results would seem to confirm that staff accord a low priority to the concept of the third stage as a major part of the childbirth process which women need to be well-informed about. Women tend to be correspondingly confused or indifferent about the third stage, desiring little part in decision making and having few, if any, opinions about how it should be managed.

CHAPTER SEVEN

Social And Behavioural Aspects of Labour: Postnatal Data

In this chapter we will look at women's experiences of the social/behavioural aspects of labour discussed in Chapter 4 and also at other aspects of interaction with staff. We will then return to the two groups of women identified in Chapter 4 who had contrasting attitudes towards control of decision making and see to what extent their experiences differed. Finally, we will look at women's actual experiences of feeling in control (or not) and how this related to the other events of their labours.

Birth companion

The majority of the sample (90%) had a birth companion with them throughout labour (antenatally 94% had wanted this).

	n	%
Yes, all of time	603	(90)
Yes, some of time	33	(5)
No, not at all	37	(5)
n = 673		

Table 7.1: Birth companion present during labour

Many women commented positively about the support given by their partner:

> 'My husband was a great help during the whole thing. I'm sure I couldn't of handled the pain as well as I did without him.'

Four per cent of the sample indicated that the involvement of their partner was, in fact, the best thing about the birth:

> 'Feeling the support of my husband made me feel that I could have gone through anything.'

'Having the support of my husband – he found it an incredible experience – it has brought us very close.'

A few women who did not have their partner with them said this was the *worst* thing:

'The worst thing was that my husband was not allowed to be with me.'

Women were appreciative when staff involved their partners:

'My husband during the delivery was encouraged to be there and not just a spare part.'

However, a few women complained about being separated both from their partner and their baby:

'I was pleased with my choice of care and amazed at the lack of intervention from staff – but wish they wouldn't split mother/father up on the night of the birth. Nothing sexual is going to happen two hours after a baby is born – I felt we were being punished by being separated – and I missed the baby who was having her stomach washed without my knowledge, in the nursery later. Can't we all be together?'

Primips were more likely than multips to have a birth companion with them throughout labour.

	Primips		Multips	
	n	%	n	%
Yes, all of the time	248	(93)	354	(88)
Yes, some of the time	14	(5)	19	(5)
No, not at all	6	(2)	31	(8)

Percentages are of women of a given parity.

Table 7.2: Birth companion present during labour by parity

Continuity of care

Twenty four per cent of the sample had met at least one of the midwives who looked after them during labour. (Antenatally, 62% had indicated that they would prefer to be looked after by a midwife they had already met, however only 18 per cent had expected this would be the case.) Where women were delivered by someone they had already met they often commented favourably on this aspect of their care:

'Because I was delivered by my community midwife who had seen me throughout my pregnancy, from nine weeks, I was treated as a person and we were treated as a couple. It was like being delivered by a friend.'

'A midwife known personally to me made all the difference on the day.'

Community midwives often made a special effort to be available even if they were officially off duty:

> 'My community midwife very kindly said that I could call her even if it was her day off or whatever time it was. We thought this was fantastic and we then didn't worry about when my labour started that I maybe wouldn't have the midwife I wanted.'

This kind of continuity was also appreciated from doctors:

> 'I asked to see the same registrar on each visit, and struck up an excellent rapport with him. When I was admitted he happened to be on duty, and actually stayed on duty longer in the morning to deliver my baby by caesarean section, this really meant a lot to my husband and I, actually knowing the person who delivered our baby.'

Even though most women had not previously met the staff who attended them during labour, 66 per cent were able to have some degree of continuity of care during labour. (Antenatally 87% had indicated a desire for continuity but only 49% had expected it.)

	n	%
Yes	445	(66)
No	224	(33)
Not sure	6	(< 1)
n = 675		

Table 7.3: At least one midwife present from start to finish

If the staff were able to quickly establish friendly and supportive relations and stay on to deliver the baby this was much appreciated:

> 'Although I had not met them before the staff managed to create a lovely family atmosphere, both my husband and I felt we had known them for years.'

Some midwives tried to stay with 'their women' as much as possible:

> 'We had the same midwife with us all the time which was wonderful. She even apologized when she had to leave to go to the toilet.'

Midwives often stayed on beyond their shift, (in at least one case five hours beyond her shift) to see the woman through to delivery:

> 'I was delivered by a student midwife and midwife who should have gone off duty some time before my baby was born, but they said it wasn't fair to pass me to strange staff and they both wanted to see if I had a daughter before they went home. Both returned to me after getting changed into coats, held my hand and wished me well.'

Women said that such continuity helped them to feel relaxed, cared for and secure:

> 'I had one midwife all the time, this was very important to me. I don't know what I would have done without her, she alone was a pain relief.'

Indeed, where continuity of care did occur, women were sometimes positively eulogistic:

> 'My community midwife who looked after me throughout my pregnancy came out to my home on a Sunday night, even though she was off duty and took us to the hospital. She delivered our little girl and stayed with us from 10 pm until about 6 am the following morning and she made my labour and the actual birth really lovely. Throughout my labour there were just the three of us – nobody else came into the room, the lights were low and when Jennifer was born the sun was coming up and the birds were singing. It couldn't have been better for us and we were really grateful to her.'

Women who did not know the staff who attended them during labour or who did not get continuity of care sometimes expressed disappointment – especially if they had been told that they could expect continuity:

> 'I was annoyed about the amount of midwives' who kept coming in saying they were going to see me for the duration. In fact [during a six hour labour] there were five midwives in all.'

> 'Midwife at antenatal told me she would deliver me. But it turned out not to be anyone I had seen before.'

Women were also upset when midwives did rush off at the end of their shifts:

> '[The worst thing about the birth was] The midwife being in a hurry, her shift just finishing and no response to our happiness. I don't think she even looked at our baby.'

However, a few women were positively glad of a change of shift if they disliked the first midwife:

> 'The first midwife was a rude, unhelpful, inconsiderate old bag. But she wasn't the midwife that delivered my baby thank christ. I was saved by the bell at nine o'clock.'

Relationship between continuity of care and parity

Multips were more likely to have already met the midwife who looked after them in labour (27% of multips compared to 19% of primips, $p < 0.05$). This is probably due to the greater continuity of care provided by the GP and satellite units. Multips were also more likely to experience continuity of care during the course of labour itself, 73 per cent compared to 55 per cent of primips ($p < 0.0001$). This may be partly due to unit differences but is also due to the fact that they had shorter labours (55% of multips had labours that were shorter than five hours as opposed to just 19% of primips).

Relationship between continuity of care and unit

Women at Little Exington were more than twice as likely to have met the midwife who attended them during labour than women at any other unit. Wychester provided the least continuity of care out of all the units – both in terms of women having already met any of the midwives and in terms of having one midwife throughout labour. These differences were independent of parity effects.

	n	%
Willowford	42	(26)
Exington Consultant	17	(19)
Exington GP	18	(35)
Little Exington	33	(75)
Wychester	20	(12)
Zedbury	24	(17)

Percentages are of women in a given unit.

$p < 0.0001$

Table 7.4: Already met any of the midwives by unit

	n	%
Willowford	122	(75)
Exington Consultant	57	(63)
Exington GP	38	(75)
Little Exington	32	(73)
Wychester	94	(57)
Zedbury	88	(61)

Percentages are of women in a given unit.

$p < 0.05$

Table 7.5: At least one midwife present from start to finish by unit

There was no relationship between continuity of care and education or social class.

Comings and goings

Over three quarters of the sample said that there were hardly any people coming in and out of their room during labour. (Antenatally, 88% preferred not to have too many comings and goings but only 62% thought their hopes would be fulfilled.)

	n	%
Yes, a lot	23	(3)
Yes, quite a few	114	(17)
No, hardly any	539	(78)
n = 676		

Table 7.6: Lots of people coming in and out during labour

Women were grateful for the privacy afforded when hardly any staff came in and out of the room:

> 'I asked that not too many people came in and out, this she did for me and even asked if I minded another sister coming to take the baby! As the baby was being born my husband had to press a bell and sure enough only one person came in to sort baby out. All in all everything was just perfect.'

Some wrote with appreciation of being left on their own with their partners to share the experience in privacy:

> 'During the first stage we (my husband and I) were left mostly to ourselves to talk and support each other which was wonderful as we were excited and wanted to be alone.'

Some women, however, were left so much on their own that they felt neglected. There appeared in some cases to be a lack of support and, perhaps, a shortage of staff:

> 'I did feel we were left for long periods of time – literally hours – without seeing anyone. In fact my husband had to go and find the nurse to tell her I'd used up one bag on the drip. And after the birth we were left. It was one and a half hours before the baby was weighed and we were given a cup of tea and before they finally got round to taking the drip out by which time my hand was really swollen and blue.'

Twenty per cent of the sample felt that there were 'a lot' or 'quite a few' people coming in and out of their room. The problems of having too many people rushing in and out were particularly associated with interventions and emergencies such as forceps deliveries, induction and acceleration (see Appendix). One woman described the feeling of being physically assaulted as lots of staff descended on her:

'The staff seemed to be in a rush to get me to theatre as the consultant had arrived. Consequently I felt I was descended on at all ends i.e. one nurse was putting a drip in my arm (and making a mess of it – finally put it in my other arm – very painful) – one nurse was shaving and then catheterizing me while the anaesthetist was putting in the epidural. I felt it was too much to adjust to all at once – I felt physically assaulted and quite frightened. Once the baby was born I went into shock and couldn't catch my breath. It was very upsetting.'

When interruptions were seen as unnecessary they were particularly resented:

'At the crucial moment the room filled with with 'sightseers' (i.e. trainees whatever they were) as it was a breech birth. There were at least ten people there and that bothered me.'

'I had hoped, as it was my second delivery, to have an intimate and private delivery. But there were so many people in with us, it made it impossible and I felt that a very special moment had been invaded by strangers. I do feel that that kind of attention was uncalled for. It happened because the machines I was attached to weren't working properly!'

Relationship between comings and goings, parity and unit

Primips were more likely than multips to feel that there were lots of people coming in and out during their labour. This is probably due to the lower intervention rates for multips as well as to differences between low risk and high risk units.

	Many people coming in and out of room					
	Yes, a lot		Yes, quite a few		No, hardly any	
	n	%	n	%	n	%
Primip	11	(4)	66	(25)	192	(71)
Multip	12	(3)	48	(12)	346	(85)

Percentages are of women of a given parity.

$p < 0.0001$

Table 7.7: Privacy by parity

There were no significant differences associated with women's education or social class. There were, however, significant differences between units. Women at Exington GP unit and Little Exington described the most privacy while women at Exington consultant unit and Zedbury described the most comings and goings during their labours.

	Many people coming in and out of room					
	Yes, a lot		Yes, quite a few		No, hardly any	
	n	%	n	%	n	%
Willowford	5	(3)	14	(9)	143	(88)
Exington Consultant	8	(9)	12	(13)	71	(78)
Exington GP	1	(2)	2	(4)	48	(94)
Little Exington	0	(0)	1	(2)	43	(98)
Wychester	3	(2)	36	(22)	126	(76)
Zedbury	5	(4)	46	(32)	93	(65)

Percentages are of women in a given unit.

$p < 0.0001$

Table 7.8: Privacy by unit

Relationship between continuity of care, privacy and outcomes

As we will see, these social aspects of birth are also important to women's sense of control during labour, their fulfilment and their overall satisfaction with the birth experience. The importance of continuity and privacy should not be underestimated.

Information

Most women (71%) felt they had been given the right amount of information and only four women (less than 1%) felt they had been given too much. However, over a quarter of the sample felt that they had been given too little information, or too little about some areas and too much about others. Twenty per cent indicated that there were specific things they wished they had known more about (see Appendix). Most comments revolved around postnatal factors such as feeding the baby (see Volume 2) or issues around pain and 'things that can go wrong'. Seventeen per cent of women felt they had been given misleading information. This information usually pertained to the same areas that they felt they had lacked information about, with the addition of antenatal diagnosis as a major problem area (see Appendix).

Decision making

Overall, 25 per cent of the sample felt that they had been in control of non-emergency decisions and only 11 per cent felt that they had had no involvement. For emergency decision making, as one would expect, women had much less involvement.

	Non-emergency decisions		Emergency* decisions	
	n	%	n	%
The staff just got on with it	74	(10)	62	(26)
The staff made the decisions but kept me informed	235	(36)	125	(53)
The staff discussed things with me before reaching a decision	183	(28)	37	(16)
The staff gave me their assessment but I was in control of the decision	165	(25)	14	(6)
Not applicable	0	(0)	421	(64) of whole sample

* For emergency decisions, the percentages given in the first four rows are of women to whom the question applied, i.e. 36 per cent of the sample.

Table 7.9: How decisions were made

Non-emergency decision making was significantly related to educational level and also to unit. It was not related to parity. Emergency decision making was not related to educational level, unit or parity.

Educational level	n	%
16 and under	144/318	(45)
17–18	98/185	(53)
19 and over	105/150	(70)

Percentages are of women of a given educational level.

$n = 653$

$p < 0.0001$.

Table 7.10: Number of women who felt that non-emergency decisions were at least discussed with them by educational level

The unit differences show women at all three Exington units to have felt less involved in decision making (35% compared to 59% for the rest of the sample). This is probably related to the lower educational level of the Exington women.

Control (internal)

The question about feeling in control of what staff were doing to you is considered in detail at the end of this chapter. Here we will look at women's answers to the three questions that we saw as being related to 'internal' control.

	n	%
Yes, most of the time	27	(4)
Yes, for some of the time	298	(44)
No, not at all	350	(52)

Table 7.11: Did you ever feel that lost control of the way you behaved during labour?

	n	%
Yes, for all or most of the time	369	(55)
Yes, for some of the time	257	(38)
No, not at all	5	(7)

Table 7.12: Did you feel in control during contractions?

It is clear from these figures that only a small minority of women felt completely out of control in these 'internal' senses and just over half of the women felt in control 'all or most of the time'. Answers to both questions showed a strong relationship with parity: multips felt more in control than primips ($p < 0.01$ for the first question, and $p < 0.001$ for the second). Neither was related to women's educational level. Differences between units were not significant when parity was controlled.

The question on making a noise during labour showed the opposite effect: answers were related to educational level but not to parity or unit.

Educational level	Yes, a lot		Yes, a bit		No, not much		Not sure	
	n	%	n	%	n	%	n	%
16 and under	33	(10)	98	(30)	190	(59)	4	(1)
17–18	17	(9)	68	(35)	106	(55)	3	(2)
19 and over	21	(14)	65	(43)	63	(42)	2	(1)
Total	71	(11)	231	(35)	359	(54)	9	(1)

Percentages are of women of a given educational level.

n = 670

$p < 0.05$.

Table 7.13: Did you make much noise during labour?

As these figures show, the most educated women were significantly more likely to say that they had made a noise during labour. This is in keeping with the antenatal findings that less educated women were more concerned about making a lot of noise. This offers further support for our belief that 'making a lot of noise' is not particularly relevant to 'internal' control. As we shall see in the following chapter, making a noise is also less related to the psychological outcome measures than the other two 'internal' control questions.

These findings on control are summarized in Table 7.14 alongside the figures given in Chapter 4 showing wants and expectations.

	% of women wanting		% of women expecting		% of women getting	
'External'						
Active part in non-emergency decisions	72	(E)	55	(E,P)	53	(E)
Active part in emergency decisions	27		17	(E)	22	(of applicable sample)
Control of what staff do to you	82	(E)	61	(E,P)	80	(P)
'Internal'						
Control of your own behaviour	77		45	(E,P)	52	(P)
Control during contractions	92		65	(P)	55	(P)
Not making a lot of noise	43	(E,P)	54	(E,P)	54	(E)

KEY: E means that there are significant differences between women of different educational levels.
P means that there are significant differences between multips and primips.

Table 7.14: Summary of 'external' and 'internal' control questions: percentage of women who wanted/expected/felt they had control

Fulfilment

Women's answers to the question 'Was the birth a fulfilling experience?' are examined in detail in Chapter 8 since this was one of our four measures of psychological outcome.

Were women's expectations and preferences met?

Having considered the overall outcomes for the sample in terms of the social and behavioural aspects of labour, we will now look at how they matched up to what women had expected or wanted.

For nine of the twelve issues considered there was a significant association between what women expected and what actually happened to them, i.e. those who expected it were more likely to get it, and vice versa. The exceptions were areas where prescience would be unlikely: having one midwife with you throughout labour, having lots of people coming in and out of the room and degree of involvement in emergency decision making. With these last two there is a potential floor effect since very few women, whatever their expectations, experienced either a lot of people coming in and out (3%) or involvement in emergency decision making (8%). The latter figure of course, includes women for whom emergency decision making did not arise. If we look only at those for whom it is applicable (36% of the whole sample), 21 per cent felt that decisions were at least discussed with them but women who expected this were no more likely than others to get it.

For the other nine issues: birth companion, midwife delivery, being delivered by a known midwife, involvement in non-emergency decision making, control of what staff were doing to you, control of own behaviour, control during contractions, making a lot of noise and fulfilment there were significant relationships between expectations and events, all at the $p < 0.001$ level (except control during contractions: $p < 0.01$). Table 7.15 shows the incidence of the various events for the extreme groups only, i.e. those who were *sure* that the event would or would not occur.

In virtually all cases the relationship is linear, i.e. women who were 'sure' were more likely to experience events than those who said 'probably' and so on. However, the point should be made that women did not automatically get what they predicted. Table 7.16 shows just two of the events, being attended by a midwife you have already met and having a fulfilling experience, to illustrate this. Overall, only 24 per cent of women were attended by a midwife that they had already met. Thus, although as the table shows there is a very strong relationship between expectations and what happens, only just over half of the women who were sure that they would be attended by a known midwife actually were. Fulfilment shows the opposite effect. Overall, 78 per cent of women said that the birth was fulfilling and the majority of those who did not expect it to be nonetheless found that it was, albeit a lower proportion than those with positive expectations. Note that the proportion of women with no expectations who experienced these events lies between those who expected it and those who did not. This is true for all of the events for which there was a significant relationship with expectations.

	Were sure they would get this aspect		Were sure they would not get this aspect	
	n	%	n	%
1. Birth companion throughout labour	418/443	(94)	4/12	(33)
2. Midwife delivery	170/204	(83)	4/9	(44)
3. Known midwife	24/47	(51)	5/53	(9)
4. One midwife throughout	42/57	(74)	7/9	(78)
5. Lots of people	0/9	(0)	2/71	(3)
6. Control of non-emergency decisions	65/145	(45)	3/25	(12)
7. Control of emergency decisions	0/19	(0)	2/132	(2)
8. Control: staff	34/81	(42)	0/3	(0)
9. Control: behaviour	29/36	(81)	5/12	(42)
10. Control during contractions	28/44	(64)	3/9	(33)
11. Make a lot of noise	6/14	(43)	2/70	(3)
12. Fulfilling experience	243/280	(87)	2/3	(67)

Table 7.15: Number or women who were 'sure' of getting or not getting aspects of labour who actually got them

	Women with particular expectations who had:			
	Already met midwife		Fulfilling experience	
Antenatal expectations	n	%	n	%
Sure would	24/47	(51)	243/280	(87)
Probably would	45/116	(39)	219/289	(76)
No expectation	38/178	(21)	53/77	(69)
Probably not	47/273	(17)	20/37	(54)
Sure not	5/53	(9)	2/3	(67)

Table 7.16: Experience of two aspects of labour by antenatal expectations

Were women's expectations better predictors than their preferences?

We observed earlier that preferences and expectations were significantly related although this was partly because women with no preferences tended not to have expectations either. In general, expectations tended to be lower than preferences which we might interpret as 'realism'. In that case we would expect expectations to be better predictors of events than preferences. In fact this did not seem to be the case. Preferences and what happens were significantly related for seven of the twelve events. The exceptions were the three areas where expectations were not significantly related to what happened, plus control of what staff were doing and control during contractions.

Table 7.17 shows the proportion of women who got what they *wanted* compared to the proportion who got what they *expected* ('sure' and 'probably' have been combined and 'no expectations' omitted).

		Got what wanted		Got what expected	
		n	%	n	%
1.	Birth companion	587/643	(91)	586/648	(90)
2.	Midwife delivery	261/340	(77)	449/578	(78)
3.	Known midwife	100/420	(24)	343/489	(70)
4.	One midwife throughout	374/580	(64)	289/489	(59)
5.	Lots of people	471/597	(79)	373/540	(69)
6.	Who makes non-emergency decisions	240/647	(37)	251/636	(39)
7.	Who makes emergency decisions*	90/235	(38)	92/235	(39)
8.	Control of staff (all or most of time)	440/559	(79)	368/506	(73)
9.	Control of behaviour	276/514	(54)	203/478	(42)
10.	Control during contractions	337/612	(55)	273/523	(52)
11.	Noise	175/289	(61)	260/485	(54)
12.	Fulfilment	465/568	(82)	472/609	(78)

*Figures given are only for women for whom emergency decision making was applicable.

Table 7.17: Preferences, expectations, events and outcomes

These figures suggest that 'realism' is actually 'pessimism' since in many cases preferences are better predictors of events than expectations. However, the differences are very small. The only event for which there is a substantial difference between the proportion getting what they wanted and the proportion getting what they expected is being attended by a known midwife. This is because the majority of women neither got it nor expected it although the majority would have liked it. Here it would seem that realism and pessimism coincide (cf. Clark, 1986).

We will now conclude this chapter by looking in more detail at the question of 'external' control. First, we will return to the women defined in Chapter 4 as those who did and did not want control over decision making.

What happened to 'high' and 'low control' women?

Pain

There were some differences between the two groups relating to pain but most did not reach statistical significance. Fifty per cent of 'Low Control' women found the pain 'exactly as expected' compared to only 37 per cent of 'High Control'. Of the rest, 'High Control' women were somewhat more likely to have found labour more painful than expected (27% compared to 17% of 'Low Control'). Neither of these differences was statistically significant. There were also differences between the two groups in their use of methods for coping with pain but again none reached the 0.05 significance level. Given the preference of 'High Control' women to avoid drugs, their relative failure to do so may account for the fact that 'High Control' women were significantly more likely to say that they were dissatisfied with the way in which they had coped with pain. On the other hand, they were also somewhat more likely to say that they were *satisfied* with how they coped with pain, while 'Low Control' women, consistent with their antenatal attitudes, were neither satisfied nor dissatisfied.

	'High Control'		'Low Control'	
	n	%	n	%
Satisfied	54	(68)	60	(64)
Neither particularly satisfied nor dissatisfied	15	(19)	32	(34)
Dissatisfied	10	(13)	2	(2)
$p < 0.01$				

Table 7.18: 'High' and 'low control' women: satisfaction with how they coped with pain

The same pattern is apparent in the answers to questions regarding specific drugs: 'High Control' women were likely to have been happy with the decision reached while 'Low Control' women had no feelings one way or the other.

Interventions

There were virtually no differences in the experiences of the groups with regard to obstetric interventions. The only one for which a significant difference was found was acceleration of labour: 18 'High Control' women (22%) were accelerated compared to only ten (11%) of 'Low Control' ($p < 0.05$). However, another four 'Low Control' women reported that they did not know whether or not their labours had been accelerated. This characteristic lack of knowledge on the part of 'Low Control' women is dramatically apparent when we look at procedures involved in the third stage of labour.

Procedure	'High Control'		'Low Control'	
	n	%	n	%
Injection	9/75	(12)	19/93	(20)
Cord cut and clamped before it finished pulsating	46/75	(61)	76/91	(84)
Controlled cord traction	11/75	(15)	41/92	(45)

Table 7.19: 'High' and 'Low Control' women: Numbers who were 'not sure' whether they experienced three common procedures in the third stage of labour

How women felt about themselves during labour

Only one of the adjectives that women could circle to describe their feelings in labour, 'involved', differentiated between the two groups. Fifty three per cent of 'High Control' women circled this compared to only 36 per cent of 'Low Control'. In particular, there were no differences between the two groups in circling 'In control' (32% of 'High' compared to 36% of 'Low') or 'Out of control' (15% of 'High' compared to 18% of 'Low'). This in turn is confirmed in the questions we included to tap 'internal' control: control of behaviour, control during contractions and making a noise. There were no differences between the two groups on any of these.

Feelings about staff

'High Control' women were significantly more likely to feel that there had been at least 'quite a few' people coming in and out of the room (25% of 'High' compared to 15% of 'Low', $p < 0.05$). This was probably not a reflection of different levels of obstetric difficulties in the two groups. The only difference in perceptions of staff according to the fifteen adjectives that women were invited to circle was 'sensitive'; 53 per cent of 'High Control' women described staff as sensitive compared to only 35 per cent of 'Low Control' ($p < 0.05$).

The only other significant difference between 'High' and 'Low Control' women in their interactions with staff was in a desire for more information. Thirty three per cent of 'High Control' women said that there were things that they would have liked to have known more about compared to just 19 per cent of 'Low' ($p < 0.05$). This is despite the fact that 'High Control' women had reported themselves to be better informed antenatally and may well be related to the differences in education between the two groups.

Decision making and 'external' control

There were significant differences between the groups in the key areas of decision making and control of what staff did during labour.

	'High Control'		'Low Control'	
	n	%	n	%
Staff got on with it	3	(4)	12	(13)
Kept informed	21	(27)	45	(50)
Discussion	25	(32)	24	(27)
Woman's own decision	30	(38)	9	(10)
$p < 0.0001$				

Table 7.20: 'High' and 'Low Control' women: how non-emergency decisions were made.

	'High Control'		'Low Control'	
	n	%	n	%
Yes, always	24	(30)	26	(28)
Most of the time	43	(53)	47	(50)
Only some of the time	13	(16)	8	(9)
No, hardly ever	1	(1)	13	(14)
$p < 0.01$				

Table 7.21: 'High' and 'Low Control' women: felt in control of what staff were doing

It is interesting to note that differences in feeling in control over what staff were doing to you are much less marked than differences in how non-emergency decisions were made, emphasizing again that these two questions are tapping somewhat different things. Since the 'High Control' women are in fact defined primarily in terms of their desire for control over decision making, the data suggest that most had their wishes met in this respect. Seventy per cent of 'High Control' women had non-emergency decisions at least discussed with them compared to only 37 per cent of 'Low Control'. However, this is not the case for emergency decision making where differences are not significant.

Postnatal differences

There were hardly any postnatal differences between 'High' and 'Low Control' women. In particular, the two groups did not differ on any of our measures of psychological outcome: satisfaction with birth, fulfilment, emotional well-being and Description of

Baby. Thus, the hypothesis that 'High Control' women would inevitably be disappointed and have poor psychological outcomes would not seem to be supported. We will however discuss this in more detail below.

One of the big postnatal differences that does exist between 'High' and 'Low Control' women is in breastfeeding. Seventy one per cent of 'High Control' women were breastfeeding at six weeks, compared to only 44 per cent of 'Low Control'. Over one third of 'Low Control' never started compared to only 7 per cent of 'High Control'.

	'High Control'		'Low control'	
	n	%	n	%
Did you breastfeed at all?				
No, not at all	7	(7)	36	(35)
Yes, still am	60	(71)	45	(44)
Yes, but stopped	18	(21)	22	(21)
$p < 0.0001$				

Table 7.22: 'High' and 'Low Control' women: breastfeeding

Although there was no overall relationship with Description of Baby, 'High Control' women were more likely to see their babies as 'sociable' ($p < 0.01$) and to describe them as 'responsive' ($p < 0.05$) and 'fascinating' ($p < 0.05$). All of these differences are consistent with those reported elsewhere for women with differing levels of education, even though, as we saw above, 'High Control' women cover the full range of educational levels, albeit with a bias towards the most educated.

'High' and 'low' control women: conclusions

This section has identified women who expressed a strong desire antenatally to be in control of decision making and those who did not. This dimension was shown to be related to level of education and many of the differences found between 'High' and 'Low Control' women were similar to those found between highly and less highly educated women. However, although the desire for control and level of education were related they were by no means synonymous; most highly educated women (79%) did not express a strong desire for control. Looked at the other way, the majority of women who did express such a desire (62%) were not highly educated. The fact that both the desire for control and a high level of education predispose towards the same attitudes is of interest but should not be written off as being 'just' an effect of education. What we have built up is a picture of women who are relatively active rather than passive, who see the birth as their responsibility as well as the staff's, who have a fairly clear idea of the sort of delivery they want and who see involvement in decision making as a necessary prerequisite for achieving this:

> 'While not being fanatical about everything being drug and technology free – I accept that it would be crazy to reject life-saving techniques and equipment purely to gratify my own expectations of experience – I would very much like to have the experience of a normal labour in a relaxed environment where I was free to move around and "do my own thing".'

The 'Low Control' women, on the other hand, are more passive, do not have particular views about what should happen during labour, and are happy to leave matters to the professionals:

> 'I have great faith in doctors and midwives knowing what to do. I think no matter how much you know and understand about birth and labour, you should not try to take over and control things yourself in case you do more harm than good.'

We have shown that there are remarkably few differences in what actually happens to these two groups of women or how they feel about it. Does that mean that the issue of control and wants and expectations in general are irrelevant? We would suggest not. On the contrary, the data already presented on wants and expectations and the following section on the experience of feeling in control (as opposed to wanting to be) give quite the opposite impression. Rather, it seems likely that the feeling of being in control is one of a number of factors which contribute to psychological outcome. Not having preferences met, as will have been the case for some of the 'High Control' women, will be a negative factor (see Chapter 8) but the feeling of control will be positive and will partly cancel this effect. 'Low Control' women, having fewer preferences, have less scope for disappointment but are also less likely to feel in control. We therefore find similar psychological outcomes for the two groups, on average.

Women who felt 'in control of what staff were doing'

Our discussion so far has focused on women who *wanted* 'external' control, primarily of decision making. We shall now look instead at an overlapping, but not identical group, women who actually felt that they *were* in control of what staff did to them. All women except those who had had an elective caesarean section were asked 'In general, did you feel in control of what the staff were doing to you during labour?'. The response options and the number of women giving each are given in Table 7.23.

	n	%
Yes, always	182	(27)
Yes, most of the time	355	(53)
Only some of the time	90	(13)
No, hardly at all	45	(7)

Table 7.23: 'In general, did you feel in control of what the staff were doing to you during labour?'

All the postnatal data were then re-analysed comparing women on the basis of their answers to this question. The results are very striking: there were highly significant differences with respect to virtually every question.

Feeling in control of staff and major independent variables

Feeling in control of what staff were doing showed no relationship with either partner's occupation or with education. There were small significant class differences when we looked at women's own occupations but these showed no consistent pattern. This is in interesting contrast to the data presented earlier for women who *wanted* control: the *desire* for control is evidently class/education related but achieving it is not. Conversely, parity was highly significantly related to the feeling of *being* in control, but was not related to the *desire* for control. Both of these findings are consistent with the results given earlier in this chapter for other social/behavioural aspects of the birth.

In control?	Primips		Multips	
	n	%	n	%
Always	49	(18)	134	(33)
Most of the time	148	(55)	207	(51)
Some of the time	53	(20)	37	(9)
Hardly at all	17	(6)	28	(7)
$p < 0.0001$				

Table 7.24: Feeling in control of what staff were doing to you by parity

There were also small but consistent differences between units. Women at the GP unit were most likely to feel in control 'always' or 'most of the time' (92%) while the other Exington women, those in the consultant unit and at Little Exington were least likely to (72% and 70%).

Obstetric procedures

Women who felt in control 'all' or 'most' of the time were much less likely to have experienced obstetric procedures. Alternatively, one could say that women who experienced various procedures were much less likely to say that they felt in control. These figures are given in Table 7.25. Women who were 'not sure' whether they had experienced a procedure were least likely to have felt in control. However, numbers were very small and they have been omitted from the table for clarity.

Procedure	Of women who did have		Of women who did not have	
	n	%	n	%
Enema	107/146	(73)	407/493	(83)
Shave	41/64	(64)	463/561	(83)
Glucose drip	94/139	(68)	412/485	(85)
Episiotomy	151/221	(68)	360/410	(88)
ARM	295/360	(82)	124/153	(81)*
Monitoring:				
continuous	127/175	(73)	387/470	(82)**
non-continuous	294/357	(82)	93/113	(82)
Induction	76/107	(71)	456/555	(81)
Acceleration	78/112	(70)	453/548	(83)
Instrumental delivery	41/65	(63)	491/691	(82)
Non-elective caesarean	17/28	(61)	520/643	(81)

Notes:

* The comparison group for those having ARM excludes women whose membranes broke early, i.e. they were not at risk of having ARM. The differences between women who did and did not have ARM are not significant.

** The comparison group for women having continuous monitoring includes both women who had some monitoring and women who had none. This difference is significant at $p < 0.01$. The comparison group for those who had non-continuous monitoring is women who had no monitoring. This difference is not significant.

All other differences are significant at $p < 0.001$ or greater with the exception of that for non-elective caesarean sections ($p = 0.07$).

Table 7.25: Proportion of women who felt in control of what staff were doing to them 'always' or 'most of the time' by their experience of different procedures

Obviously, one might expect that women who have labours that are in some way difficult would be more likely to have things done to them by staff and so potentially be less likely to feel in control of what is done to them. This is supported by the fact that women with long labours (> 12 hours) were much less likely to say that they had felt in control. There were, however, no differences between women whose babies were admitted to a Special Care Baby Unit and those who were not. In any case it is clear that difficulties in labour can be only one contributory factor to feeling in control. Women who are shaved, for example, are just as likely to report a lack of feeling in control as women who had instrumental deliveries. This suggests that it is the experience of the procedures, or how they are carried out, which are important to women's feeling of control. An interesting, and highly significant, difference to note in this context is between women who had episiotomies and women who tore. As Table 7.25 shows, only 68 per cent of women who had episiotomies felt in control all or most of the time. The comparable figures for women who tore and those with an intact perineum were 86 per cent and 88 per cent, i.e. virtually identical. None of the other questions to do with suturing were related to control (e.g. who sutured, use of local anaesthetic).

However, of the women who were sutured, those who reported themselves to be less in control were significantly more likely to have subsequent problems with their stitches ($p < 0.005$). The link between feeling in control of staff and avoiding an episiotomy might be that having an episiotomy leads women to feel that they have lost control over what staff are doing to them. Alternatively, feeling out of control of what staff do to them might reflect a type of care which includes interventions such as episiotomies, and also leads to women not being able to get comfortable, for example, thus decreasing the chance of an intact perineum. Perhaps related to the experience of interventions was the ability to get comfortable in labour which was very strongly related to feeling in control of staff: if women could not get comfortable they were much less likely to feel in control of staff.

Comfortable?	In control?			
	All/most of the time		Only some/hardly any of the time	
	n	%	n	%
Yes, all the time	290	(92)	25	(8)
Some of the time	190	(75)	65	(26)
No, hardly ever	55	(56)	43	(44)

$p < 0.0001$

Percentages are of women in a given row

Table 7.26: Feeling in control of what staff were doing by being able to get comfortable in labour

Control and other social/behavioural aspects of labour

Nearly all of the questions to do with the social/behavioural aspects of labour were significantly related to feeling in control. Whether or not women had previously met at least one of the midwives who looked after them was not but having one midwife throughout labour was, as was being delivered by a midwife rather than a doctor. Both of these would, of course, be related to relatively short, trouble-free labours. Similarly, we find that women who were seen by a doctor during labour, even if not delivered by a doctor, felt significantly less in control. One of the biggest differences relates to the number of people coming in and out of the room. The figure given in Table 7.27 combines 'quite a few' and 'a lot'. Taken separately, the point is made still more strongly; only 44 per cent of those who felt that there were 'a lot' of people coming in and out felt in control most or all of the time compared with 85 per cent of those who said that there were 'hardly any'. Once again, this is something that is likely to relate to long or difficult labours. Only 69 per cent of women who experienced some sort of emergency felt in control 'always' or 'most of the time' compared with 87 per cent of those who did not. Nevertheless, it is evident that women who had difficulties with their labours were still able to feel in control of what staff were doing to them, particularly if they were involved in decision making.

	Of women who had		Of women who did not have	
	n	%	n	%
One midwife throughout	368/442	(83)	165/221	(75)
Midwife delivery	438/522	(84)	81/122	(66)*
Saw a doctor during labour	286/386	(74)	249/283	(88)
'Quite a few' or 'a lot' of people coming in and out	81/136	(60)	455/534	(85)

All differences are significant at $p < 0.005$ or greater.

* Includes only women delivered by a doctor. Those delivered by students etc. are not included.

Table 7.27: Proportion of women who felt in control of what staff were doing to them 'always' or 'most of the time' by aspects of staffing during labour

Further evidence that the feeling of being in control of what staff were doing is not simply a function of the difficulty of the labour comes from the adjectives women used to describe staff. Of the fifteen adjectives available to women, every one was significantly related to feeling in control of what staff did. Thus, women who described staff as any one of rushed, insensitive, unhelpful, off-hand, rude, inconsiderate, bossy or condescending felt significantly less in control than women who did not use these words. Conversely, women who experienced staff as humorous, sensitive, considerate, supportive, polite, warm or informative felt more in control. While it may be the case that certain obstetric problems may oblige staff to behave in ways that appear 'rushed' or 'bossy', difficult labours should also give staff greater scope for appearing, for example, 'sensitive' and 'supportive'. Further analysis could establish whether or not there is a direct relationship between difficult labours and perceptions of staff (see Chapter 10). Pending this our assumption would be that a woman's perception of the staff is a major determinant of her feeling of control (or vice versa) over and above any contribution made by the difficulties of the labour.

	Of women who had this degree of involvement in non-emergency decisions		Of women who had this degree of involvement in emergency decisions	
	n	%	n	%
Staff got on with it	38/73	(52)	35/60	(58)
Kept informed	172/235	(73)	81/124	(65)
Discussed things	159/183	(87)	28/37	(76)
Women's own decision	154/164	(94)	13/14	(93)

Table 7.28: Proportion of women who felt in control of what staff were doing to them 'always' or 'most of the time' by involvement in decision-making

Linking to the perception of staff as 'informative', we found that the amount and quality of information women felt they had been given were also strongly related to feeling in control of what staff did. Eighty six per cent of women who felt they had had the right amount of information also felt in control 'always' or 'most of the time', compared with only 64 per cent of those who did not feel that they had had the right amount of information ($p < 0.0001$). Similarly, not feeling in control was associated with wanting to have known more about some aspect of childbirth ($p < 0.05$) and with having been given misleading or confusing information ($p < 0.01$).

Pain and women's overall descriptions of labour

Again fifteen adjectives were available to women to describe their feelings during labour. Twelve of these were significantly related to feeling in control of what staff were doing. Women who described themselves as any one of out of control, dopey, frightened, powerless, detached or helpless, felt less in control of what staff were doing. Conversely, women who felt calm, confident, excited, involved, in control, or alert were much more likely to feel in control of staff. We are not, of course, able to say anything about cause and effect but it seems reasonable to imagine that a woman who feels in control of what staff are doing to her has more scope for feeling calm, confident, etc. while one who does not may well feel frightened and powerless. Others of these adjectives, for example, involved, detached, dopey, alert are more likely to relate to the use of drugs, particularly sleeping pills and Pethidine and are less likely to be causally related to not being in control of what staff were doing. In fact, women who had Pethidine felt themselves to be significantly less in control of staff as did women who had epidurals. In neither case was the reported effectiveness of the pain relief related to control. However, feeling under pressure to use it was strongly related and this was also true for Gas and Air. The use of breathing and relaxation exercises shows the opposite pattern; those who used them most felt most in control of staff and feeling in control of staff was related in turn to how helpful women actually found breathing and relaxation as a pain-relieving technique. Overall, women who were dissatisfied with their own response to pain were least likely to say that they had felt in control of staff while those who were satisfied felt most in control. Consistent with this, women who found that the pain differed from their expectations felt less in control, but, interestingly, the women least likely to report feeling in control were those who said that they had had no expectations about the pain.

It is perhaps not surprising, in the light of these findings, to discover that feeling in control of staff is significantly related to reports of 'internal' control: control of behaviour, control during contractions and how much noise women felt they made. Once again, we cannot postulate cause and effect; the most likely possibility is that external events which lead to loss of 'external' control also lead to loss of 'internal' control.

	In control of staff?			
In control of behaviour?	All/most of the time		Only some/hardly any of the time	
	n	%	n	%
Yes, all the time	301	(87)	47	(14)
Yes, some of the time	226	(76)	70	(24)
No, not at all	9	(35)	17	(65)

Percentages are of women in a given row.

$p < 0.0001$.

Table 7.29: Feeling in control of what staff were doing by feeling in control of own behaviour

	In control of staff?			
In control during contractions?	All/most of the time		Only some/hardly any of the time	
	n	%	n	%
Yes, all of the time	330	(90)	37	(10)
Yes, some of the time	178	(70)	77	(30)
No, not at all	25	(57)	19	(43)

Percentages are of women in a given row.

$p < 0.0001$.

Table 7.30: Feeling in control of what staff were doing by feeling in control during contractions

	In control of staff?			
Made a noise?	All/most of the time		Only some/hardly any of the time	
	n	%	n	%
No, not much	300	(84)	58	(16)
Yes, a bit	187	(81)	43	(19)
Yes, a lot	46	(65)	25	(35)
Not sure	3	(30)	7	(70)

Percentages are of women in a given row.

$p < 0.0001$.

Table 7.31: Feeling in control of what staff were doing by making a noise

Outcome variables

We found earlier that there were very few differences in outcomes between those women who asserted a high desire for control over decision making and those who did not. We postulated, however, that the sense of actually being (or not being) in control of what staff did would prove important and this seems to be borne out by our findings. In terms of fulfilment, for example, 84 per cent of those who felt in control all or most of the time felt fulfilled while this was true for only 60 per cent of those who felt in control only some of the time or not at all ($p < 0.0001$). Satisfaction with the birth shows a strong linear relationship with control as Table 7.32 shows.

Felt in control?	Mean satisfaction score
Yes, always	8.5
Yes, most of the time	7.7
Only some of the time	6.1
No, hardly at all	5.9
n = 658	
p < 0.0001	

Table 7.32: Mean marks out of ten for satisfaction with the birth by feeling in control of what staff were doing to you.

As we shall see later, women who felt in control of staff also had significantly higher emotional well-being scores. There was, however, no relationship between feeling in control of what staff were doing and the proportion of negative adjectives used to describe the baby.

The results reported in this section make it clear that, far from being a peripheral issue of interest only to a handful of middle class 'NCT types', feeling in control is central to women's experience of childbirth. Subsequent analysis has shown very similar results for 'internal' control; both are important, but, as we have seen, they tend to go together. The implications of these findings will be discussed further in the following two chapters.

CHAPTER EIGHT

Psychological Outcomes

This chapter explores the relationship between women's hopes and expectations of the birth, their actual experiences and their postnatal psychological outcome. We focused on four outcome measures – fulfilment, satisfaction, Description of Baby and emotional well-being. Each of these measures is discussed separately.

Fulfilment

As has been discussed earlier (in Chapter 4), the majority of women hoped and expected the experience of giving birth to be fulfilling. Only 19 women said 'don't know what this means' in response to the question about fulfilment.

Postnatally, most women (88%) felt they could identify with the idea of birth being 'fulfilling' or 'not fulfilling'. Only nine women said they did not know what was meant by 'finding the birth fulfilling'. In fact, eight of these had claimed antenatally that they did know what it would mean to have a fulfilling experience of childbirth.

	n	%
Yes	546	(77)
No	76	(11)
Not sure	65	(9)
Don't know what it means	9	(1)
No response	14	(2)
n = 710		

Table 8.1: Was birth fulfilling?

The women who said they had found birth fulfilling often added jubilant comments describing their feelings of fulfilment due to having a 'good' birth experience, or doing something as wonderful as producing a baby:

> 'I am still elated and have kept the excited feeling from the actual birth day. I think everything has been great simply because I had a good delivery with no medical intervention, no forceps, episiotomy etc., etc.'

> 'The whole process of conception, pregnancy and birth still amazes me. It's truly remarkable and truly wonderful.'

'Definitely fulfilling, I felt I had justified my role of being a woman.'

Some of the women who (antenatally or postnatally) said that they could not relate to the concept of childbirth being fulfilling, explicitly stated that they wanted a baby but had no expectation that the experience of childbirth itself could be fulfilling:

'... we wanted a baby, not a birth...'

' I don't think birth is fulfilling, only the moment you have the baby.'

'Giving birth is not, for me, satisfying as an experience in itself – I forgot that I was having a baby at all! Once the pain had gone it *was* a very moving experience to see our daughter for the first time.'

It is also possible that some women who ticked 'Yes it was fulfilling' felt that it was only fulfilling because of the baby itself, and certainly many women who seemed to have had negative experiences of labour (very painful, lots of interventions, negative descriptions of how they felt, etc.) still said they found birth fulfilling. One woman, for instance, who had a forceps delivery, indicated that birth had been fulfilling and added:

'Only in that it produced a beautiful baby – healthy and all: It was not personally fulfilling because I never "pushed" the baby out.'

However, as the comment shows, this woman still had a concept of childbirth as potentially personally fulfilling.

Fulfilment and the independent variables

There were no relationships between fulfilment and parity, class or education. There were, however, differences between units in fulfilment. Only 62 per cent of the women at Little Exington found the birth 'fulfilling' as opposed to between 77 per cent and 86 per cent of those at other units (antenatally, the women at Little Exington were also less likely to expect birth to be fulfilling).

	Yes		No		Not sure what this means		Don't know	
	n	%	n	%	n	%	n	%
Willowford	136	(81)	16	(10)	15	(9)	2	(1)
Exington Consultant	72	(79)	11	(12)	6	(7)	2	(2)
Exington GP unit	44	(86)	3	(6)	3	(6)	1	(2)
Little Exington	28	(62)	8	(18)	9	(20)	0	0
Wychester	135	(80)	18	(11)	14	(8)	1	(<1)
Zedbury	118	(77)	16	(11)	16	(11)	2	(2)

Percentages are of women giving birth in each unit.

$p < 0.05$

Table 8.2: Was the birth a fulfilling experience by unit

Fulfilment and interventions

Women were more likely to find the whole experience 'fulfilling' if they had a vaginal delivery rather than a caesarean section. Even so, just over half of the women who had caesarean sections described the experience as 'fulfilling'. These were predominantly women who had had caesarean sections under epidurals, whereas women who had caesarean sections under general anaesthetic were least likely to feel fulfilled (see also Garel et al., 1987).

Fulfilling?	Had caesarean		Did not have caesarean	
	n	%	n	%
Yes	27	(52)	518	(82)
No	18	(35)	58	(9)
Not sure	7	(14)	58	(9)

Percentages are of women in a given column.

$p < 0.0001$

Table 8.3: Was birth fulfilling by whether or not had caesarean section

Fulfilling?	Epidural		General anaesthetic	
	n	%	n	%
Yes	19	(68)	8	(33)
No/not sure	9	(32)	16	(67)

Percentages are of women in a given column.

$p < 0.05$

Table 8.4: Was the birth fulfilling by type of anaesthetic for caesarean section

It should be noted, therefore, that having a caesarean section does not necessarily preclude finding the experience fulfilling and that an epidural increases the chances of fulfilment.

Fulfilment was also clearly associated with all other interventions (except ARM, acceleration, induction and monitoring), and with the total number of interventions experienced. This latter effect is, however, weakened considerably when parity is controlled for.

Women who had instrumental deliveries expressed very low rates of fulfilment – almost as low as the rate for caesarean sections. As one woman commented:

> 'The forceps delivery was such a distressful experience for me that it has destroyed any pleasurable memories or feelings of fulfilment that I might otherwise have.'

Fulfilling?	Had instrumental delivery		Did not have instrumental delivery	
	n	%	n	%
Yes	38	(59)	487	(82)
No/not sure	27	(42)	104	(18)

Percentages are of women in a given column.

$p < 0.0001$

Table 8.5: Was the birth a fulfilling experience by instrumental delivery

'Minor' interventions were also significantly related to fulfilment, as Table 8.6 shows.

	Did have		Did not have		Significance p<
	n	%	n	%	
Enema	(106/145)	73	(399/485)	82	0.05
Shave	(38/62)	61	(461/553)	83	0.0001
Glucose drip	(98/136)	72	(402/479)	84	0.01
Episiotomy	(158/217)	73	(347/405)*	86	0.0001
ARM	(286/353)	81	(234/287)	82	NS
Electronic fetal monitoring	(419/525)	80	(88/111)	79	NS

* Women who tore and women with intact perineums were equally likely to find birth fulfilling.

Table 8.6: Percentage of women who found the birth fulfilling by experience of 'minor' interventions

Women who were 'not sure' whether or not they had experienced a procedure have been omitted from the table; they, in fact, were generally the least likely to have found birth fulfilling. The lack of association between fulfilment and monitoring confirms the other findings showing that many women do not experience monitoring in the same way as other interventions. It is interesting that women who were shaved (a so-called 'trivial' or 'minor' intervention) were almost as likely to be unfulfilled as those who had forceps. We would have to explore our data further to explain the lack of association between ARM, acceleration and induction and fulfilment. Perhaps this may be due to the fact that these interventions are medically significant and potentially helpful (unlike, for example, shaving).

Fulfilment and pain

Women who found the pain different from what they expected were more likely to say they did not find the experience of birth fulfilling. However, there was no association with whether they found the pain more painful than expected. One hundred and forty women volunteered that they found labour more painful than expected but 76 per cent of these said the experience was fulfilling as did 80 per cent of those who did not find that labour was more painful than expected (a non-significant difference).

	Pain as expected?					
Fulfilling?	No, not at all		In some ways		Yes, exactly	
	n	%	n	%	n	%
Yes	95	(73)	197	(78)	220	(86)
No/Not sure	35	(27)	54	(22)	37	(14)

Percentages are of women in a given column.

n = 638 $p < 0.05$

[The 14 women who said they had 'no expectations' were excluded from this analysis, as were those women who had elective sections.]

Table 8.7: Was pain in labour as expected by was birth a fulfilling experience

There was, though, a clear association between fulfilment and how satisfied women were with the way they responded to the pain.

Fulfilling?	Satisfied		Neither satisfied nor dissatisfied		Dissatisfied	
	n	%	n	%	n	%
Yes	399	(88)	94	(67)	31	(56)
No/Not sure	57	(13)	46	(33)	24	(44)

Percentages are of women in a given column.

n = 651

$p < 0.0001$

Table 8.8: Satisfaction with response to pain by was birth fulfilling experience?

Use of pain-relieving drugs

Whether or not women used gas and air was not associated with fulfilment but women who used Pethidine and those who had an epidural were less fulfilled than those who did not ($p < 0.05$).

Also, not surprisingly, women's feelings about having had or not having had any particular drug were associated with fulfilment. Women who were pleased with what happened were more likely to say they were fulfilled than those who were not pleased with what happened. Similarly, women who felt under pressure from staff about drugs were less fulfilled than those who did not feel under any pressure.

Fulfilment and feelings during labour

Fulfilment was most strikingly associated with women's descriptions of how they felt during labour. Women who ticked the words: calm, confident, in control, excited and involved to describe how they felt during labour were more likely to feel fulfilled than those who did not. On the other hand, women who described themselves as frightened, helpless, out of control, overwhelmed, powerless, dopey and detached were more likely to describe the experience as unfulfilling. The only adjectives which were not significantly associated with fulfilment were 'powerful', 'challenged' and 'alert'.

Feeling that the birth was a fulfilling experience was closely tied to women's feelings about the labour itself. It was not just a question of the fulfilment of achieving motherhood and obtaining the end product of the baby.

Fulfilment and 'internal' control

Being fulfilled was significantly associated with feeling in control during contractions ($p < 0.0001$) and feeling in control of one's own behaviour during labour ($p < 0.05$). It was not, however, associated with feeling one made a lot of noise during labour. Making a lot of noise is not necessarily equated in women's minds with losing control of themselves and does not affect their experience of fulfilment. This had also been apparent from women's antenatal views on making a noise.

Fulfilment and treatment by staff

Fulfilment was associated with four of the adjectives used to describe staff. Women who described the staff as humorous, polite and warm were more likely than other women to feel the birth had been a fulfilling experience, whereas women who described staff as 'rushed' were least likely to feel fulfilled. Fulfilment was also related to women's responses to the open-ended invitation at the end of the questionnaire to describe the care they received. Women whose comments were coded as 'eulogistic' were the most likely to describe the experience of giving birth as fulfilling and those whose comments were coded as 'generally negative' were the least likely (86% compared to 55%).

Other aspects of staff care

Fulfilment was also related to other aspects of care such as continuity and privacy. Although there was no association between fulfilment and whether or not a woman had previously met the midwife who looked after her during delivery, there was a clear association with continuity of care during labour itself. Eighty three per cent of the women who had at least one midwife who stayed with them throughout labour found the experience fulfilling as opposed to 75 per cent of the women who did not experience continuity of care.

	Continuity of care			
Fulfilling?	Yes		No	
	n	%	n	%
Yes	361	(83)	163	(75)
No/not sure	74	(17)	55	(25)

Percentages are of women in a given column.

$p < 0.05$

Table 8.9: Fulfilment by continuity of care

A lot of people coming in and out of the room during labour was significantly associated with finding birth unfulfilling. Over a third of the women who felt there were a lot of people coming in and out during their labour said the experience was not fulfilling or were unsure whether it was or not, as opposed to less than a fifth of those who felt they had had more privacy. Both fulfilment and privacy, however, were independently associated with having interventions, which may confound this finding.

Fulfilling?	A lot of people		Quite a few		No, hardly any	
	n	%	n	%	n	%
Yes	14	(61)	81	(72)	433	(83)
No/not sure	9	(39)	31	(28)	91	(18)

Percentages are of women in a given column

$p < 0.0001$

Table 8.10: Fulfilment by many people coming in and out during labour

Whether a woman's companion was present was also associated with fulfilment. The least fulfilled women were those who only had their birth companion with them *some* of the time. This reflects the fact that women who did not have a companion present at all were the women who did not want or expect antenatally to have a companion present. The women who only had a companion present some of the time, on the other hand, had usually wanted and expected to have their companion with them throughout labour but were denied this (e.g. companion sent out of room, staff saying woman was not in labour and sending companion home).

Fulfilling?	Companion present all the time		Companion present some of the time		Companion not present	
	n	%	n	%	n	%
Yes	481	(82)	20	(63)	24	(71)
No	58	(10)	10	(31)	2	(6)
Not sure	51	(9)	2	(6)	8	(24)

Percentages are of women in a given column.

$p < 0.0001$

Table 8.11: Fulfilment by presence of birth companion

Being able to get into the most comfortable position possible was associated with feelings of fulfilment. Women who were always able to get comfortable were much more likely to feel that birth had been fulfilling than those who were only able to get comfortable some of the time or who could hardly ever get comfortable (87% versus 77% versus 65%; $p < 0.0001$).

Fulfilment and 'external' control

Women who felt in control of what staff did to them were much more fulfilled than those who did not ($p < 0.0001$). It is striking that only half of those who hardly ever felt in control of what staff did to them described the birth experience as 'fulfilling' as opposed to 91 per cent of those who were always in control of what staff did to them.

Fulfilling?	Yes, always		Yes, most of the time		Only sometimes		No, hardly at all	
	n	%	n	%	n	%	n	%
Yes	163	(91)	283	(82)	59	(67)	22	(51)
No/not sure	16	(9)	64	(18)	29	(33)	21	(49)

Percentages are of women in a given column.

$p < 0.0001$

Table 8.12: Fulfilment by were you in control of what staff did to you?

Non-emergency decision making was also related to fulfilment. Women who felt they were kept informed, had decisions discussed with them or who actually felt in control over non-emergency decisions were equally fulfilled. Women who felt the staff just got on with it without even informing them were significantly less likely to feel the experience had been fulfilling.

Fulfilling?	Staff just did it		Staff kept me informed, discussed decisions or I was in control	
	n	%	n	%
Yes	49	(70)	465	(81)
No/not sure	21	(30)	107	(19)

Percentages are of women in a given column.

$p < 0.05$

Table 8.13: Fulfilment by non-emergency decision making

The relationship between fulfilment and control over non-emergency decisions only becomes significant when the degrees of control are amalgamated to contrast women who felt the staff 'just did it' with everyone else. It is also worth noting that more women felt they were generally in control of what staff did to them than felt in control of decisions – the former, as we will see, also seems to be of more importance to outcomes such as emotional well-being and satisfaction. Control in this sense is a way of experiencing care and reflects an attitude of the staff rather than any detailed choice over what is actually done and input into decision making *per se*. What seems to be important is *how* things are done rather than *what* is done.

As one would expect, the most fulfilled women were those who felt the question about emergency decisions was irrelevant to them, as there had been no emergency. There were no other significant differences.

Fulfilment and information

Feeling that they had been provided with complete and accurate information was associated with women's feelings of fulfilment. Women who felt they had been given the right amount of information were more fulfilled than the other women (84% compared to 67%, $p < 0.0001$). Similarly, women who wished they had known more about some aspect were less fulfilled than other women (64% compared to 84%, $p < 0.0001$) as were those who felt they had been given misleading information (69% compared to 82%, $p < 0.005$).

Antenatal predictors of fulfilment

The only clearcut antenatal predictor of postnatal fulfilment was a woman's initial feelings on finding that she was pregnant. Women who expressed unhappiness about being pregnant were less likely to describe the birth as a fulfilling experience than other women. (There were some other associations with antenatal data that were just significant but these do not present a clearcut picture.)

Fulfilment and other postnatal outcomes

Finding the birth a fulfilling experience was positively associated with the other outcome measures: satisfaction, emotional well-being and Description of Baby. There was no association with breastfeeding or any of the other questions designed to tap the relationship with the baby.

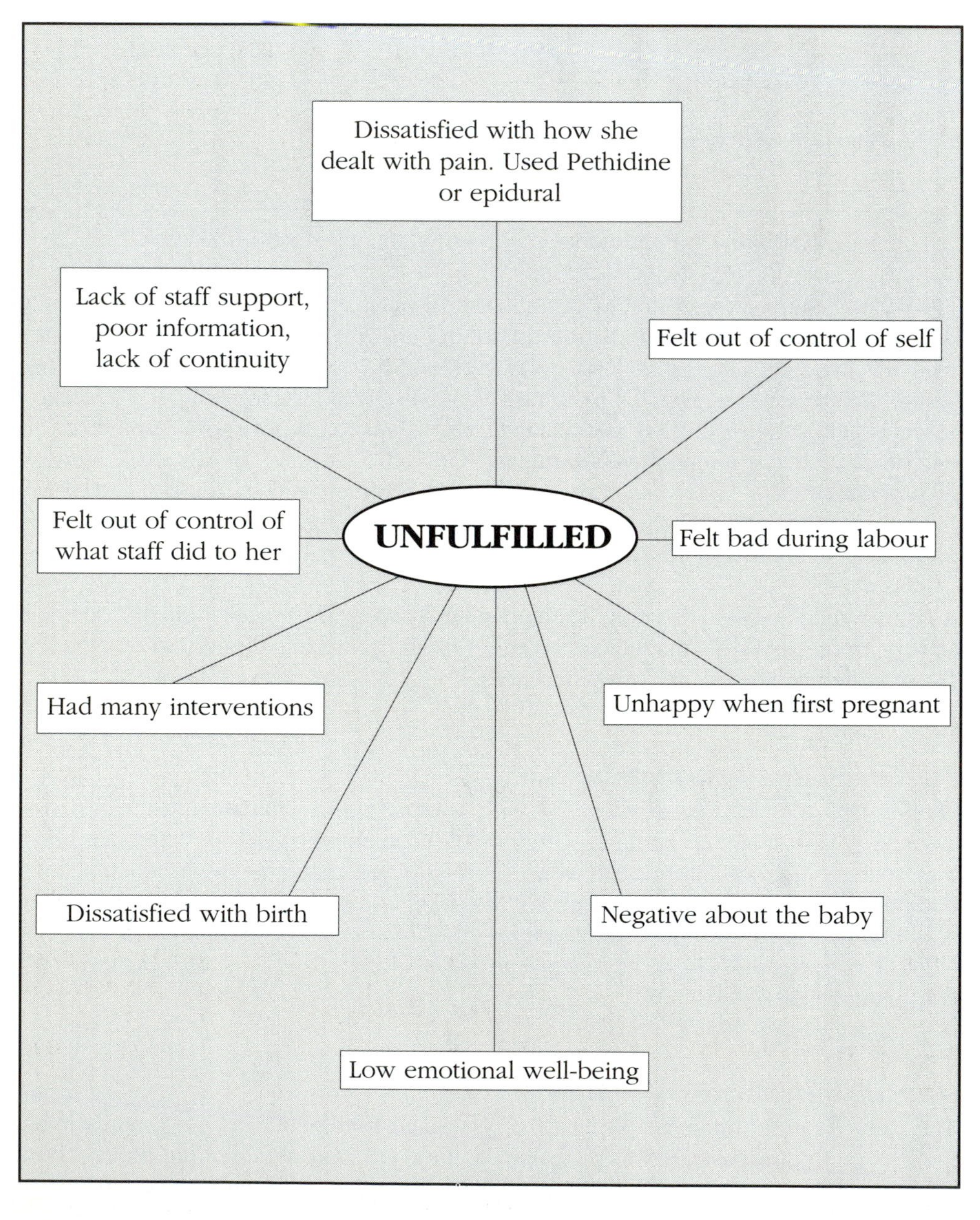

Lack of fulfilment

Satisfaction with birth

One of our four psychological outcome variables was women's satisfaction with the experience of birth six weeks after the event. At the end of the postnatal questionnaire we asked women:

> To sum up we would like you to tell us how satisfactory an experience the birth was by giving it a mark out of ten. Ten-out-of-ten would mean an absolutely wonderful experience that could not have been better, nought-out-of-ten would mean a thoroughly unsatisfactory experience with nothing good to be said for it. Please mark in this box how many points out of ten you would give your birth.
>
> Marks out of 10 ☐

Women responded as follows:

Satisfaction (Marks out of 10)	Number of women	% of sample
0	19	(3)
1	5	(<1)
2	11	(2)
3	13	(2)
4	9	(1)
5	64	(9)
6	44	(6)
7	82	(12)
8	180	(26)
9	136	(20)
10	129	(19)

Clearly, the majority were very satisfied with their experience of birth, with two thirds giving it a score of eight, nine or ten. This is the finding we would expect from other studies and from the discussion in Chapter 1 which highlighted the ceiling effects of global questions about satisfaction. Even so, it is important to note that the question is picking up over 17 per cent of women, i.e. a sixth of the sample, who only gave a score of five marks or less, which is particularly meaningful in the context of this marked tendency towards high scores.

Analysis of variance

As the distribution of scores was highly skewed towards the upper end, the data were transformed by squaring, thus improving normality. An analysis of variance was carried out to test the relationships between satisfaction with birth as the dependent variable as measured by marks out of ten, and particular aspects of the birth experience as independent variables (see also Chapter 10 for subsequent multivariate analysis).

Results

Of the major independent variables considered in this study (parity, unit, education, women's class, partner's class), parity, unit and women's social class were significantly related to satisfaction with birth.

Variable	n	Transformed mean (marks out of 10)[2]	Significance (F test)
Parity			
primips	269	58	p = 0.001
multips	423	65	
Unit:			
Willowford	167	66	
Exington consultant	96	60	
Exington GP	45	72	
Little Exington	43	60	p < 0.05
Wychester	168	61	
Zedbury	148	58	
Woman's social class			
I + II	262	58	
IIIN + IIIM	341	63	p < 0.05
IV + V	71	68	

Table 8.14: Satisfaction with birth by parity, unit and social class

Multips were more satisfied than primips. Women who gave birth at Exington GP unit were the most satisfied in our sample. The explanation for this might be thought to lie in the fact that 43 out of the 45 women who gave birth there were multips. However, when we control for parity and look at multips only, significant differences in their satisfaction scores remain, with women who gave birth at Exington GP unit and Willowford remaining the most satisfied. Unit differences among primips are not significant except that primips who gave birth at Zedbury had notably lower scores than everyone else. In this context, it is important to keep in mind the low non-instrumental vaginal delivery rate for primips in Zedbury (see Chapter 6).

Women in the higher social classes were the most dissatisfied and those in the lowest the most satisfied. However, the relationship is not a particularly strong one, only just reaching significance.

Since parity is strongly related to many of the variables we looked at in relation to satisfaction with birth, we carried out two-way analyses of variance to control for the effects of parity. In practically all cases, parity and the other variable under consideration were seen to exert independent significant effects on satisfaction. These effects are clarified where relevant.

Satisfaction with birth and obstetric interventions

CAESAREAN SECTION

As one would expect, having a vaginal delivery rather than a caesarean section was strongly related to satisfaction with birth ($p < 0.0001$). Whether the section was planned and how far in advance also affected how satisfied women were ($p < 0.05$). Women who had 'true' elective sections were the most satisfied, followed by women who had a caesarean section after being permitted a trial of labour. Women who were least satisfied as gauged by their scores for marks out of ten, were:

- women booked for electives who went into spontaneous labour and were then operated on as emergencies,
- women who had emergency sections,
- women who had elective sections at such short notice that they were not psychologically prepared.

Women who had caesarean sections under epidural anaesthesia were much more satisfied than those who had general anaesthesia.

	n	Transformed mean (marks out of 10)^2	Significance (F test)
Caesarean section	55	41	$p < 0.0001$
Vaginal delivery	636	64	
Type of section:			
Elective	25	54	
After a trial of labour	7	48	
Elective but went into labour first	4	37	$p < 0.05$
Emergency	15	25	
Elective at very short notice	4	7	
Anaesthetic:			
General	25	25	$p < 0.001$
Epidural	30	54	

Table 8.15: Satisfaction with birth by caesarean section

Other interventions

All the interventions whether 'major' or 'minor' in nature were significantly associated with women's satisfaction with their birth, the great majority very strongly so (see Appendix B19). For most interventions, the pattern of association was straightforward: women who said that they had had the intervention were less satisfied than those who did not (enema, shave, glucose drip, episiotomy, fetal heart monitoring, chemical induction and acceleration, forceps delivery and syntometrine). Two-way analysis of variance shows that these relationships were independent of parity effects. There was, however, a tendency for effects to be stronger for multips than for primips. Scores with regard to fetal heart monitoring were linear in that women who had none were more satisfied than those monitored intermittently, and those monitored continuously were the least satisfied. These are somewhat surprising findings given the positive attitude towards monitoring shown by women antenatally (see Chapter 6).

Women whose membranes broke spontaneously during established labour were more satisfied than women whose membranes were broken artificially. Women whose membranes broke spontaneously before labour began had even lower scores, but this is primarily a parity effect. Satisfaction was also related to when ARM was performed in terms of dilatation ($p < 0.01$). Women whose waters were broken later in labour (seven or more centimetres dilated) were more satisfied than those whose waters were broken earlier in labour. Disagreement between the women and the staff was related to satisfaction ($p < 0.05$) as was how happy they were with having/not having an ARM ($p < 0.01$). Women who had been able to participate in a discussion with staff about the disagreement and reach a mutually acceptable decision were the most satisfied.

Number of interventions

The number of interventions experienced by women was significantly associated with how satisfied they were with the experience of birth. The most satisfied women were those who had only one intervention or none at all. Dissatisfaction increased linearly with the number of interventions that were carried out so that the least satisfied women were those who had experienced five or more interventions. The relationship between the number of interventions and satisfaction was independent of parity.

Number of interventions	n	Transformed mean (marks out of 10)[2]	Significance
None	28	72	$p < 0.0001$ (F test and Pearson's correlation coefficient)
1	160	72	
2	172	67	
3	106	64	
4	98	51	
5 or more	90	47	

Table 8.16: Satisfaction with birth by the number of interventions experienced

Other 'medical' aspects of birth

Women whose babies were admitted to a special care unit after birth were less satisfied than other women ($p < 0.05$). Shorter labours were associated with high satisfaction scores and long labours (over 12 hours) with lower satisfaction ($p < 0.0001$). Both these findings are likely to be related to difficult labours and be thus associated in turn with a higher intervention rate. Indeed seeing a doctor during labour, also indicative of obstetric difficulties, was also related to lower satisfaction ($p < 0.0001$).

Satisfaction, pain and pain relief

Women who found that the pain in labour was exactly as they had expected it to be, were more satisfied than those who did not find this to be the case (this was particularly true for primips).

Was pain as expected	n	Transformed mean (marks out of 10)²	Significance (F test)
Yes, exactly	258	70	
Yes, in some ways	251	61	p < 0.0001
No, not at all	132	53	
No expectations	13	63	

Table 8.17: Satisfaction with birth by whether pain was as expected

Satisfaction was related to use of breathing and relaxation exercises ($p < 0.01$) and to how helpful women found such exercises ($p < 0.0001$). These relationships are independent of parity effects. Women who used the exercises all the time were the most satisfied followed by women who did not use them at all. The least satisfied women only used the exercises for part of the time. Women who said the exercises only helped a bit, or not at all, were the least satisfied and these are on the whole the same women who used such techniques for only part of the labour.

Women's overall feelings about the way they responded to the pain were very strongly related to their satisfaction with the experience of birth.

Feelings regarding response to pain	n	Transformed mean (marks out of 10)²	Significance (F test)
Satisfied	454	69	
Neither satisfied nor dissatisfied	142	53	p < 0.0001
Dissatisfied	57	38	

Table 8.18: Satisfaction with birth by response to pain

Use of pain-relieving drugs

Satisfaction with birth was related to women's use of gas and air ($p < 0.01$), Pethidine ($p < 0.0001$) and epidural anaesthesia ($p < 0.001$). In each case, the women who used the drugs were less satisfied with birth than those who did not. When we look at satisfaction in relation to how many drugs were used and in what combination, we find that the most dissatisfied women were those who had both Pethidine and an epidural (whether or not gas and air was also used). The most satisfied women were those who used no drugs at all, followed by those who only used gas and air. Women who found that the gas and air, and Pethidine had been very effective were more satisfied than other women, but there was no significant association between satisfaction and effectiveness of epidural anaesthesia.

Women who felt under pressure from staff to either have or not have pain-relieving drugs were less satisfied than those who did not feel under pressure. Satisfaction was related to women's feelings about the decision to have or not to have Pethidine and about having/not having an epidural, but not to feelings about gas and air. Those who felt positive about the decision or who had no particular feelings about it were more satisfied than those who felt unhappy or who had mixed feelings. Two-way analysis of variance showed that pain and pain relief were related to satisfaction independently of parity effects.

These findings are not surprising and are fairly consistent with the results for fulfilment. It might be said that findings such as women are more satisfied when they do not feel under pressure from staff are self-evident. However, such results underline the need for staff to discuss the issue of drugs with women in labour with sensitivity and respect for women's views on the subject.

Feelings during labour

Thirteen out of the 15 adjectives offered as descriptions of feelings during labour were very strongly associated with satisfaction. Women who were more satisfied felt calm, confident, excited, powerful, involved, in control and alert. Women who were less satisfied felt out of control, dopey, frightened, detached, helpless and powerless. Two of these – alert and powerful – were significant at the $p < 0.001$ level; all the others were significant at the $p < 0.0001$ level.

Comfortable position

Whether women were able to get into comfortable positions, or the most comfortable position possible, was strongly related to overall satisfaction with birth ($p < 0.0001$). Those who were hardly ever able to get comfortable gave lower scores for satisfaction.

Satisfaction and 'internal' control

Satisfaction was also significantly related to both of the major aspects of 'internal' control that we looked at: control of behaviour in labour, and control during contractions. Thus, the women who were able to maintain control of their behaviour throughout were the most satisfied, and the women who were not in control any of the time were the least satisfied. The same pattern is evident for being able to maintain control during contractions. There was also a relationship with the other question that we included to tap 'internal' control: how much noise women felt they made. The more noise a woman felt she was making, the less she was satisfied. Those who were not sure how much noise they made were the least satisfied – this is likely to be related to use of pain-relieving drugs and their side-effects on women's awareness.

'Internal' Control Variable	n	Transformed mean (marks out of 10)[2]	Significance (F test)
Lose control of behaviour?			
All the time	24	44	
Some of the time	294	57	p < 0.0001
Not at all	342	69	
In control during contractions?			
All the time	360	70	
Some of the time	253	55	p < 0.0001
Not at all	43	48	
Make much noise?			
Yes, a lot	70	51	
Yes, a bit	229	60	p < 0.0001
No, not much	350	67	
Not sure	10	46	

Table 8.19: Satisfaction with birth by 'internal' control

Satisfaction and 'external' control

Satisfaction with birth was significantly related to two aspects of 'external' control: the general feeling of being in control of what staff were doing and specific control over non-emergency decision making (see Table 8.20). Women who felt most in control were the most satisfied.

'External' Control Variable	n	Transformed mean (marks out of 10)[2]	Significance (F test)
Non-emergency decisions:			
Staff just did it	72	58	
I was kept informed	233	61	p < 0.05
Staff discussed with me first	179	62	
I was in control	161	68	
Control of what staff did:			
Yes, always	180	76	
Yes, most of the time	347	63	p < 0.0001
Only some of the time	87	43	
No, hardly at all	44	44	

Table 8.20: Satisfaction with birth by 'external' control

The results for 'internal' and 'external' control clearly demonstrate the positive effects of maintaining control both over one's own body and over external factors on women's overall satisfaction with the experience of birth.

Information

There were significant relationships between satisfaction with birth and the amount of information women said they had been given ($p < 0.0001$), wishing they had had more information prior to giving birth ($p < 0.0001$) and feeling they had been given misleading information ($p < 0.0001$). The results for misleading information are significant for multips only. Women who had been given the 'right amount' of information and who had not been told anything misleading were clearly more satisfied. Information is in many ways a pre-requisite for 'external' control since having adequate information forms part of the basis upon which decisions can be made.

Adjectives used to describe the staff

Ten out of the fifteen adjectives offered as descriptions of the staff were significantly related to women's satisfaction with the birth. Half of these described the staff positively (humorous, considerate, polite, warm and informative) and half negatively (insensitive, offhand, inconsiderate, bossy and condescending). Those women who saw the staff in positive terms felt more satisfied whilst those who saw them in negative terms felt less satisfied. Clearly the staff's attitude towards women was very important in their overall assessment of how pleased they were with the birth. Likewise, women's overall comments on the care they received at the hospital made at the end of the questionnaire were related to satisfaction.

Overall comments on care	n	Transformed mean (marks out of 10)[2]	Significance (F test)
Eulogy, excellent care	187	68	
Generally positive	69	62	$p < 0.001$
Mixed – positive and negative	57	57	
Generally negative	30	45	

Table 8.21: Satisfaction with birth by overall comments on care

Continuity of care

Women were more satisfied with the birth experience when there was at least one midwife with them for the duration of the labour ($p < 0.0001$). This was particularly true for multips. However, satisfaction was not related to having met the midwives antenatally.

The number of people present during labour was negatively related to satisfaction irrespective of parity ($p < 0.0001$). Again, lots of different people coming in and out is likely to be indicative of obstetric problems but may sometimes be due to insensitivity on the part of the staff.

These results mirror those already presented above with regard to fulfilment. Similarly, women whose birth companions were with them during only part of labour were less satisfied than either those whose companions were with them throughout or those who did not have a companion with them at all.

Antenatal predictors of satisfaction

Choice in where a woman was booked for delivery proved to be significantly associated with her overall satisfaction with birth ($p < 0.05$). Women who felt they had had a clear choice were more satisfied than those who did not. This does suggest that having choice about where to give birth is important but it may also be that women who are more easily satisfied are more likely to feel they have been given a choice.

There is an interesting association between antenatal class attendance and satisfaction with birth: women who at the time of the questionnaire (36 weeks pregnant) had attended classes were more dissatisfied than anybody else ($p < 0.01$). However, this association may well be explained by the fact that antenatal class attendance was strongly related to parity, education and social class; primips and well-educated women were far more likely to have attended classes than multips and less educated women. Women who described the classes they had attended as 'very good' were more satisfied than the women who did not ($p < 0.001$). Again, this might well be a reflection of how good the classes actually were, but it may also be simply a measure of how easily satisfied women were.

Confidence in relating to the staff was related to satisfaction. Women who felt they were always able to discuss things with staff had the highest satisfaction scores ($p < 0.01$). Likewise, the women who felt they were as assertive with staff as they wanted to be had higher scores than the women who did not feel as assertive as they wanted to be ($p < 0.001$).

Women who had been warned by their doctor that their delivery might not be straightforward were less satisfied ($p = 0.05$), perhaps because this expectation had been realized.

Feelings about continuous electronic fetal monitoring were related to satisfaction ($p < 0.05$). Women who quite liked or definitely wanted continuous monitoring were the most satisfied, and women who did not know enough to choose or who definitely did not want continuous monitoring were the least satisfied.

Several questions about antenatal expectations of pain during labour were significantly related to satisfaction with birth. Anxiety about the pain was associated with lower levels of satisfaction ($p < 0.01$), while women who said they would ideally prefer a drug-free labour were more satisfied than those who wanted drugs to control the pain ($p = 0.05$). The women who wanted a drug-free labour were less worried by the thought of the pain than those who wanted drugs. Indeed, the question on how painful women expected labour to be without drugs, was also related to satisfaction with birth ($p < 0.05$). Women who expected labour to be very painful or unbearably painful had lower satisfaction scores than those who did not expect this. In addition, expectations of the helpfulness of breathing and relaxation exercises were related to satisfaction ($p < 0.001$). The more helpful women expected the exercises to be, the more satisfied they were. We thus have the very important finding that high expectations do not inevitably lead to disappointment. On the contrary the most optimistic women are consistently most satisfied. This would seem to run contrary to the stereotype described in Chapter 1, and will be discussed further below.

Satisfaction and other postnatal outcomes

SATISFACTION AND FULFILMENT

These two outcome variables are very strongly related ($p < 0.0001$). Women who did not find birth fulfilling, or did not know what this meant, had much lower satisfaction scores.

SATISFACTION AND RELATIONSHIP WITH THE BABY

Relationship with baby is discussed in detail later in this chapter. Satisfaction with birth was not related to either the sex of the baby or to whether or not the mother breastfed the baby. It was related to whether the mother saw the baby as a sociable person ($p < 0.05$) but not in a very clear cut manner. Women who said the baby either was or was not a sociable person scored higher than those who said the baby was just starting to be sociable. However, there was no relationship between satisfaction and whether the woman felt her baby knew her, preferred her, how organized/disorganized life had been since the baby was born or who determined the routines of the household.

Five out of the 16 adjectives offered as descriptions of the baby were significantly related to satisfaction – women who perceived their baby as demanding ($p < 0.05$) and exhausting ($p < 0.001$) reported less satisfaction with the birth, whilst those who thought their baby was cuddly ($p < 0.01$), talkative ($p < 0.05$) and contented ($p < 0.05$) said that they were more satisfied. The adjective 'demanding' was no longer significant when the effects of parity were controlled.

The composite variable Description of Baby which measures the proportion of negative adjectives women used to describe their babies, was significantly related to satisfaction with birth ($p < 0.01$). Overall, then satisfaction with birth was related to how positively women described their babies, and the relationship was independent of both parity and class.

SATISFACTION AND EMOTIONAL WELL-BEING

Emotional well-being is discussed in detail later in this chapter. The question 'Have you been feeling at all depressed?' does not quite reach significance ($p = 0.06$). Women who were not at all depressed or only mildly so had higher satisfaction scores, but the differences were not very marked. Women who wanted things to be different, for example to have more time, rated the birth as less satisfying than those who were happy with the state of things. As so often, the 'not sure' women came out worst of all – they were the least satisfied ($p < 0.05$).

Four out of the six Edinburgh Postnatal Depression Scale items were associated with satisfaction. The most satisfied women were more likely to say they had looked forward to things as much as ever in the past week ($p < 0.05$) and were less likely to say things had been getting on top of them ($p < 0.05$), that they had problems sleeping because they were unhappy ($p < 0.01$) or that they had felt sad or miserable during the past week ($p < 0.01$). However, when we look at the composite Emotional Well-Being Factor, we find that it is not significantly associated with birth satisfaction as tested by analysis of variance although there is correlation through the upper range of scores (see discussion at the end of the chapter).

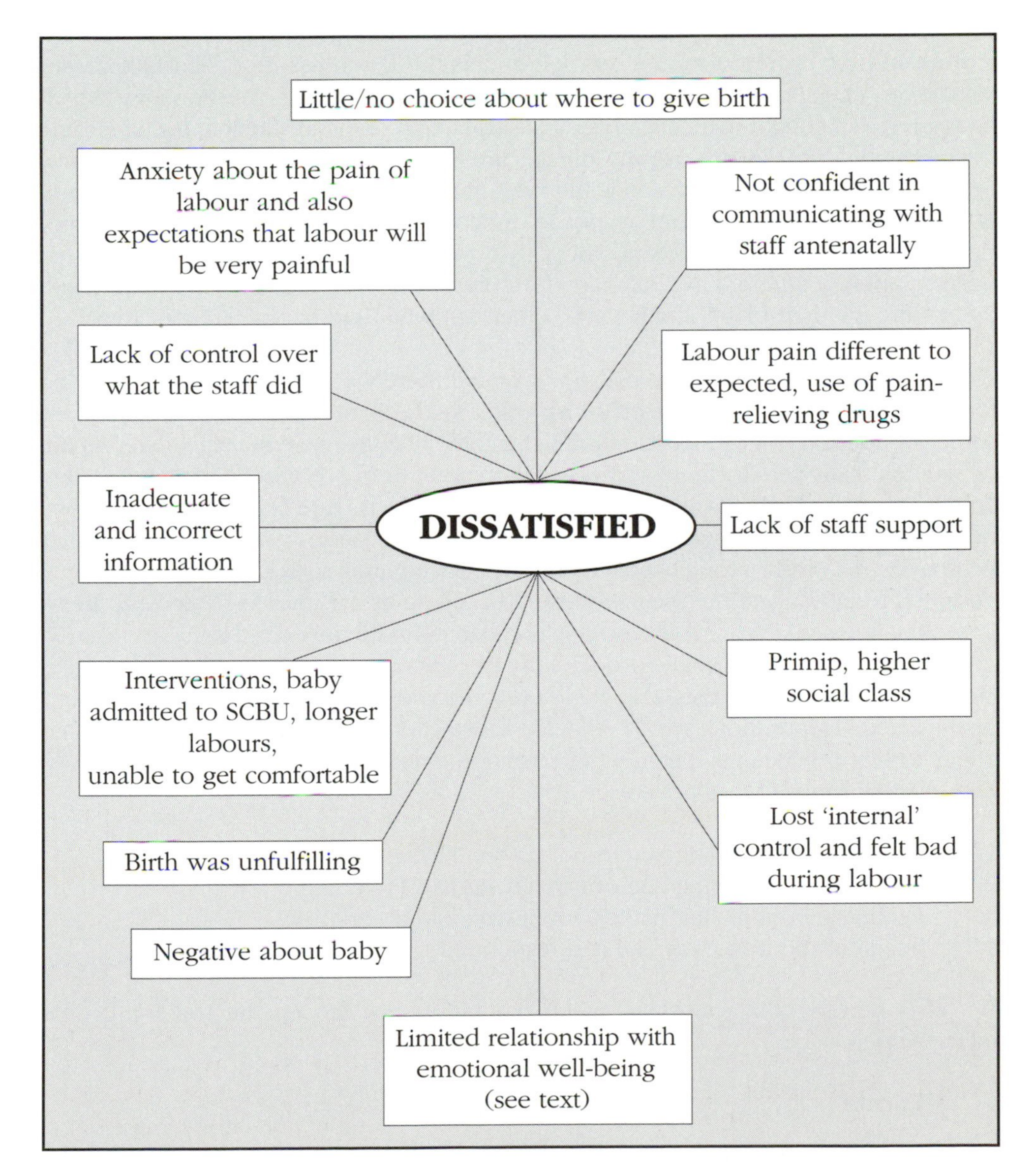

Dissatisfaction

Satisfaction factor analysis

Introduction

The problem with our measure of satisfaction with birth is a tendency for particular areas of dissatisfaction to be masked in the expression of feelings of relief, gratitude, happiness and so on which are elicited by a general question about satisfaction. This was discussed in Chapter 1 in relation to other research. Whilst this tendency may be less marked if the question is asked some time after birth rather than a few hours or days afterwards, it may also be that dissatisfaction with experiences of labour and delivery recede with time.

We were aware of this problem from the outset and although satisfaction with birth as expressed by a score out of ten was selected as the key measure of satisfaction, we also asked specific questions at earlier points in the postnatal questionnaire which attempted to highlight particular aspects of satisfaction or dissatisfaction, e.g. regarding interventions. We did not use the phrase 'are you satisfied' except in one instance regarding women's feelings about the way they responded to the pain of labour, where they were offered three response categories of satisfied, neither satisfied nor dissatisfied, and dissatisfied. In all other cases, we asked women whether they felt that what happened *should* have happened, or about their feelings on what happened. Essentially we tried to get at whether women felt what had happened was 'right'.

Our next step was to attempt to discover whether there was in fact a single underlying factor which determined women's responses to these questions, for example, are some women simply more easily satisfied than others? If this were the main determinant of women's answers to these individual questions then we would expect a strong correlation between them all. If, on the other hand, the picture is less simple, then we might expect that the answers to some subgroups of questions would cluster together without there being a strong overall correlation. Factor analysis is a statistical technique designed to investigate precisely this question. All items are intercorrelated and those groups of items which are most strongly correlated are identified as having a common underlying factor. (The analysis does not, of course, tell you what the underlying factor *is*, merely that it exists.) We therefore carried out a factor analysis on women's responses to 14 questions which reflected satisfaction or lack of it. The areas asked about were pain, feelings regarding intervention decisions and treatment by the staff. The four pain related questions were:

1. Feelings about having had or not having had gas and air
2. Feelings about having had or not having had Pethidine
3. Feelings about having had or not having had an epidural
4. Feelings about the way she had responded to the pain of labour.

We also asked about satisfaction with having or not having the following nine interventions:

5. Enema
6. Shave
7. Glucose drip
8. Episiotomy

9. Electronic fetal monitoring
10. Artificial rupture of membranes (ARM)
11. Induction
12. Acceleration.
13. Instrumental delivery.

Finally, we included one specific question about staff care:

14. Overall comments on treatment by the staff.

The 61 women who had caesarean sections were excluded from this analysis on the assumption that having a caesarean section is a major confounding factor for psychological outcome, further complicated by the fact that some women were psychologically prepared because an elective section had been planned, whilst others had emergency sections.

Factor analysis results

The analysis produced four factors, each representing a different area of satisfaction/ dissatisfaction. The details of the eigenvalues and factor loadings for each variable making up the factors after Varimax rotation are given in Appendix C2.

The formation of each factor is shown below.

Factor 1. Satisfaction regarding 'major' interventions

A group of mainly 'major' interventions cluster to yield the first factor, which accounts for 16.5 per cent of the variance. It is important to remember that we are not talking about satisfaction with the interventions themselves, but about whether women felt satisfied with what happened, whether or not they received these interventions. Factor 1 is linked to the following variables: satisfaction regarding induction, acceleration, forceps, glucose drip and episiotomy. These seem a logical combination of interventions to cluster together. Satisfaction with coping with pain also loads on this factor, although not as strongly as it does on Factor 2.

Factor 2. Satisfaction regarding pain and pain relief

Aspects of how women felt about how they coped with the pain cluster to yield the second factor which accounts for a further 8.6 per cent of the variance. The four variables which load on Factor 2 are: how women felt about using/not using Pethidine, their overall satisfaction with how they responded to the pain, how they felt about having/not having an epidural and about having/not having gas and air.

Factor 3. Satisfaction regarding 'minor' interventions

Factor 3 accounts for a further 8.3 per cent of the variance and is revealed by a group of mainly 'minor' interventions: shave, enema, glucose drip and ARM. Glucose drip loads on both Factor 1 and Factor 3, which suggests it straddles the boundary between major and minor interventions and may be viewed as either major or minor or perhaps as both. Note that, on the whole, women's feelings about the 'rightness' of having or not having particular interventions do fall into two groups which correspond to our earlier, relatively arbitrary, groups of interventions as 'major' and 'minor'. The fascinating exceptions are monitoring, which does not cluster with other interventions at all, and episiotomy. Women's feelings about episiotomy cluster with their feelings about major, not minor, interventions, reiterating the point that this procedure should not be undertaken lightly.

Factor 4. Satisfaction with staff care/monitoring

Two variables load on Factor 4: satisfaction with the way women were treated by the staff and satisfaction with the extent to which they had electronic fetal monitoring. The fact that these two variables go together suggests that women see electronic monitoring as an aspect of staff care, or that the process of monitoring requires staff to be in close contact with the women, something women may experience as caring. Factor 4 accounts for an additional 7.6 per cent of the variance. Taken together the four factors explain 41 per cent of the total variance.

Independent variables

The factors related differently to the main independent variables. Only Factors 1 and 2 (satisfaction with having/not having major interventions and satisfaction with pain and pain relief) were significantly associated with parity, with multips being more satisfied than primips. It is interesting to note that Factor 3 (satisfaction with having/not having minor interventions) is independent of parity, as tested by analysis of variance. Only Factor 3 was related to unit: women who gave birth at the three Exington units were least satisfied, women who gave birth at Zedbury were the most satisfied. This finding is the reverse of the result for overall satisfaction (i.e. satisfaction with the birth experience) where women at Zedbury were the least satisfied and those at Exington GP unit were the most satisfied. Given that overall satisfaction is related to not having interventions we might have expected the higher score on Factor 3 at Zedbury to be associated with a low rate of minor interventions there. Zedbury does not in fact have a low minor intervention rate so the explanation may be that staff there are particularly good at presenting minor interventions in a way women find acceptable. Factors 2 and 4 (satisfaction with pain and pain relief and satisfaction with care/monitoring) were related to education: the more educated women were the least satisfied. Finally, Factors 1, 3 and 4 were related to women's social class. However, whereas for Factor 4 women in the highest social groups were the least satisfied (as for overall satisfaction), they were the *most* satisfied as far as Factors 1 and 3 were concerned. As already noted, both Factor 1 and Factor 3 were to do with having/not having interventions and how women felt about this. Working class women did not in fact have more interventions nor did they feel that they should have had, so it is difficult to explain their dissatisfaction unless it is a reflection of some lack of involvement in the decision making process. Table 8.22 summarizes these relationships.

Independent Variable	Factor	Significance (F test)
Parity	Factor 1	$p < 0.01$
	Factor 2	$p < 0.001$
	Satisfaction with birth	$p < 0.001$
Unit	Factor 3	$p < 0.01$
	Satisfaction with birth	$p < 0.05$
Education	Factor 2	$p < 0.01$
	Factor 4	$p < 0.05$
Woman's social class	Factor 1	$p < 0.05$
	Factor 3	$p < 0.05$
	Factor 4	$p < 0.05$
	Satisfaction with birth	$p < 0.05$

Table 8.22: Satisfaction Factors by the main independent variables

'External' control

Turning now to other important variables, control over what the staff were doing was significantly related to all four satisfaction factors. In each case, the women who were most satisfied were those who were always in control followed by those who were in control most of the time. However, for Factors 1, 2 and 3, the women who were most dissatisfied were those who were in control for only some of the time rather than those who were never or hardly ever in control. We would suggest that the explanation for this may lie in difficulties that arose during labour requiring obstetrical intervention or pain relief that women ideally did not want. In such a situation, especially where negotiation was poor, women who *had* felt in control would feel that that control had been summarily removed from them. In the case of Factor 4, the staff care and monitoring factor, there was a linear relationship between the degree of control a woman reported and how satisfied she was: women who were hardly ever in control of what the staff did were the most dissatisfied.

Factors 1, 2 and 3 were significantly associated with whether women felt in control of emergency decision making, but each in a somewhat different way. No factor was significantly related to control of non-emergency decision making.

All the factors were related to information: women who had received what they felt to be the correct amount of information and accurate information were the most satisfied.

'Internal' control

All aspects of having 'internal' control (control of behaviour, control during contractions and the amount of noise women made) were related to Factors 1, 2 and 4 (satisfaction with major intervention decisions, pain and pain relief, and satisfaction with aspects of staff care). However, none were related to Factor 3 – satisfaction with minor intervention decisions. In each instance, women who remained in control or did not make much noise were the most satisfied. Women who were not sure of how much noise they made were the most dissatisfied, followed by those who made a lot of noise.

Interventions

Satisfaction with whether a woman had or did not have major interventions (Factor 1) was inversely related to all the interventions, with the exception of shaves and ARM, i.e. women who had interventions were less satisfied. Satisfaction with how a woman coped with pain and with using/not using pain relieving drugs (Factor 2) was inversely related to all the interventions with the exceptions of shaves and inductions. Satisfaction with having or not having minor interventions (Factor 3) was inversely related to all the interventions with the exceptions of monitoring and instrumental delivery. Even where relationships were not significant, the trend was always in the same direction – women who did not have the interventions were more satisfied. Factors 1, 2 and 3 were all inversely related to the total number of interventions experienced. Satisfaction with aspects of staff care (Factor 4) was not related to any of the interventions with the sole exception of ARM. Thus, it seems that having interventions does not lead women to feel dissatisfied with how they are treated by staff. Instead, women assess the quality of care separately from the interventions that are carried out.

It needs to be remembered that there is likely to be a parity effect in the significant relationships between Factors 1 and 2 and interventions. Further analysis is required in order to determine whether a relationship still exists once the effects of parity have been controlled.

Tables 8.23–8.26 summarize the relationships between the four factors and particular aspects of labour.

Psychological outcomes

Each factor was significantly associated with the score out of ten for overall satisfaction with birth. These associations were significant both by a test of analysis of variance and by Pearson's correlation coefficient. Factor 3 (satisfaction with having/not having minor interventions) was less strongly related to overall satisfaction with birth than the other three factors.

The relationships with the other psychological outcome variables are as follows: Factors 1 and 2 were related to fulfilment, Factors 3 and 4 were not (as tested by analysis of variance). Thus fulfilment was related to only two aspects of satisfaction: how women felt about having/not having major interventions and how they felt about pain and pain-relieving drugs. Although we already knew that fulfilment was related to overall satisfaction, factor analysis has enabled us to get a clearer idea of precisely which aspects of satisfaction relate to fulfilment.

Using Pearson's correlation coefficient, emotional well-being was found to be significantly correlated with Factors 1 and 3 but not Factors 2 and 4, i.e. it was related to how women felt about having or not having various interventions, both major and minor, but not to satisfaction with coping with pain or with staff care.

The only factor related to the composite Descriptions of Baby variable was Factor 3, but the relationship was not linear (analysis of variance). The individual adjectives describing the baby also showed little or no relationship with any factor.

Summary

The aim of carrying out the satisfaction factor analysis was to try to pinpoint possible aspects of satisfaction/dissatisfaction that may be masked by the global question on satisfaction with the birth experience. Furthermore, we wished to see if the global question related to certain dimensions of satisfaction rather than others.

The factor analysis produced four distinct factors which do distinguish between different aspects of satisfaction/dissatisfaction. Two of these reflect women's feelings about having/not having major and minor interventions, another deals with pain and pain relief while the fourth reflects feelings about monitoring and (other) aspects of the care received from staff. Each factor is significantly related to the global satisfaction with birth question. Thus, we can conclude that women's overall satisfaction with birth, as expressed by the mark they gave it out of ten, does reflect the various dimensions of satisfaction as represented by the factors.

The four factors do relate to somewhat different variables, although there are also features that they have in common. Factors 1 and 2, in particular, seem to pick up on the same variables. Factors 3 and 4 have in common a very weak relationship with pain and pain relief, a weak or no relationship with Description of Baby, and no relationship with parity, length of labour or fulfilment (unlike Factors 1 and 2).

Control over what the staff did, the amount and accuracy of information received and being able to get into the most comfortable position possible were all significantly related to each satisfaction factor, and can therefore be seen as key ingredients in women's satisfaction. (They were all also significantly related to overall satisfaction with birth.) Additionally, each aspect of 'internal' control was related to Factors 1, 2 and 4 and also to overall satisfaction with birth, although Factor 3 was completely unrelated to 'internal' control.

Finally, a very important finding that we wish to draw out of these results is that emotional well-being is related to Factors 1 and 3, that is to satisfaction with having/not having interventions, although it is unrelated to having the interventions themselves (see section on emotional well-being). Thus, the context in which decisions about interventions are made is seen to be highly important since it is women's perceptions of the necessity or the 'rightness' of intervention which seems to be critical to their emotional well-being rather than the experience of the interventions per se. Women who felt that the right thing happened, that the right decision was made to intervene or not, were significantly happier.

Factor	Significant Relationships (F Test)
FACTOR 1 Satisfaction with having or not having major interventions	**Pain and pain relief** Effectiveness of gas and air Feelings about using/not using gas and air Use of and feelings about Pethidine Use of and feelings about epidurals Use of breathing and relaxation exercises Overall response to pain **Internal control** Control over behaviour Control during contractions Amount of noise made **Relationship with staff** Only significant adjective – BOSSY Not related to general comments on care **Feelings during labour** Related to eight adjectives, which mostly describe aspects of control: calm, confident, involved, alert, in control, powerless, helpless, out of control **Interventions** All except shaves and ARM **Length of labour** **External control** Emergency decision making Control of what the staff did Amount of information Accurate information **Comfortable position** – able to get into **Relationship with baby** Little association with baby adjectives – 'fascinating' & 'responsive' – just significant **Psychological outcomes** Related to satisfaction with birth, fulfilment, emotional well-being. Not related to Description of Baby

Table 8.23

Factor	Significant Relationships (F Test)
FACTOR 2 Satisfaction with pain and pain relief	**Pain and pain relief** Pain in labour conformed to expectations All aspects of using gas and air, Pethidine and epidurals Use of and usefulness of breathing and relaxation exercises Overall response to pain **Internal control** Control over behaviour and contractions Amount of noise made **Relationship with staff** Related to eight adjectives: insensitive, off hand, inconsiderate, bossy, condescending, sensitive, warm, considerate. Not related to general comments on care by staff. **Feelings during labour** Related to nearly all the adjectives offered **Interventions** All except shaves and inductions **Length of labour** **External control** Emergency decision making Control of what the staff did Amount and accuracy of information **Comfortable position** **Relationship with baby** Not very marked relationship. Only associated with four adjectives: placid, stubborn, demanding, unresponsive. **Psychological outcomes** Related to satisfaction with birth and fulfilment. Not related to emotional well-being or Description of Baby.

Table 8.24

Factor	Significant Relationships (F test)
FACTOR 3 Satisfaction with having or not having minor interventions	**Pain and pain relief** Weak relationship overall. Only related to feelings about using/not using gas and air and epidural. Not related to use of drugs. Related to overall response to pain (p = 0.05) **Internal control** Not related to any aspect of internal control **Relationship with staff** Related to some, mainly positive, adjectives of staff behaviour: humorous, sensitive, insensitive, polite, supportive, informative. Related to general comments on staff care **Feelings during labour** Not related to adjectives describing feelings. **Interventions** All except monitoring and forceps Not related to **length of labour** **External control** Emergency decision making Control of what the staff did Amount and accuracy of information **Comfortable position** **Relationship with baby** Little association with adjectives – only 'fascinating' and 'responsive' **Psychological outcomes** Related to satisfaction with birth and emotional well-being. Non linear relationship with Description of Baby. Not related to fulfilment.

Table 8.25

Factor	Significant Relationships (F test)
FACTOR 4 Satisfaction with aspects of staff care and monitoring	**Pain and pain relief** Very weak relationship with pain and pain relief Only aspect significant: feelings about having/not having Pethidine. Related to overall response to pain **Internal control** Related to control of behaviour and contractions Related to amount of noise made **Relationship with staff** Strongly related to all adjectives describing the staff Strongly related to general comments on staff care **Feelings during labour** Related to eight adjectives which mostly describe aspects of control: calm, confident, involved, in control, alert, powerless, helpless, out of control (exactly the same as Factor 1) **Interventions** No relationship except with ARM **Length of labour:** no relationship **External control** Related to control over what staff did Amount and accuracy of information **Comfortable position** **Relationship with baby** No relationship with any adjectives **Psychological outcomes** Related to satisfaction with birth Not related to fulfilment, Description of Baby or emotional well-being

Table 8.26

Description of baby

To get some idea of how women perceived their babies we asked them to circle all the adjectives in a given list which described their baby, as well as giving them the option to add their own descriptions. The question format, showing the percentages of the sample that circled each adjective, is shown below.

'Could you please circle all the words below which describe your baby.

Placid (35%)	Alert (92%)	Demanding (42%)	Unresponsive (<1%)
Responsive (77%)	Stubborn (15%)	Cuddly (76%)	Draining (11%)
Grizzly (13%)	Fascinating (61%)	Exhausting (26%)	Determined (33%)
Talkative (41%)	Angry (7%)	Fretful (7%)	Contented (75%)

Is there anything else that you would like to tell us about your baby?'

The most popular adjectives were 'alert', 'responsive', 'cuddly' and 'contented'. Women were least likely to describe their babies as 'unresponsive', 'fretful' or 'angry'. Women were also very ready to add glowing comments about their babies. 'He's wonderful, a really little angel', 'She's beautiful, but I'm biased!'. They were less ready to add negative comments.

For ease of presentation we divided the sample into three groups: the women who did not circle any negative adjectives, the women whose adjectives were at least 60 per cent positive and the women who gave a lower proportion of positive adjectives than this. We have called these three groups 'positive', 'mixed' and 'negative' about the baby. (We used the proportion of negative adjectives circled to control for differences caused by differences in the overall number of words circled.) Obviously, this is rather a blunt instrument and not all the adjectives can be clearly identified as positive or negative or may be of equal positive or negative weight. For the purposes of this analysis, however, we defined as 'negative' the following adjectives: 'angry', 'fretful', 'grizzly', 'exhausting', 'stubborn', 'draining', 'unresponsive' and 'demanding'.

'Negative' does not refer to the quality of relationship with the baby *per se* but refers to the proportion of negative adjectives used to describe the baby.

Description of baby and other perceptions of baby

Women who saw their babies as sociable and those who said their babies knew them were more positive about their babies than the other women ($p < 0.0001$ and $p < 0.001$ respectively) (see Appendix B22).

There was no association between Description of Baby and whether women felt their babies preferred them to other people.

Description of baby and parity

Multips were more likely to describe their babies as placid (42% compared to 23%). Primips were more likely to see their babies as demanding (57% compared to 32%), stubborn (23% compared to 10%), grizzly (19% compared to 10%), exhausting (33% compared to 22%), determined (44% compared to 27%) and angry (11% compared to 5%). They were, however, also more likely to see their babies as fascinating (71% compared to 56%). Not surprisingly given these differences on individual items, primips also came out as much more negative about their babies overall.

Parity	Positive		Mixed		Negative	
	n	%	n	%	n	%
Primips	62	(22)	127	(46)	87	(32)
Multips	215	(50)	135	(32)	76	(18)

Percentages are of women of a given parity

$p < 0.0001$

Table 8.27: Description of Baby by parity

Primips and multips were equally likely to see the baby as a sociable person or to feel that their baby knew them or preferred them to other people.

Primips came across differently in their qualitative comments as well. It was primips who seemed most stunned by the changes having a baby had made to their lives:

> 'I have never felt so trapped in all my life. The sudden responsibility for another little, totally dependent human being is overwhelming.'

> 'I can't do what I want to do anymore, everything revolves around my daughter. I didn't think it would be as bad as all this.'

Primips, in particular, talked about feeling inadequate, unsure of their own ability to care for a baby and helpless in the face of their babies' tears:

> 'Sometimes I feel I cannot, or rather am not able to look after my baby well enough, for instance, if she is crying and I cannot find the reason I feel useless.'

All data discussed in the following section has been analysed to ensure that it is independent of parity unless specified otherwise.

Description of baby and the events of labour

CONTROL

There was no association between Description of Baby and how involved women had felt in emergency or non-emergency decision making, nor with whether or not they felt in control of what staff did to them. Multips who felt in control of their own behaviour were more positive about their babies, but this was not true for primips.

Description of baby and feelings during labour

The only relationship between feelings during labour and Description of Baby was that multips who described themselves as 'involved' during labour were more positive about their babies than multips who did not circle this adjective ($p < 0.05$) and multips who described themselves as 'detached' during labour were less positive about their babies than other multips ($p < 0.01$). For multips, then, it would seem that the degree of involvement or detachment experienced during labour is associated with how they perceive their babies. There was also an association for both primips and multips with feeling 'challenged' during labour. Women who did not circle this adjective were more often purely positive about their babies than those who did circle it (53% compared to 41%; $p < 0.05$). Feeling 'challenged' during labour is thus associated with a more negative description of the baby. Women who were always able to get comfortable were less negative about their babies than other women ($p < 0.01$) (see Appendix B21). However when broken down by parity the effect only holds for multips.

Description of baby and interventions

Women who had caesarean sections were more negative about their babies than those who had vaginal deliveries. There were, however, no differences associated with whether the operation was planned in advance or with what type of anaesthesia was used.

	Positive		Mixed		Negative	
	n	%	n	%	n	%
Caesarean section	19	(32)	19	(32)	22	(37)
Vaginal delivery	262	(41)	243	(38)	139	(22)

Percentages are of women in a given row

$p < 0.05$

Table 8.28: Description of Baby by caesarean section

Description of Baby was not associated with any of the other individual interventions considered, nor was there any straightforward relationship with the total number of interventions experienced.

Description of baby and pain

Women who found the pain unexpected in some way were more negative about their babies than those who found it exactly as they expected. This relationship was independent of parity effects but when looked at by educational level we found that the association remained statistically significant only for those women who left school at 16 or under. There was no association between Description of Baby and the use of pain relieving drugs.

Pain as expected	Positive		Mixed		Negative	
	n	%	n	%	n	%
No, not at all	47	(36)	53	(40)	32	(24)
Yes, in some way	89	(35)	109	(43)	56	(22)
Yes exactly	130	(49)	83	(31)	52	(20)

Percentages are of women in a given row.

$p < 0.05$

Table 8.29: Description of Baby by pain as expected

Description of baby and birth companions

Women who only had their birth companion with them some of the time (as discussed earlier, these were mainly women who had wanted their companion with them throughout labour) were the most negative about their babies. This finding holds true independently for both multips and primips. It is also interesting to note that those who had no birth companion were overwhelmingly positive about their babies.

	Positive		Mixed		Negative	
	n	%	n	%	n	%
Yes, all of the time	232	(39)	240	(40)	127	(21)
Yes, some of the time	10	(30)	7	(21)	16	(49)
No, not at all	26	(72)	6	(17)	4	(11)

Percentages are of women in a given row.

$p < 0.0001$

Table 8.30: Description of Baby by birth companion

Description of baby and information

Women who felt they had been given the right amount of information were more positive about their babies than other women.

Right amount of information?	Positive		Mixed		Negative	
	n	%	n	%	n	%
Yes	211	(42)	189	(38)	101	(20)
No	67	(34)	71	(36)	59	(30)

Percentages are of women in a given row

$p < 0.05$

Table 8.31: Description of Baby by amount of information

Similarly, women who felt that they had known enough antenatally or did not feel they had been given misleading information were also more likely to be positive about their babies.

Wish you had known more	Positive		Mixed		Negative	
	n	%	n	%	n	%
Yes	41	(29)	58	(42)	40	(29)
No	236	(43)	196	(36)	117	(21)

Percentages are of women in a given row

$p < 0.05$

Table 8.32: Description of Baby by lack of information

Given misleading information	Positive		Mixed		Negative	
	n	%	n	%	n	%
Yes	37	(31)	40	(34)	41	(35)
No	236	(41)	216	(38)	120	(21)

Percentages are of women in a given row

$p < 0.01$

Table 8.33: Description of Baby by misleading information

These women are probably focusing in the main on information given about postnatal factors (e.g. breastfeeding and life with a new baby), 'no one gives you any idea of how responsible you are for a new baby, the buck stops here', rather than about labour itself. A fact which would support this suggestion is that Description of Baby was unrelated to any of the questions we asked antenatally about information. However, some of the comments about inadequate information also related to unexpected aspects of the labour such as having an emergency caesarean section or finding the pain different from what was expected.

Description of baby and description of staff

Women's descriptions of their babies did not relate to any of the staff variables such as overall assessment of staff care, or continuity of care and nor did it relate to 14 out of the 15 adjectives women were offered to describe the staff. The one adjective that they *did* relate to was 'informative'. Women who found the staff informative were more positive about their babies ($p < 0.05$). This echoes the link we have found between all the direct information questions and women's descriptions of their babies. Information is a central issue. In fact, many of the criticisms of staff being uninformative or giving conflicting advice revolved around the subject of breastfeeding and, as the following section shows, breastfeeding was also strongly associated with Description of Baby.

Description of baby and breastfeeding

(see also Volume 2, Chapter 9)

Women who had tried but given up breastfeeding their baby, circled most negative adjectives about their babies while women who had never tried to breastfeed were the most positive.

	Positive		Mixed		Negative	
	n	%	n	%	n	%
Did not breastfeed	90	(55)	44	(27)	31	(19)
Still breastfeeding	140	(37)	154	(41)	83	(22)
Breastfed but stopped	50	(31)	64	(39)	49	(30)

Percentages are of women in a given row

$p < 0.0001$

NB. This finding is confounded by the different feeding practices of multips and primips. When broken down by parity the pattern remains true for multips but is not significant for primips (see Appendix B20).

Table 8.34: Description of Baby by breastfeeding

When we look at the specific adjectives used to describe the baby, we find that women who had tried but given up breastfeeding were more likely than women who had never breastfed to describe their babies as stubborn, determined, demanding and exhausting. Women who were still breastfeeding were also more likely than those who had never tried to breastfeed to describe their baby as determined, demanding and exhausting. However, they were not more likely to describe their baby as stubborn. Women wrote about the process of trying to breastfeed as very time-consuming and problems with feeding tied in with feelings of inadequacy and resentment of the way the baby had changed their lives. It is not, therefore, surprising that women who tried to breastfeed their babies were more likely to describe their babies in negative terms. The negative feelings were particularly noticeable in comments made by women who felt they had failed to breastfeed:

> 'To make things worse, I had so wanted to breastfeed but because of the shock of the Caesarean my milk never arrived. This made me feel even worse of a failure, and I spent a week trying to feed a desperately hungry baby and, dare I say it, gradually beginning to wish that I had never had him because he cried continually, night and day.'

The negative adjectives seem clearly related to women's engagement with the babies in the struggle to breastfeed. On the positive side, women who tried to breastfeed (whether or not they were still breastfeeding by six weeks) were more likely to describe their babies as 'fascinating'. The first few weeks of breastfeeding are often the most fraught and we might have found a group of women still breastfeeding who were more positive about their babies had we approached them at a later stage. When women were able to establish successful breastfeeding this could be a source of satisfaction and relief:

> 'I enjoy her very much. I think a lot of it is that she corresponds to accepted ideals fairly well, i.e. feeds 3–4 hourly and has a long sleep at night and is awake all evening. Her older sister didn't and I felt overwhelmed and a failure as a consequence.'

> 'I feel very at ease with my baby, he is very easy to please and settles down very well when he has been fed.'

It should also be noted that it was the women who were breastfeeding, followed by those who had tried but given up, who were more likely to see their baby as 'a sociable person' ($p < 0.0001$) and to feel that their baby preferred them to other people ($p < 0.05$). The women who bottlefed their babies seemed in some ways more distanced from them.

Description of baby and organization

Women who were most positive about their babies were also most likely to describe life since the birth as organized and more likely to feel that they determined the overall daily routine ($p < 0.001$). They were less likely to say they wanted things to be different ($p < 0.0001$). These factors were all independent of parity except that the link between being negative about the baby and feeling out of control of the daily routine only held true for multips.

	Positive		Mixed		Negative	
	n	%	n	%	n	%
Totally/fairly disorganized	65	(24)	108	(41)	93	(35)
Neither	33	(39)	36	(43)	15	(18)
Fairly/very organized	183	(52)	118	(33)	54	(15)

Percentages are of women in a given row.

$p < 0.0001$

Table 8.35: Description of Baby by organization of life

It was clear that some women felt trapped by their babies. One woman who felt her baby controlled the day and who described her baby as stubborn, draining, demanding and determined wrote:

> 'I feel the entire day and my life revolves around him. If not actually feeding, changing etc. (I am) preparing to do so or thinking how to stop him crying, panicking etc.'

Antenatal predictors of description of baby

Women who felt cheerful during their pregnancy were more likely to describe their baby positively ($p < 0.01$). Women who antenatally expressed a preference for 'natural' labour (e.g. would ideally prefer a drug-free labour, rejected epidurals and said they would try for a vaginal delivery even if it was almost certain that they would need a caesarean section) were also more positive about their babies. Attending antenatal classes was, however, a factor associated with negative descriptions of their babies (a fact that is probably associated with the parity and education differences in class attendance). Similarly, women who were in paid employment during pregnancy were more negative about their babies ($p < 0.0001$), but this was purely an effect of parity and there are no differences when parity was controlled for. The majority of women in paid work were primips.

Description of baby and emotional well-being

Women's descriptions of their babies were clearly related to their own emotional well-being as measured by their EWB score ($p < 0.0001$). Women who were more positive about their babies were more likely to say there were more good days than bad ($p < 0.0001$), and that they looked forward with enjoyment to things as much as ever ($p < 0.0001$). They were less likely to say they had been feeling depressed ($p < 0.0001$), or anxious ($p < 0.0001$), panicky ($p < 0.0001$) or that they had been feeling sad ($p < 0.0001$) or so unhappy that they had difficulty sleeping ($p < 0.05$). They were also less likely to say that things have been getting on top of them ($p < 0.0001$).

In summary, being negative about the baby is related more to postnatal factors such as breastfeeding and how life is organized (or not) than to the experience of labour and birth itself. In addition, being negative about the baby is associated with not being happy during the pregnancy and with low postnatal emotional well-being – an association which could logically be causal in either direction.

The link between parity and Description of Baby is particularly interesting as it seems to be additional to primips' and multips' different experiences of labour. Where the factors discussed above are confounded by parity (e.g. getting comfortable) the association remains true for multips but not for primips. It seems that there is something so overwhelming about the nature of first time motherhood that (regardless of most of the events during labour) primips describe their babies more negatively than multips.

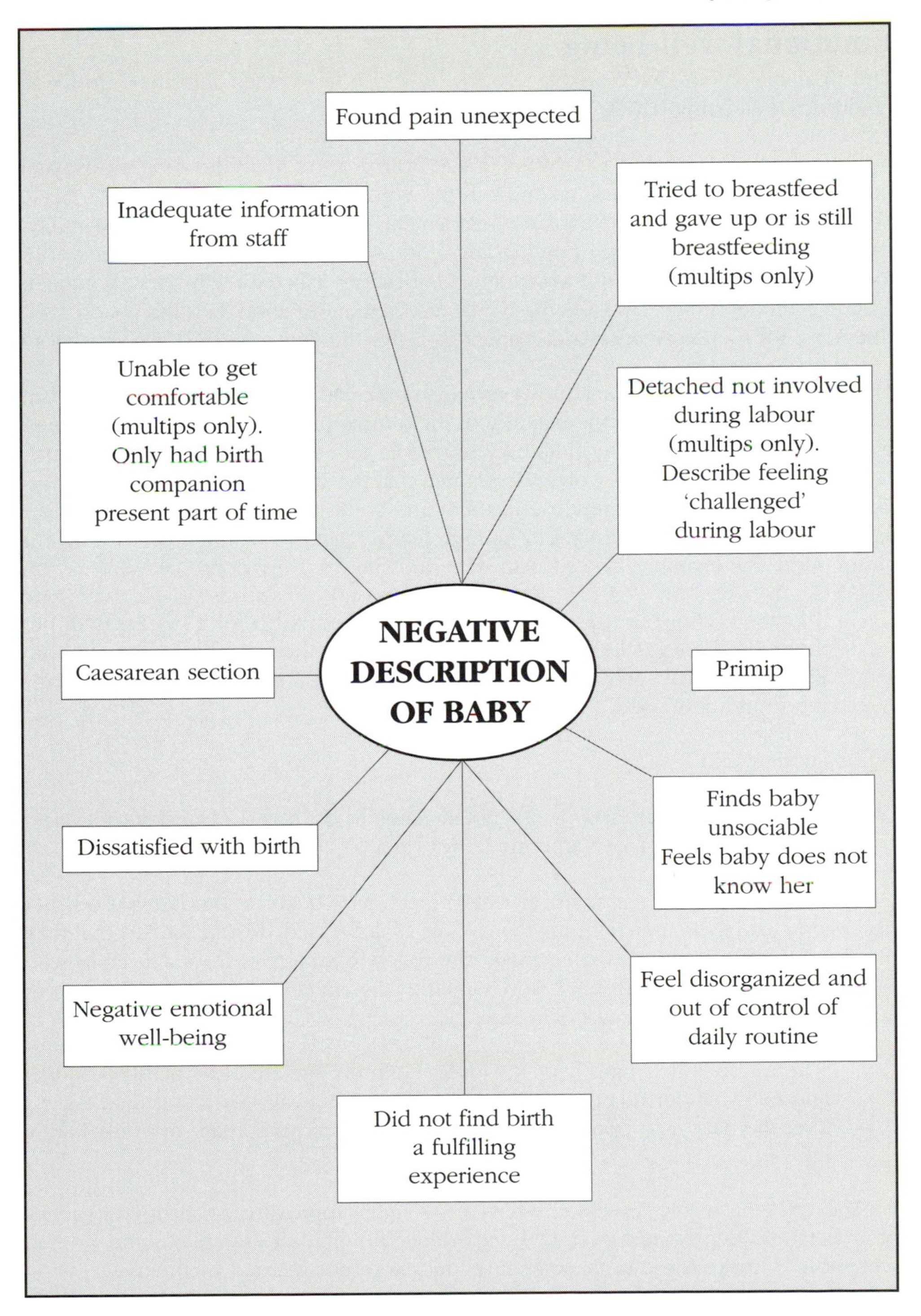

Negative description of baby

Emotional well-being

The final major outcome variable used to assess how women felt after birth was emotional well-being (EWB).

An Emotional Well-Being Factor was derived from a factor analysis of eight postnatal questions. Six questions were taken from the Edinburgh Postnatal Depression Scale and concerned women's experience of enjoyment, anxiety, fear/panic, coping ability, difficulty in sleeping because of unhappiness, and sadness/misery over the week prior to filling in the questionnaire. Two additional questions asked directly 'Have you been feeling at all depressed?' and 'On the whole are there more good days than bad?'. (See Chapter 2 for the explanation and Appendix C1 for the details of the factor analysis.)

The response to the individual questions which make up the EWB factor are shown in Table 8.36. This shows that the majority of the sample had experienced some degree of depression since the birth of the baby and nine per cent said they had been 'quite' or 'very' depressed. Several women explained that the cause of such depression was due to the death of someone close to them and were keen to stress that it was not related to the birth or the baby itself, perhaps fearing that this would otherwise be our assumption. For example, one woman who said she was very depressed wrote:

> 'I have no complaints about my baby. I could not wish for a better child, but these last three weeks I had have to watch my mother dying in such pain from leukaemia. That's why I have had to tick the ones I have ticked which makes me sound depressed.'

While another said:

> 'My depressions are *in myself* – not attached to days as such and do not affect my friendship and love with my baby.'

However, experiencing a stressful life event such as a death in the family does not necessarily lead to women defining themselves as depressed, despite the fact that they may come over to others as depressed. The following quote is from a woman who said she was 'not at all depressed', and highlights the limitations of single questions in tapping into complicated emotional feelings:

> 'There's not much apart from my lovely children. We are older parents (40-ish) and many of our relatives are ill or have passed away. My father died 9 days after the baby was born. He hasn't seen her. Our children are our only family life.'

Feelings of being 'mildly depressed' which may roughly approximate Oakley's categories of anxiety and depressed mood were experienced by half the sample. Some women were able to make sense of these feelings and were not worried by them, accepting them as a 'normal' part of early motherhood:

> 'Feelings of worry or anxiety or depression occur mildly and I can definitely attribute them to being tired most of the time. I am confident this will pass and do not resent it. I was prepared for how I would feel.'

Variable		n	%
Been feeling depressed since birth?			
No, not at all		292	(41)
Mildly		352	(50)
Yes, quite		49	(7)
Yes, very		16	(2)
	Total	709	(100)
More good days than bad?			
Yes, more good days		594	(84)
Half and half		95	(13)
No, more bad days		16	(2)
	Total	705	(100)
Looked forward with enjoyment to things during the last week?			
As much as I ever did		487	(69)
Rather less than I used to		171	(24)
Definitely less than I used to		31	(4)
Hardly at all		18	(3)
	Total	707	(100)
Anxious or worried for no good reason? *			
No, not at all		307	(43)
Hardly ever		173	(24)
Yes, sometimes		203	(29)
Yes, very often		26	(4)
	Total	709	(100)
Scared or panicky for no very good reason? *			
Yes, quite a lot		10	(1)
Yes, sometimes		95	(13)
No, not much		151	(21)
No, not at all		453	(64)
	Total	709	(100)
Things have been getting on top of me *			
Yes, not coping at all most of the time		7	(1)
Yes, not coping as well as usual sometimes		173	(24)
No, coping quite well most of the time		379	(53)
No, coping as well as ever		150	(21)
	Total	709	(100)

Difficulty in sleeping because so unhappy *			
Yes, most of the time		12	(2)
Yes, sometimes		29	(4)
Not very often		67	(9)
No, not at all		601	(85)
	Total	709	(100)
Felt sad or miserable during the last week *			
Yes, most of the time		13	(2)
Yes, quite often		72	(10)
Not very often		322	(46)
No, not at all		299	(42)
	Total	706	(100)

* Question applied to feelings during the previous week

Table 8.36: Responses to individual questions assessing Emotional well-being

Emotional Well-Being Factor (EWB) – Data analysis

As only a minority of women had low emotional well-being scores across the range of questions, the factor scores were highly skewed towards the upper end of the distribution. The data were transformed by cubing to improve normality and analysis of variance was then performed to test the relationships between the EWB factor and the postnatal data. Thus, the mean transformed factor score was the measure of emotional well-being employed in the analysis.

Results

None of the major independent variables considered (parity, unit, woman's social class, partner's social class, education) were related to emotional well-being.

Emotional well-being and obstetric interventions

CAESAREAN SECTION

Research has shown a link between having a caesarean section and experiencing postnatal depression, or generally feeling worse emotionally after birth (Oakley and Richards, 1988). In our sample, an analysis of variance on the EWB scores did not find a significant difference between women who had had a caesarean section and women who had not. However, a chi-square analysis on the non-transformed EWB scores divided into five discrete categories ranging from high to low emotional well-being did find a significant difference ($p < 0.01$), in the expected direction. Thus, 24 per cent of women who had a caesarean section fell into the low EWB group, compared to only ten per cent of those who had not, while seven per cent of women who had a section fell into the high EWB group compared to 11 per cent of those who had not.

	Low EWB (i.e. bottom 11% of scores)	High EWB (i.e. top 11% of scores)	Total no. of women who had/did not have a caesarean section
No. women who had a caesarean section	14	4	59
% of women who had a caesarean section	24	7	
No. of women who did not have a caesarean section	60	72	632
% of women who did not have a caesarean section	10	11	

Table 8.37: Low/high EWB by caesarean section and vaginal delivery

Other interventions

No other obstetric interventions were significantly related to EWB. There was also no relationship between the number of interventions experienced and EWB. This is a very important finding in the context of Oakley's (1980) conclusion that medium to high levels of intervention were associated with depression and is supported by Elliott et al. (1984) who also found no relationship between the amount of intervention used and depression.

Previously, in the analysis of the four satisfaction factors we found that Factors 1 and 3 (satisfaction with having/not having major and minor interventions) were significantly related to EWB. Thus we arrive at the critical discovery that while emotional well-being is unrelated to interventions themselves, it is related to how women feel about having or not having interventions (as was suggested by Elliott et al., 1984). The importance of the kind of communication that takes place between staff and women in a situation where there is a question on the part of one or the other about the necessity to intervene, is highlighted.

Other 'medical' aspects of labour

Emotional well-being was not related to any other variable which may be indicative of medical problems or events during labour: being seen by a doctor during labour, being delivered by a doctor, the length of labour or whether the baby was admitted to a Special Care Baby Unit.

Pain and pain relief

There does not appear to be a strong or coherent relationship between emotional well-being and the use of pain-relieving drugs in labour. Women who used Pethidine had lower EWB scores than those who did not; women who were not sure about whether they had used Pethidine had the lowest scores of all ($p < 0.05$). The effectiveness of gas and air was significantly related to emotional well-being ($p < 0.01$); however, it was women who said the drug was not effective who had the highest scores, followed by those who said it was very effective. Feeling under pressure from staff to have either gas and air or an epidural was significantly related to emotional well-being ($p < 0.05$) but again, not in a very straightforward way. While in each case women who felt under pressure to have these drugs had the lowest EWB scores, women who had felt encouraged by staff *not* to have gas and air and women who had felt under actual pressure *not* to have an epidural had the highest scores. This may be because such encouragement/pressure was experienced by women as supporting their own wishes not to have these drugs.

Women's feelings about their overall response to the pain of labour was not related to emotional well-being. Feeling dissatisfied with the way they coped with the pain was not therefore directly related to feeling unhappy postnatally.

Emotional well-being and 'external' control

Emotional well-being was not related to the two specific aspects of 'external' control – decision making in emergency and non-emergency situations. However, the question 'Did you feel in control of what the staff were doing to you during labour' was related to emotional well-being ($p < 0.001$). Women who said they were always in control had the highest EWB scores followed by those who felt they were in control most of the time. Women who were only in control some of the time or hardly at all had the lowest scores. These results again demonstrate that being in control of the staff and being involved in decision making are two quite separate issues and mean different things to women, although it tends to be assumed in the literature that they are essentially the same thing.

Table 8.38 shows the degree of control reported by women in the two extreme categories of high EWB and low EWB.

Control of staff	Low EWB		High EWB		All women*
	n	%	n	%	
Always	12	(7)	29	(17)	176
Most of the time	31	(9)	34	(10)	347
Only some of the time	13	(15)	5	(6)	81
Hardly at all	9	(21)	4	(9)	44

* Percentages are of all women reporting each degree of control. Only those with extreme EWB scores are shown.

Table 8.38: Low/High EWB by being in control of staff

Information

Information was a predictor of emotional well-being as it was for the other psychological outcome variables. Women who felt they had been given the 'right amount' of information had significantly higher EWB scores than those who did not ($p < 0.01$), whilst women who wished they had known more prior to giving birth and who had been given misleading information had significantly lower EWB scores ($p < 0.01$).

Adjectives used to describe the staff

The only adjectives that differentiated between women with high and low EWB scores were 'informative' ($p < 0.05$), 'bossy' ($p < 0.001$) and 'rushed' ($p < 0.001$). The adjectives 'bossy' and 'rushed' are likely to be interrelated in that the first could well be a consequence of the second. Overall, the way women perceived the staff's attitude during the time they were in hospital was not important in terms of their subsequent emotional well-being. This conclusion is supported by the lack of any relationship between EWB and women's overall comments about the care they received at the hospital. Furthermore, continuity of care, which might also be seen as a dimension of staff care/attitude is unrelated to emotional well-being as is Satisfaction Factor 4 (satisfaction with aspects of staff care/monitoring).

Emotional well-being and 'internal' control

EWB was significantly related to both of the major aspects of 'internal' control that we asked about. Women who most felt able to maintain control over their behaviour had the highest EWB scores, whilst those who were not able to maintain control any of the time had the lowest scores ($p < 0.001$). The same pattern is evident for control during contractions ($p < 0.01$). The amount of noise women felt they made during labour was also related to emotional well-being ($p < 0.05$), in exactly the same way as was described for satisfaction with birth.

The results for both 'internal' and 'external' control demonstrate their importance for women's emotional well-being in the weeks following birth, and again make clear that the sense of being in control is not simply a function of lack of objective problems during labour, since these are not associated with EWB.

Other factors to do with the experience of labour

Women who were hardly ever able to get into the most comfortable position possible had the lowest EWB scores ($p < 0.001$), as did women who lacked privacy because there were lots of different people coming in and out of the room ($p < 0.05$).

Feelings during labour

Five adjectives describing feelings during labour were related to emotional well-being. Women who felt 'out of control', 'frightened' and 'helpless' had lower EWB scores while women who felt 'in control' and 'confident' had higher scores. All these relationships were significant at the $p < 0.01$ level. In addition, 'powerless' was another negative adjective related to emotional well-being, though it just missed significance ($p = 0.0525$).

Emotional well-being and the relationship with the baby

On the basis of both the individual variables and the composite measure 'Descriptions of Baby', the way women felt about and saw their babies would seem to be strongly related to emotional well-being. Women who felt that their baby was not yet a sociable person or who did not know whether the baby was a sociable person had lower EWB scores ($p < 0.05$), whilst the fourteen women who six weeks after giving birth said that their baby did not know them yet, had much lower EWB scores than women who felt their babies did know them. (When the scores were divided into five categories, ten of the women whose babies did not know them yet fell into the low or moderately low EWB groups, and none into the high EWB group.) There was a highly significant, linear relationship between how organized/disorganized life had been since the birth of the baby and women's emotional well-being ($p < 0.0001$). Women who felt life had been totally disorganized since the baby was born had the lowest EWB scores, followed by women who felt life had been fairly disorganized. To illustrate this further, it is worthwhile to look at the non-transformed EWB scores divided into five categories. Table 8.39 shows the results for women who fell into the low EWB and high EWB groups.

Organized life?	Low EWB		High EWB		All women*
	n	%	n	%	
Totally disorganized	11	(27)	1	(2)	41
Fairly disorganized	33	(15)	9	(4)	217
Neither	8	(10)	13	(16)	84
Fairly organized	24	(7)	43	(13)	326
Very organized	0		10	(42)	24

* Percentages are the proportion of women whose life was totally disorganized, fairly disorganized etc. The 3 intermediate categories of EWB have been omitted.

Table 8.39: Emotional well-being by organization of life

Emotional well-being was not related to whether women breastfed or not.

Seven negative adjectives describing the baby were related to low emotional well-being: grizzly and stubborn at the $p < 0.001$ level, and exhausting, angry, fretful, demanding and draining at the $p < 0.0001$ level. Women who saw their babies as fascinating ($p < 0.001$), cuddly ($p < 0.01$) and determined ($p < 0.05$) had higher EWB scores.

The composite variable Description of Baby was significantly related to emotional well-being ($p < 0.0001$). Women who perceived their babies negatively had lower EWB scores. It seems likely that, on balance, women's low emotional well-being is responsible for their negative feelings towards their babies rather than the other way around. However, we can only hypothesize the direction of the relationship and it may easily be that women with difficult babies have low emotional well-being as a result. The relationship between perceptions of the baby and emotional well-being is complex and interwoven, and each factor may feed the other in circular fashion (see also Chapter 10).

Other psychological outcomes

The individual components of the EWB factor (see introduction to this section) are, as one would expect, all highly related to the factor itself. In addition, women who wanted things to be different (in terms of their daily routine), or who could not even say if they wanted them to be different, had lower EWB scores than those who were happy with things as they were ($p < 0.0001$). Social support from friends and family was also very important. We asked: 'Is there anyone that you can talk to about how you have been feeling since the birth of your baby?'.

Women who replied by ticking the response categories 'No, there isn't anyone I can really talk to' and 'I don't particularly want to talk about how I feel' had the lowest EWB scores, while women who said 'There isn't anything I feel I need to talk about' followed by those who replied 'Yes, and they are very supportive' had the highest scores ($p < 0.0001$). Implicit in the responses of the women with the lowest emotional well-being scores would seem to be the feeling of being alone with problems or concerns.

Fulfilment

The women who did not find birth a fulfilling experience or were not sure if it was had lower EWB scores than women who found it fulfilling.

Satisfaction with birth

The relationship between satisfaction (marks out of ten) and EWB is an interesting one (women who had caesarean sections were excluded from this analysis). Overall most women were satisfied and only a few women had low EWB. We find a low but significant correlation between the two outcome measures using both Pearson's correlation coefficient and Spearman's Correlation Coefficient ($r = 0.1$, $p < 0.01$, two-tailed, in both cases), although when broken down by parity the finding does not hold for primips. However, when we carry out an analysis of variance on the data broken down into the 11 levels of satisfaction (0 to 10 inclusive), we find no significant relationship. This is because the correlation only holds for the top range of satisfaction scores: 5–10. For women with low satisfaction scores (0–4) the relationship, if anything, goes in the opposite direction. The 11 women who gave the birth 0 out of 10 (a score defined on the questionnaire as 'a thoroughly unsatisfactory experience with nothing good to be said for it') had the *highest* average EWB score in the whole sample. The lack of a linear relationship with EWB scores throughout the range of satisfaction scores has important implications; it tells us that women who have thoroughly unsatisfactory births do not necessarily suffer low emotional well-being, and also that women who feel unhappy postnatally do not necessarily project this retrospectively onto their birth experience by giving it a very low mark out of 10.

Antenatal predictors of emotional well-being

Two questions about women's mood were asked at the time women were approximately 30 weeks pregnant. One was about how they felt when they first discovered they were pregnant and the other about overall mood during the pregnancy. Both questions proved to be significantly related to women's postnatal mood (EWB). Women who were quite unhappy or very unhappy on discovering they were pregnant had the lowest EWB scores, followed by women who seemed indifferent, i.e. they said they had no particular feelings on the subject ($p < 0.01$). Again, women who on the whole had felt depressed or worried and anxious while they were pregnant had much lower scores postnatally than those who had been cheerful. Women who oscillated between high and low moods had interim EWB scores ($p < 0.0001$).

One particularly interesting finding was that women who had been in paid employment during pregnancy had significantly *higher* EWB scores than women who had not. A two-way analysis of variance showed that this result was independent of parity. This runs contrary to the hypothesis that primips who have been working prior to the birth are particularly vulnerable.

Marital status seemed to be related to EWB – women who were single, separated or widowed had much lower scores than other women, but the numbers were too small to reach significance. One woman who had been widowed in pregnancy wrote:

> 'I have felt very lost and alone without my husband to give me a hug when I need one. Also when my baby needs one.'

Having a choice in where the baby was born was also important for EWB in that those who felt they had no say in where they were booked for delivery had lower scores than those who felt they did have a choice ($p = 0.05$). The women who felt they had less say were also less satisfied with the experience of birth ($p < 0.05$).

Information and feeling confident in communicating with staff were significantly associated with EWB. The more women felt they were able to discuss things fully with the staff, the higher were their EWB scores ($p < 0.0001$). Similarly, women who felt they were as assertive as they wanted to be had high EWB scores whereas those who felt they were hardly ever assertive had low scores ($p < 0.0001$). The antenatal information question was an important predictor as was the postnatal question. Women who felt that they had received the 'right amount' of information at the time of the second questionnaire (approximately 36 weeks) had higher EWB scores than those who felt they had not ($p < 0.001$). This theme was repeated for a number of the more specific antenatal questions to do with knowledge/information. Women who felt that they did not know enough about the third stage of labour to have any preference on it had significantly lower EWB scores than other women ($p < 0.001$). Similarly the more women said they knew about acceleration the higher their EWB scores ($p < 0.05$). How women felt antenatally about having an enema and being shaved was related to EWB; the women who did not know enough to choose but also those who definitely did not want these interventions had the lowest EWB scores.

Anxiety about the pain of labour was strongly related to EWB ($p < 0.0001$). The women who were not at all worried had much higher scores. A similar but weaker relationship between general anxiety about pain in everyday life and EWB was no longer significant when both of these questions were included in a 2-way analysis of variance.

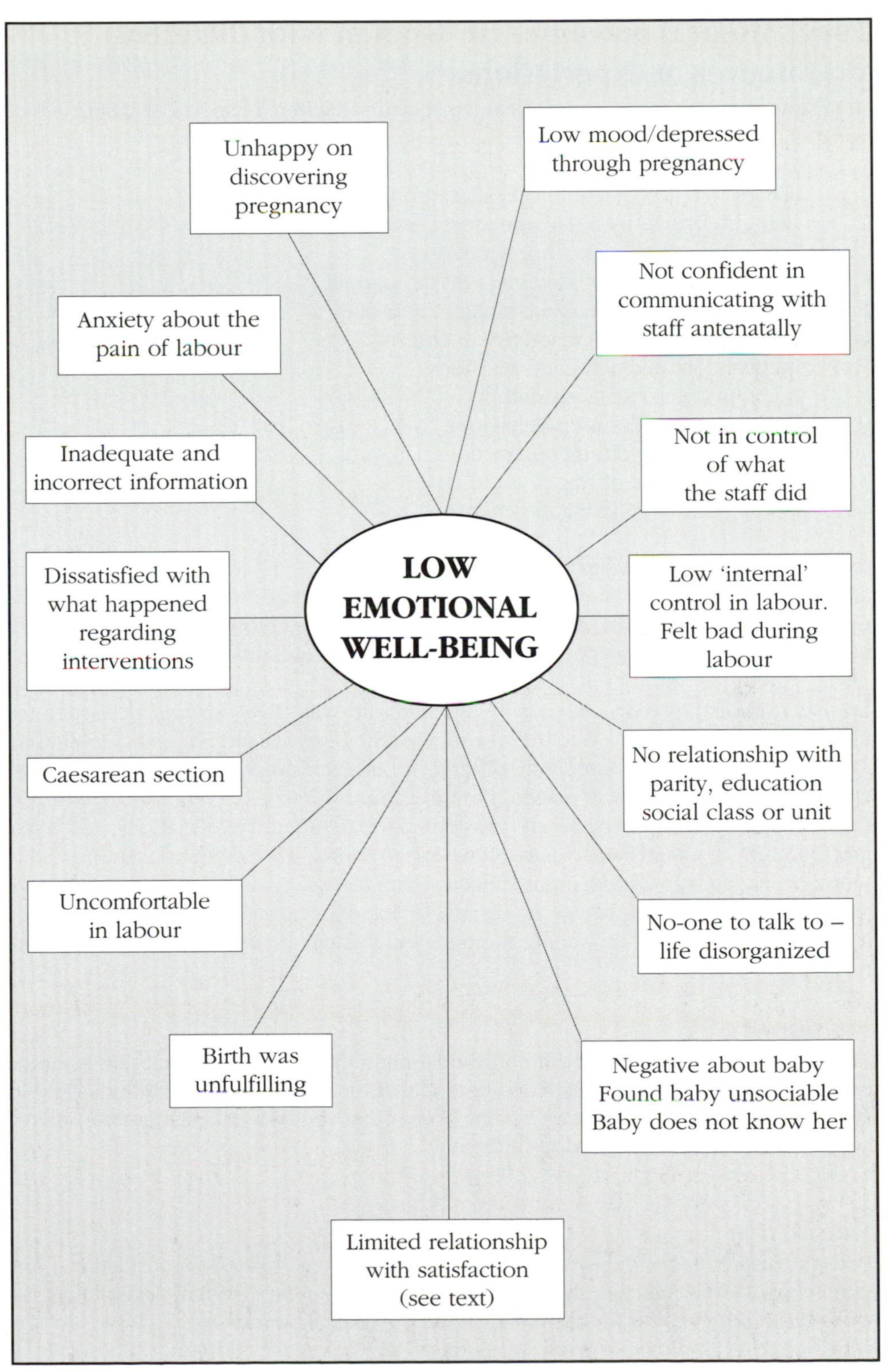

Low emotional well-being

Psychological outcomes for women with different preferences or expectations

In Chapters 4 and 7 we discussed twelve social/behavioural aspects of labour which were:

1. Having a birth companion present throughout
2. Being delivered by a midwife as opposed to a doctor
3. Being looked after by a known midwife
4. Being looked after by one midwife throughout
5. Not having lots of people coming in and out
6. Involvement in non-emergency decisions
7. Involvement in emergency decisions
8. Being in control of what staff do
9. Being in control of own behaviour
10. Being in control during contractions
11. Not making a lot of noise
12. Finding birth a fulfilling experience.

By looking at the relationship between women's antenatal preferences and expectations and the four psychological outcome measures we were able to examine some of the hypotheses detailed in Chapter 2 and also to look at the stereotype of the woman with high expectations who sets herself up for disappointment and postnatal depression.

For each of the 12 events, antenatally, women said what they *wanted* to happen (or how important the issue was to them) and what they *expected* to happen (see Chapter 4). These answers were frequently different from each other, i.e. what they wanted was not always what they expected. For the current purposes, women who expected that a given event *would* occur are considered to have 'high' expectations, and those who thought it would not to have 'low' expectations. This definition ignores what women actually wanted to happen, which is also the way in which other studies have defined expectations. However, it is arguable that expectations should be considered in relation to what women want to happen, and this will be done later in this section.

Fulfilment

Expecting that birth would be fulfilling and feeling that it was important that it should be so, were both positively related to finding that birth actually was fulfilling. This has already been reported in Chapter 7. None of the other wants or expectations considered here were significantly related to fulfilment.

Satisfaction

Both the desire for and expectation of fulfilment were also related to satisfaction in the same ways as for fulfilment; the greater the desire for, or expectation of, fulfilment the more satisfying the birth was reported to be ($p < 0.001$ in both cases). This is consistent with our other findings showing strong links between satisfaction and fulfilment.

For feeling in control during contractions and for being in control of what staff do to you, expecting to be in control was associated with high scores and not expecting to be with low scores ($p < 0.001$ and $p < 0.05$ respectively). There was no consistent pattern to the scores of women with no expectations.

Description of baby

None of the twelve wants/expectations were systematically related to the words which women chose to describe their babies.

Emotional well-being

Emotional well-being was significantly related to five of the expectations considered in this section. In every case high expectations were associated with high emotional well-being and low expectations with low emotional well-being, although the relationship was not always completely linear. Like the findings for the other psychological outcomes, this runs contrary to the stereotype predicting disappointment and depression for women with high expectations. The five expectations were:

- Being looked after by a midwife you had already met ($p < 0.05$)
- Degree of involvement in non-emergency decision making ($p < 0.001$)
- Losing control of your behaviour ($p < 0.01$)
- Feeling in control during contractions ($p < 0.05$)
- Fulfilment ($p < 0.05$).

Women with no expectations tended to have average or low scores but there was no consistent pattern. They never had higher than average scores which runs counter to the hypotheses outlined in Chapter 2. In other words, keeping an open mind about what might happen during labour is *not* necessarily associated with positive outcome.

This may mean that for 'open mindedness' to be a useful psychological mechanism (i.e. to protect against disappointment), it is necessary that women should genuinely not mind what happens to them rather than simply having no expectations. The 'no expectations' group will have included women who did actually care about the various issues along with those who did not. Most women with no preferences, however, did not have expectations either and it may be that this sub-group is the one that we should be looking at. Similarly, we hypothesized that a 'low' expectation, as defined so far, is really only low if it is contrary to what you want. The final analysis of the social/behavioural data therefore took the combination of wants and expectations into account.

Expectations controlled for what women wanted and what happened

For this analysis we concentrated on the majority of women, those who said that they would 'definitely' or 'quite like' the specified events to occur, and subdivided them into those who expected their preference to be met and those who did not (combining the 'definitely' and 'probably' categories. This gives us two groups:

- 'wanted and expected' = high expectations
- wanted but did not expect' = low expectations.

These two groups were then compared with a third group, those who 'did not mind'. Women who did not want the specified event or who wanted it but had no expectations, were omitted from these analyses. We then looked at what had actually happened, i.e. did the desired event occur? The results broadly confirm the cruder analysis given in Chapter 7: women with high expectations were more likely to have their wishes met than women with low expectations. The women who did not mind usually fell midway between the two. The only events where the relationship was not significant were having lots of people coming in and out ($p = 0.07$, relationship in the expected direction), and control of staff ($p = 0.2$, relationship in the expected direction). Emergency decision making could not be tested because numbers in individual cells were too small.

Psychological outcomes for women with high/low expectations who did/did not get what they wanted

Having subdivided the sample in the way just described we were able to run two-way analyses of variance with 'expectations' and 'what happened' as main effects. This was done for those three of the outcome measures which could be treated as continuous variables (satisfaction with birth, Description of Baby and emotional well-being). Fulfilment was investigated by using a Chi-square analysis controlling for 'what happened'.

These analyses allowed us to test directly several of the hypotheses outlined in Chapter 2, in particular, the hypothesis that women with particular preferences and high expectations who did not get what they wanted were more likely to be disappointed and have negative psychological outcomes than women who either had no preferences or had low expectations. This is a more sophisticated way of analysing the data than that already reported because it removes the confounding effect of women with different expectations having different preferences.

The effect of *experiencing* the social/behavioural events has been discussed in detail earlier in this chapter. Briefly, virtually all were related to satisfaction and to fulfilment. Hardly any, on the other hand, were related to the composite variable Description of Baby, while both' internal' control and control of what staff were doing to you, as well as birth being a fulfilling experience were related to postnatal emotional well-being.

As far as expectations are concerned, there were a number of interesting findings. Fulfilment and Description of Baby, as before, showed little association with expectations except that Description of Baby was significantly related to low expectations of being in control of behaviour ($p < 0.05$). However, both satisfaction with birth and emotional well-being showed a number of significant associations with antenatal expectations which are summarized in Table 8.40.

	Satisfaction		Emotional well-being	
	Expecting	Experiencing	Expecting	Experiencing
1. Birth companion	ns	$p < 0.05$	ns	ns
2. Midwife delivery	ns	$p < 0.001$	ns	ns
3. Known midwife	$p < 0.01$	ns	$p < 0.05$	ns
4. One midwife throughout	$p < 0.01$	$p < 0.001$	ns	ns
5. Not lots of people	ns ($p < 0.06$)	$p < 0.001$	ns	$p < 0.05$
6. Making non-emergency decisions	$p < 0.05$	$p < 0.05$	ns	ns
7. Making emergency decisions:	omitted, numbers too small for analysis			
8. Control: staff	$p < 0.01$	$p < 0.001$	ns	p0.001
9. Control: behaviour	ns	$p < 0.001$	$p < 0.001$	p0.001
10. Control: contractions	$p < 0.05$	$p < 0.001$	$p < 0.01$	ns
11. Not making noise	ns	$p < 0.01$	ns	ns
12. Fulfilment	ns	$p < 0.001$	ns	$p < 0.05$

Notes

1. The events 1–12 refer to the questions numbered 1–12 discussed above and in Chapters 4 and 7.
2. The 'expecting' comparison is between high expectations, low expectations and no preferences as described in the text.
3. When 'expecting' was significant, low expectations always had the worst outcome. When 'experiencing' was significant, the women who did not have the experience had the worst outcome.

Table 8.40: Summary of significant relationships between a) expecting and b) experiencing twelve social/behavioural aspects of labour and i) satisfaction and ii) emotional well-being

The most important finding, as our earlier analysis suggested, is that in every single case where there is a significant difference between women with high and low expectations it is the women with high expectations who have the better psychological outcome and the women with low expectations who have the worst. This is in direct contradiction to the popular idea of women with high expectations setting themselves up for failure and postnatal depression. The other important point is that the relationship between *expectations* and psychological outcome is independent of the relationship between *events* and psychological outcomes. There are four cases where events are not significant at all although expectations are, but, even in the other cases, there are no significant interactions. What this means in practical terms is that the difference in, say, the satisfaction of women who did and did not experience a particular aspect of labour is just as great whether they expected it or not. Similarly, the difference between women who did and did not *expect* events is just the same whether they experienced them or not. This is a critical finding. To make it more concrete, Table 8.41 gives the example of control of behaviour and emotional well-being. It shows that women who 'didn't mind' (i.e. said that the issue was not important to them) had the highest emotional well-being scores and women with low expectations the lowest. This was true whether they lost control or not. Similarly, women who lost control had lower emotional well-being scores than those who did not whatever their wants/expectations.

	Was in control		Was not in control	
		n		n
Wanted to be and expected to be	+0.24	163	-0.09	89
Wanted to be and did not expect to be	-0.15	47	-0.41	72
Issue not important	+0.69	13	+0.03	14

The scores shown in the table are emotional well-being scores (EWB) transformed to a standard normal variable (mean = zero, standard deviation = 1). Positive scores indicate high EWB and negative, low EWB. A two-way analysis of variance shows both main effects significant at $p < 0.0001$ but there was no interaction effect.

Table 8.41: Being in control of the way you behave. Wants/expectations by outcome and emotional well-being

Thus, the idea that low expectations might be a protection against disappointment continues to receive no support; it was the women with *low* expectations who did not get what they wanted who had the worst outcome.

It is also interesting to see that women to whom the issue was unimportant still had better outcomes if they were in control than if they were not (i.e. control is good for you). It would therefore appear that not minding is not a total protection against the effects of not having control. However, the fact that women who 'didn't mind' antenatally consistently had good psychological outcomes whenever wants/expectations were significant requires explanation. These outcomes were often better than those of women with high expectations whose wishes were met, and they were never significantly lower. This, coupled with the consistently poor outcomes of the women with low expectations, suggests that the issues go rather deeper than the particular events that our questions examine, especially when only expectations proved to be significantly related to psychological outcomes and events were not. An example is the expectation of being looked after by a midwife that you have already met. Whether or not this actually happened proved to be unrelated to either satisfaction or emotional well-being but what women said antenatally was significantly related to both of these outcome variables. The first possible explanation is that women's stated preferences/ expectations are a reflection of their antenatal psychological mood. We have seen elsewhere that poor antenatal psychological status predicts poor psychological outcome. It could therefore be that women who are feeling low antenatally say that they do not expect their wishes to be met for this reason. It is not that they care any less about the issues, they simply have a jaundiced view of the world. This hypothesis would fit the data presented so far. Examination of answers to the relevant antenatal questions does not, however, offer very much support for the hypothesis; few of the relevant Chi-square tests were significant, although there are problems of small numbers since the majority of women claimed to be in good spirits antenatally. Perhaps a more likely explanation is that women's stated preference/expectations relate to more permanent personality characteristics. For example, those with low expectations may be rather dour people who are not easily satisfied, while those who say they do not mind, really *are* more likely to be easily satisfied. The data would seem to support the idea suggested earlier that it is the 'don't mind' women rather than those with low expectations who are protecting themselves from disappointment. That they do actually mind, at least about some events, would seem to be indicated by their higher scores when they did experience the event in question. There are, however, other explanations and we are now in the realm of speculation (see also Chapter 10).

Summary of the inter-relationship between preferences, expectations, events and psychological outcome

These are highly complex inter-relationships to examine. Preferences/expectations do not appear to be closely related to fulfilment or to Description of Baby but there are some significant relationships with satisfaction and emotional well-being. These are independent of whether or not women actually got what they wanted/expected. Women who did not expect to have their preferences met had consistently worse psychological outcomes in those cases where there were significant differences. Women who 'didn't mind' often had the best outcomes.

CHAPTER NINE

Discussion

This final chapter will not attempt to summarize all of our findings but will draw together some of the threads that have emerged and examine their implications.

Assessment of psychological outcome

This study has been unusual in using four measures of psychological outcome by which we hoped to differentiate particular aspects of women's feelings after birth. Two of these measures, fulfilment and satisfaction, concern women's feelings about the birth itself, and as one would expect, are strongly related to intrapartum events. The other two, emotional well-being (EWB) and Description of Baby, are reflections of how women are finding their lives after the birth and have more obvious long term implications. These latter two measures are also related to some intrapartum events but reflect the social context in which women find themselves to a much greater extent.

There are significant relationships between each of the measures, but not to such a degree that they would all seem to be measuring the same thing. This is also clear from the fact that each of the measures is related to a different pattern of events.

The two outcome variables which seem the most similar are fulfilment and satisfaction with birth. To some extent fulfilment, which was important to nearly all the women irrespective of education or parity, was a component of satisfaction. More women were fulfilled and dissatisfied than vice versa. In fact, most women, again independently of education or parity, did find birth a fulfilling experience.

The impression gained is that most women are predisposed towards finding birth fulfilling (see Chapter 4) and the factors associated with *lack* of fulfilment are therefore of particular interest. Some of the strongest associations were with the adjectives that women used to describe themselves in labour, such as 'powerless', 'detached' and 'helpless'. These were also associated with a feeling of lack of control, both 'internal' and 'external'. Other related factors were a range of obstetric interventions, both major and minor, the use of pain-relieving drugs, lack of continuity of care during labour and feeling ill-informed.

All of these factors related to satisfaction with birth as well, but satisfaction covered a wider compass. Our study supports all others in this field in finding that women are predisposed to be satisfied with the experience of birth. We have, however, succeeded in pinpointing elements of dissatisfaction that might otherwise not have surfaced, firstly, by allowing women to give an overall score on a scale from zero to ten and, secondly, by having 14 additional questions which assessed satisfaction with particular aspects of labour and delivery. The factor analysis carried out on these data makes it clear that individual components of satisfaction and dissatisfaction can be identified. Its most important contribution to our findings has been to highlight the importance of women believing that the 'right thing' happened with respect to obstetric interventions, both major and minor, whether they had such interventions or not.

The overall measure of satisfaction with the birth related to most of the events of labour. It also related to expectations of labour in a way that fulfilment did not, but with the somewhat surprising finding that women with low expectations were less satisfied. Also, most importantly, it related to parity, which fulfilment did not. That primips should be less satisfied is consistent with the fact that they have a worse time in labour. What is surprising is that so many of them did feel fulfilled.

Our measure of emotional well-being was a non-clinical attempt to detect depression in the six week period since the birth. The fact that we did not use a standard psychiatric measure should not be considered a problem. Eight questions were used to assess EWB, including six items from the Edinburgh Postnatal Depression Scale. A factor analysis showed that a single factor accounted for 45.5 per cent of the variance. We would suggest that our EWB measure is detecting something comparable to what other studies have called postnatal depression. By using a continuous measure we have avoided the necessity for an arbitrary cut off dividing women into 'depressed' and 'not depressed' and are able to examine factors associated with the full range of scores.

The final outcome measure, Description of Baby, was intended to reflect something of the mother-infant relationship, which, clearly, we could not assess first-hand using postal questionnaires. It was the measure that was most closely related to EWB ($p < 0.0001$). This could be causal, insofar as depressed women were more likely to be negative about their babies. Of course the relationship could work the other way: women who are negative about their babies become depressed.

The most striking link between the two outcome variables is their very strong association with postnatal factors which are essentially to do with the social organization of women's lives at home and with the mother-baby relationship. Women were more negative about their babies and had lower EWB scores when they said that life was very disorganized, that they had no-one to talk to who understood, that at six weeks old their baby was not yet a sociable person and that their baby did not know them yet. We also found that Description of Baby was related to breastfeeding. Contrary perhaps to expectation, it was women who had never attempted to breastfeed who were the most positive about their babies. Possible reasons for these findings were discussed in Chapter 8.

EWB tended to be associated with more aspects of labour than Description of Baby, but, as we have already observed, much of what happened during labour was unrelated to these two outcomes. The other main difference between them is that Description of

Baby was very strongly related to parity ($p < 0.0001$) and was also related to education ($p < 0.01$), while EWB was not related to any of the independent variables considered.

There were, in addition, antenatal questions which proved to be related to outcome. How women felt on first discovering that they were pregnant was related to both fulfilment and EWB, while overall feelings during pregnancy were related to all the outcome measures except fulfilment. Clearly then, *antenatal* emotional well-being is responsible for some of the variation in psychological outcome. It may also account for some of the differences in the more subjective areas of women's reports, such as whether they thought the staff were nice and how they felt in labour. In other words, women who are unhappy antenatally are likely to continue to be unhappy during and after birth and their reports of their experiences are coloured accordingly. However, the number of women who reported feeling unhappy antenatally is too small to be a major factor in explaining our results. There is, though, corroboration from two additional sources for the idea that women who are likely to have poor outcomes can be predicted from their antenatal mood. Firstly, women with low expectations of having certain preferences met were less satisfied and less fulfilled than other women, even if they got what they wanted. Secondly, women who were anxious about the pain of labour had lower postnatal EWB scores.

Interestingly, the other group of antenatal questions which related to psychological outcome (particularly satisfaction and EWB) were those to do with information and communication with staff which, we have seen, were also critical areas in the postnatal reports. This suggests either that i) these issues are genuinely important in determining how women feel, to the extent that antenatal events can influence postnatal outcomes, or that ii) there are subgroups of women who are easily satisfied/dissatisfied and who therefore gave 'satisfied'/'dissatisfied' answers throughout all the questionnaires. In practice, it seems likely that elements of both of these explanations are true. It is not, however, the case that the most dissatisfied women had the lowest EWB scores, or vice versa, which is what one would expect if unhappy or pessimistic women were being globally negative.

Our conclusion is that our four measures of psychological outcome are measuring distinct aspects of women's feelings after birth. Some degree of negative postnatal feeling is simply a continuation of negative affect during pregnancy and some is probably predictable from more basic personality traits such as whether women tend to be hard to please, or are pessimistic, or anxious. Nevertheless, events during labour, as well as independent variables such as parity and education, do have a part to play. We will now discuss these factors further within the context of the hypotheses presented in Chapter 2.

As we saw in Chapter 1, the research literature generates a number of hypotheses about determinants of psychological outcome. These were formalized in Chapter 2 and will be re-examined here as a framework for discussing some of the major themes of this report: wants and expectations, control, parity, social class/education and interventions.

Wants/expectations

The first three hypotheses concerned wants and expectations and their implications for psychological outcome. Hypothesis 1 stated that:

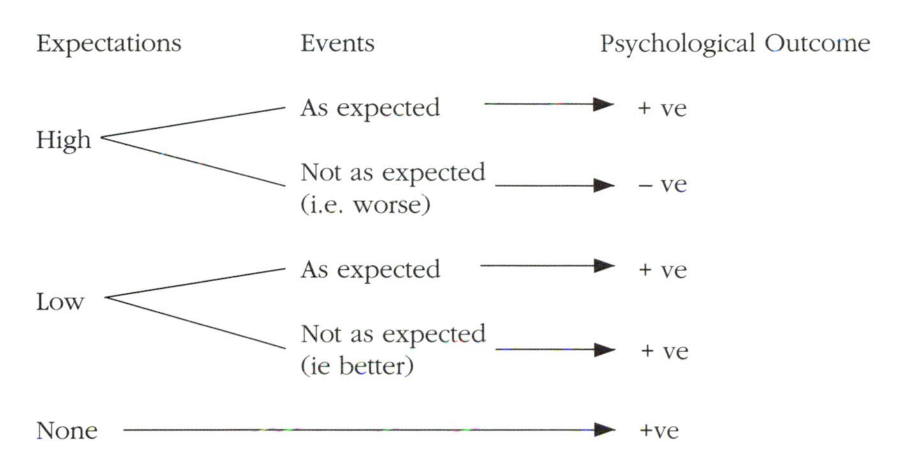

This hypothesis assumes that negative outcome is the result of not having high expectations met. Therefore, if you have either low expectations or no expectations you cannot be disappointed and will have a positive outcome. Our results do not support this hypothesis. In Chapter 8, in particular, we have seen that,

i) expectations are generally only related to two of the four outcome measures: satisfaction and, to a lesser extent emotional well-being,

ii) where expectations are related to psychological outcome the relationship is always:

High expectation ⟶ + ve outcome

Low expectation ⟶ – ve outcome

No expectations ⟶ average/low outcome, no consistent pattern

These findings, however, have not taken account of whether or not women's expectations were met, nor of their preferences. These aspects were considered in the more detailed analyses at the end of Chapter 8 and relate also to the second of our hypotheses which stated that:

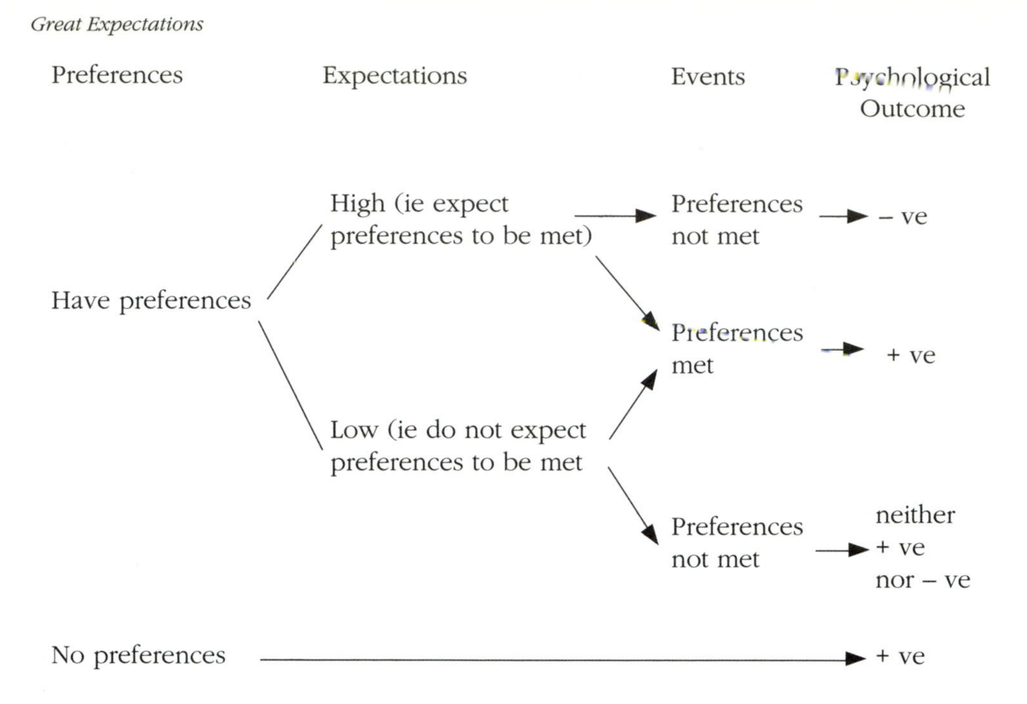

Here it is assumed that expectations are only of importance if preferences are not met, although the underlying logic is similar to that of Hypothesis 1. Hypothesis 3 was a variant on this which placed more emphasis on preferences by predicting that outcomes would be poor if preferences were not met, whatever the expectations.

What we found in practice for expectations and preferences concerning the social and behavioural aspects of labour was:

i) as above, fulfilment and Description of Baby are only weakly related to experiencing social/behavioural aspects of labour, or to wanting them or expecting them,

ii) satisfaction and emotional well-being are related to a number of social/ behavioural aspects but *experiencing* the event in question and *expecting* it or wanting it have independent effects on these outcome measures such that:

experiencing a particular aspect of labour (e.g. being in control of your behaviour)	$>$	not experiencing it
wanting and expecting that aspect	$>$	wanting and *not* expecting it
having no preferences	$\geqslant$	wanting and expecting

where $>$ means better psychological outcome and $\geqslant$ means better than or equal to.

Thus, Hypothesis 3 rather than Hypothesis 2 is supported insofar as women whose preferences are not met have worse outcomes whatever their expectations. However, what none of the hypotheses predicted was that women who do not expect to have their preferences met actually have worse psychological outcomes than women who *do* expect this. Most strikingly, this is true both when the desired event occurs and when it does not. The worst outcomes are therefore for women who do not expect their preferences to be met and who are proved right. Note also that women with no preferences tend to have positive outcomes, which is consistent with the second hypothesis. Nevertheless, whenever there is a significant effect of experiencing a particular aspect of labour, it applies equally to these 'don't minds'. In other words, notwithstanding their apparent lack of preference, such women do have better outcomes if they experience the event in question than if they do not.

Data presented in Chapter 8 on expectations of pain confirm this pattern of findings. Women who expect labour to be very or extremely painful, who are anxious about the pain, and who would prefer the most pain-free labour that drugs can give them are less satisfied than women who are more optimistic. Anxiety about pain in labour is also associated with low emotional well-being. Thus, the conclusion would seem to be that pessimism is associated with poor psychological outcomes, and that being proved right only makes things worse. The other noteworthy finding is that all the aspects of care investigated such as having one midwife present throughout and not having lots of people coming in and out, are associated with higher satisfaction scores for all subgroups of women, whether or not they wanted them and whether or not they expected them.

Parity

Hypothesis 4 predicted worse psychological outcomes for primips on the grounds that their expectations would be less realistic and that unmet expectations lead to negative outcomes. We have indeed found worse outcomes for primips on two out of four measures. Although primips were just as likely to feel fulfilled and no more likely to suffer low emotional well-being than multips, they were less satisfied with the birth as a whole and were more negative about their babies. It is not however clear that the reason for this is the one postulated by the hypothesis. We have already seen that higher expectations are not necessarily associated with poor outcomes and we also saw in Chapters 4 and 5 that primips do not necessarily have higher expectations. Where we did find parity differences it was often because primips were more likely to say that they had no expectations. They were not, in general, expecting labour to be less painful than multips were and it was, as one might expect, multips who were more likely to approach labour with confidence in their own knowledge and opinions. Multips were also more likely to express preferences about interventions and drugs than primips, and to have confidence in their own ability to maintain 'internal' control. However, primips did have higher expectations of being in control of what staff did to them and of being involved in non-emergency decisions – both questions about which multips were more cynical. Clearly, any hypothesis which talks generally about 'expectations' needs also to consider: expectations of what?

The main point to note, however, is that whatever their expectations, primips actually have a much worse time giving birth. They were more likely to say that they felt overwhelmed, dopey, frightened, detached and helpless during labour while multips were more likely to say that they felt alert, calm, confident and in control. Primips were also more likely to be surprised by some aspect of the pain and more likely to use Pethidine and epidurals. They had longer labours, more interventions, were given less privacy and continuity of care, and felt less in control of what staff did to them. It is for these reasons, not because they had particularly high expectations, that the gap between expectations and events is greater for primips. The same point has also been made by Booth and Meltzoff (1984) as we noted in Chapter 1, although their primips did in fact have very high expectations of 'internal' control. However, even if primips had had lower expectations, it is unlikely that they would have had better psychological outcomes since, as we have seen, low expectations were associated with poorer psychological outcome. In fact, it seems possible that expectations are less relevant to primip outcomes than our hypotheses have suggested. In addition, the tendency of primips to be more negative about their babies is not as strongly related to the events of labour as one might expect suggesting that this very clear finding has more to do with the shock of first-time motherhood. This is an area where we would hope to be able to explore our data further in the future. Meanwhile, we would stress that there does seem to be a 'primip factor' which leads first-time mothers to be less satisfied than multips and more negative about their babies even when they have apparently similar experiences. This was demonstrated by using two-way analysis of variance to re-examine some of the associations between the events of labour and satisfaction with birth (see Chapter 8). To confirm this impression and to explore it further it would, however, be necessary to control for *all* the events of birth, which is not a practical possibility in this case (see, however, Chapter 10).

Control

Hypotheses 5 and 6 were both concerned with control. Hypothesis 5 stated that wanting control and not getting it is bad for you:

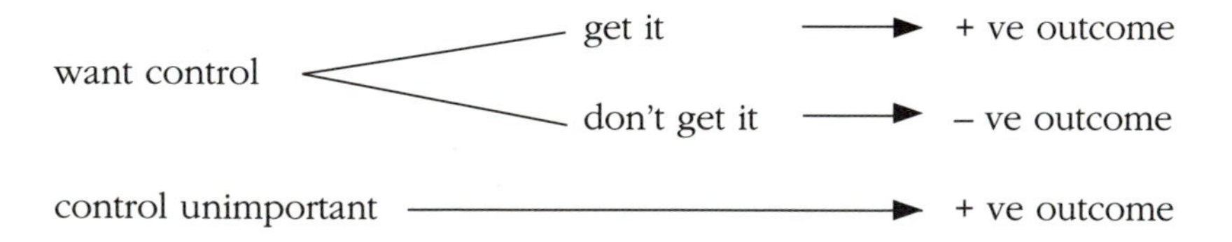

Hypothesis 6 effectively said that not feeling in control is bad for you whether you wanted it or not. These hypotheses were tested on our data using control in the 'external' sense, although similar analyses could be done on the questions concerning 'internal' control. In Chapter 4 we defined two extreme subgroups of women: those who consistently expressed a desire for control over decision making ('High Control') and those who never did ('Low Control'). These two groups were found to differ antenatally in a number of ways particularly in their preferences for drug use and other aspects of labour. They also differed in terms of their level of education as predicted by Hypothesis 7.

Postnatally, we found that 'High Control' women did indeed experience more involvement in non-emergency decision making and were also more likely to have felt in control of what staff did to them. However, there were hardly any other reported differences in the events of labour and no significant differences between the two groups on any of the four outcome measures. We did not compare the two groups controlling for what actually happened to them, but we did compare women on the basis of their answer to the single question concerning feeling in control of what staff were doing. This tended to support Hypothesis 5: women who had said that the issue was unimportant had the highest satisfaction scores, women who wanted control and did not get it had the lowest scores. However, this was only true for satisfaction and not for any of the other three psychological outcome measures. Also, the 'don't mind' women who did not feel in control were less satisfied than those who did. This leads us on to Hypothesis 6 which also seems to be supported by our data: not feeling in control *is* bad for you. Women who did not feel in control were less satisfied, less likely to feel fulfilled and had lower postnatal emotional well-being. This was true independently of their antenatal desires or expectations of control. Of course, this could be partly because women who had long or difficult labours were less likely to feel in control and were also less likely to have positive psychological outcomes. However, feeling in control of what staff are doing is not simply a function of the difficulties of labour. Some women who experienced major interventions or who had long labours were still able to feel in control while other women who had none of these problems did not. The fact that it is the feeling of being in control rather than the experience of interventions that relates so strongly to psychological outcomes emphasizes this point.

So what does it mean to 'feel in control' of what staff are doing to you? This was one of three questions designed to tap into the idea of 'external' control. The other two concerned emergency and non-emergency decision making. It was the desire for control over decision making in five different areas of childbirth that we concentrated on antenatally in order to define 'High' and 'Low Control' women. However, it became apparent that 'feeling in control of what staff do to you' and having a high level of involvement in decision making are not synonymous. The answers that women gave both antenatally and postnatally show that decision making is only one specific aspect of 'external' control and is perhaps of less relevance to less educated women than to well-educated women. In fact, many more women felt in control of what staff were doing to them than felt that they had had an active part in decision making. The answers that women gave suggest that 'feeling in control of what staff do to you' relates much more broadly to the sort of relationship that they felt that they had with the staff: whether they felt they had some potential influence over events or whether things were simply done to them, as these two quotations illustrate:

> 'The staff were marvellous and treated us as a couple having our first baby rather than treating me as a lump of meat.'

> 'The consultant didn't even reply to my questions – but carried on with what he was doing to me – [he] treated me like a piece of meat.'

The phrase 'treated like a lump of meat' (or 'piece of meat', or 'slab of meat') may seem somewhat hackneyed. It does, however, seem to capture the essence of what women mean when they talk about control in childbirth. This is further illustrated by answers to the question 'Were you able to get into the positions that were most comfortable for you during labour and delivery?'. Answers were not only strongly related to the feeling of being in control of what staff were doing but, most strikingly, were related to every one of the four psychological outcome measures. In other words, not being able to get comfortable was associated with being dissatisfied, unfulfilled, having low emotional well-being and describing the baby in negative terms. It is obviously, therefore, a very important issue and for many women there was a clear link with control. They could not get comfortable precisely because the staff, the drugs or the equipment were depriving them of that fundamental degree of control over their own bodies. It is in this sense that 'external' control is important to most women rather than in the sense of women issuing orders to the staff, as some of the obstetricians quoted in Chapter 1 seemed to imply. This also explains why birth plans proved to be such a relatively unimportant issue to most of the women in our study (see Volume 2, Chapter 3) while control clearly was not.

The idea of not being able to get comfortable because of the effects of drugs takes us to the borders of 'internal' control. As we saw in Chapter 7, there was a strong relationship between experiencing 'external' and 'internal' control. In the same way that we tried to approach 'external' control via different possible interpretations, we also asked three questions about 'internal' control: control of one's behaviour, control during contractions and making a lot of noise. Our original expectation was that 'behaviour' and 'making a noise' would yield similar responses but this was not the case. On the contrary, making a lot of noise was relatively unimportant to a large number of women, particularly well-educated ones, while the other interpretations of 'internal' control were important to most women and were not related to education. Concern over making a noise was *negatively* related to a strong desire for control over decision making which may again be a reflection of the priorities of women of different levels of education and social class. Making a noise was not related to finding birth fulfilling, unlike the other 'internal' control questions. All three questions were, however, associated with satisfaction and emotional well-being in the same way as 'external' control was. As we saw in Chapter 7, the two senses of control often went together.

Our conclusion is that both 'internal' and 'external' control are important not only to women's experience of the birth but also to their subsequent emotional well-being. Obviously, there are some (unavoidable?) obstetric circumstances which make it less likely that a woman will feel in control. However, our data also make it clear that 'minor' interventions and psychosocial aspects of labour such as shaves, enemas, lack of continuity of care, unsupportive staff and lack of information are similarly associated with loss of control. These are aspects of which staff should be aware.

Education/social class

Out of three possible indicators of social class (women's educational level, women's highest ever occupation and partner's current occupation), partner's occupation proved to be almost totally irrelevant to our findings and, consequently, we have ignored it. (It was, in fact, unrelated to any of the four psychological outcome variables.) Women's social class, although a far superior predictor of outcome to partner's social class, nevertheless had the familiar problem of small numbers in the two extreme categories, class I and class V, while over three quarters of the women fell into classes II and IIIN. Hence, its usefulness was hampered by its lack of sensitivity. Furthermore, results when presented in six social class categories were often non-linear. Amalgamation of the categories into high (I and II), medium (IIIN and IIIM) and low (IV and V) achieved linearity and a more even spread of numbers, but at the expense of the disappearance of important differences between classes IV and V. Women's educational level yielded three distinct groups – basic education, some further education up to age 18, and higher education – which lent themselves to meaningful analysis. We have concentrated on education as the best predictor of differences: in most instances, relationships were more significant by education than by woman's social class.

Women's approach to labour

Well-educated women were more knowledgeable about labour and delivery and were generally more confident in how they approached childbirth. They were much more likely than less educated women to have attended antenatal classes, to be well-informed about the advantages/disadvantages of pain-relieving drugs and to say that they were knowledgeable about the third stage of labour. They also put greater emphasis on the importance of being well-informed about childbirth, and were more likely to have written a birth plan. Well-educated women were more likely to both want and expect control in decision making and control over what the staff did to them, supporting Hypotheses 7 and 8. They were more likely to have views about interventions (on the whole preferring to avoid them), whereas less educated women more often said they did not know enough to make a choice, as they also did about drugs. The more highly educated women were, however, not anti-intervention *per se*. For example, they were in favour of intermittent fetal heart monitoring whilst wishing to avoid continuous monitoring. Maintaining 'internal' control was not more important to highly educated women, although they were more confident than less educated women of their ability to control their behaviour during childbirth. Interestingly, while highly educated women were no more likely to say that they were always as assertive as they wanted to be when talking to professionals, women in social classes I and II were.

Contrary to expectations, well-educated and middle class women were no more committed to the ideal of a drug-free labour than other women. However, well-educated women were concerned to avoid Pethidine, instead being much more prepared to use breathing and relaxation exercises and other alternative methods to control the pain of labour.

A particular aspect of the negative 'NCT type' stereotype discussed in Chapter 1 is that she places an unwarranted degree of importance on childbirth as a fulfilling experience. In fact, highly educated women were not more likely to think birth should be fulfilling or to expect that it definitely would be: it was less educated women who had the highest expectations of birth as a fulfilling experience. Postnatally, the vast majority of women said that they found birth fulfilling and there were no differences between women of different levels of education.

Education and outcome

Women's educational level was unrelated to the interventions that they experienced during labour. However, women in the higher social classes (I and II) were more likely to be given an episiotomy.

Women's experience of 'external' control did differ according to educational level insofar as more educated women felt they had had greater input into non-emergency decisions. However, they did not feel any more in control of what the staff did.

Use of pain-relieving drugs also varied according to educational level: highly educated women were less likely to use Pethidine, were more likely to employ alternative methods and to find breathing and relaxation exercises helpful. Importantly, they were no more likely to be dissatisfied with the way they dealt with the pain.

Level of education was not associated with psychological outcome except for the variable relating to the baby, Description of Baby. Well-educated women were more negative about their babies than less educated women and also more often said they wanted things to be different. However, well-educated women were more likely to say that their baby was already a sociable person at six weeks after birth and to describe the baby as 'fascinating' and 'responsive'.

The profile drawn here of the well-educated (and higher social class) woman in our sample tends to support the positive rather than the negative aspects of the stereotype of the well-educated, middle class 'NCT type' presented in Chapter 1. As described in the positive stereotype, she wants to be and is relatively well informed about labour and delivery, is aware of the side effects of drugs and wants to be in control of decision making. Unlike the negative stereotype, she does not have overly high expectations either about pain and her ability to deal with it, or about her chances of retaining 'external' control. Furthermore, she does not have an intellectual approach to labour which renders her unable to 'let go' and leads her to place undue importance on maintaining 'internal' control during labour. Finally, she is not more likely to focus on birth as a fulfilling experience in itself than anyone else and is not more likely to end up unfulfilled, dissatisfied, and – most critical of all in terms of the stereotype – no more likely to end up postnatally depressed.

Aspects of the stereotype of the working class, less educated women are also refuted by our data. Far form being unconcerned with birth as a fulfilling experience, it was as important to her as it was to the more educated and middle class woman. Futhermore, although she was less likely to want and expect 'external' control, she was far from abdicating all responsibility to the staff as suggested by the stereotype. The great majority of less educated women still wanted to be involved to some degree. although they had lower expectations of gaining such involvement than the well educated middle class women, and indeed did experience less involvement in decision making.

Interventions

Our final two hypotheses concerned interventions. Hypothesis 9 stated that major interventions would be more likely to lead to poor psychological outcomes than minor ones, while Hypothesis 10 predicted that the more interventions that a woman had (whether major or minor), the worse her psychological outcome. Neither hypothesis is fully supported.

Women who had any of the interventions considered were less *satisfied* than women who did not have them, and there was no indication that dissatisfaction was higher for women who had major interventions than for those who had minor ones. There was also a significant relationship between satisfaction and the total number of interventions experienced, supporting Hypothesis 10.

The link between interventions and psychological outcomes becomes more complex when we look at our other three measures. Fulfilment, which tends to show similar patterns to satisfaction, is not related to the experience of acceleration, induction, ARM or electronic fetal monitoring, although it is related to all the other interventions and also to the total number experienced. Women who had caesarean sections, particularly unplanned ones, were more likely to be negative about their babies and to have lower emotional well-being. However, no other intervention was associated with emotional well-being or Description of Baby, the two outcome measures which relate more to women's feelings *after* the birth rather than *about* the birth. Furthermore, the total number of interventions was unrelated to emotional well-being, and only affected multips descriptions of their babies. This is in contrast to Oakley's (1980) finding of a relationship between a medium/high level of intervention and both depression and medium/poor feelings towards the baby and Jacoby's (1987) finding of a relationship between the number of procedures experienced and depression. (It is important to remember that Oakely's study dealt only with primiparous women.) Our study supports the findings of Elliott et al. (1984) who also failed to find a link between the number of interventions and depression despite basing their intervention score on Oakley's method, which we did not. This suggests that the differing results are not an artefact of the method of assessing the level of intervention.

From this one might conclude that the experience of obstetric interventions, apart from caesarean section, has few ill-effects, or at least not ones which are detectable by our measures six weeks after birth. However, this conclusion is challenged by the results of our satisfaction factor analysis (see Chapter 8). This showed that the two factors concerning satisfaction with major and minor interventions (i.e. 'did the right thing happen?') were both significantly related to emotional well-being and also to Description of Baby, even though the experience of the interventions themselves was not.

Such a result could simply mean that unhappy women are more likely to be dissatisfied with what happened to them (as we have already suggested more generally) but this explanation is unlikely for two reasons. First, such a relationship between low emotional well-being and low satisfaction with the whole birth experience was not found overall (see Chapter 8). Second, it was only the two satisfaction factors which concerned interventions that were related to Emotional well-being. If there were a general effect of unhappy women expressing retrospective dissatisfaction we would expect all four of the satisfaction factors to be related to emotional well-being. Given that this is not the case, our conclusion would be that having interventions *per se* does not make women unhappy but having interventions that they do not think that they should have had does. Thus, interventions *do* have implications for women's emotional well-being in a context which brings us back to the recurring themes of information and control, both of which were also related to three out of four outcome measures.

Staff issues

Much has been written about the importance of staff support and this issue was obviously important to the women in our study. The relationship each woman established with an individual midwife was important as was having one midwife present throughout labour. Women who received continuity of care in labour were much more satisfied with the birth experience than those who did not. Privacy was similarly important and was related both to satisfaction and to emotional well-being.

The attitude of the staff was related to psychological outcome. Women who described the staff as humorous, considerate, polite, warm and informative had positive outcomes. 'Informative' turned out to be a key word. Women who described the staff as informative were more satisfied, more positive about their babies and had greater emotional well-being than did other women.

Information was important at every stage: before, during and after labour. Women who indicated on the antenatal questionnaire that they felt they could discuss things fully with staff and felt they had been given the right amount of information were happier than other women postnatally. Women who felt they had at the very least been kept informed of non-emergency decisions during labour were more likely to feel that birth had been a fulfilling experience, to be satisfied and to be positive about the baby than other women. The women who said postnatally that they had been given the right amount of information, that there was nothing they wanted to know more about and that the information had been neither incomplete nor confusing, came out well on all four outcome measures. Information about the labour itself was welcomed both at the time and when looking back (especially if anything 'went wrong'). Women particularly wanted information about the postnatal period (especially breastfeeding).

Points for staff

- Caesarean sections are associated with a lack of fulfilment, as are instrumental deliveries. They are also associated with dissatisfaction with birth, negative descriptions of the baby and low emotional well-being.

- So-called 'minor' interventions like shaves or enemas, especially when perceived as unnecessary, can have major implications for women – they should not be given lightly.

- Contrary to obstetric lore we found that episiotomies are not necessarily better than tears. Having an episiotomy, unlike tearing, is associated with a sense of loss of control over what staff are doing to you and a lack of fulfilment postnatally. Suturing should be done with minimum delay and maximum care.

- Enabling women to move round and get as comfortable as possible is an important aspect of staff care during labour. Being able to get as comfortable as possible is positively associated both with having an intact perineum and psychological outcome measures.

- Supporting women in their wish to avoid pain-relieving drugs, especially Pethidine and epidurals, may help them to have more positive psychological outcomes. Women should not be pressurized to use pain-relieving drugs.

- Lack of continuity of care in labour inhibits the development of an intimate relationship and is associated with lack of fulfilment and dissatisfaction with the birth.

- Sending birth companions out of the room has a negative effect on women in labour.

- Women who feel informed about and involved in the management of labour and are able to retain some degree of 'external' as well as 'internal' control have better outcomes. The quality of staff care and *how* things are done are as important as *what* is done.

- Caring postnatal support and clear, skillful and *consistent* guidance for women trying to establish breastfeeding is vital in helping women in the first days and weeks of motherhood.

The stereotypes revisited

We all use internal models and sets of assumptions in the way we think about and interact with other people. When we do not know them personally we are more ready to make judgements on the basis of the way they look or the way they talk. These assumptions may be based on media representations, our previous experiences with people we perceive to be similar and our own 'in-group' stereotypes about 'such people'. Our review of the maternity care debates at the beginning of this report showed how stereotypes about pregnant women may be used to support generalizations about how the maternity services should operate (see Chapter 1). Our earlier research (Green et al., 1986) also showed how such stereotypes operate on the labour ward and form part of the ward 'ethos' and we suggested ways in which they might effect the care women receive. Staff may draw conclusions from, for instance, a woman's apparent educational level or what type of antenatal class (if any) she has attended. This may lead them to assume that they know what a particular woman wants and what is good for her. Indeed, we would suggest, that it is inevitable that staff will sometimes rely on stereotypes when working on a busy labour ward, especially if they do not have the chance to get to know the woman during labour. Stereotypes are a tool staff use to react quickly to a changing situation to approach a variety of women with different hopes and wishes. There is, however, a danger that they may become a substitute for communication between a woman and her caregivers. Furthermore, the kind of stereotypes evident among staff are often inappropriate and misleading. Many aspects of the most commonly expressed stereotypes did not hold true for the women in our sample. As noted earlier:

- the less educated and working class women did not want to hand over all control to the staff;
- working class women and middle class women were equally likely to subscribe to the ideal of avoiding drugs during labour;
- women who hoped to cope without drugs were not naive about the pain;
- having high expectations does not necessarily lead to feelings of failure and dissatisfaction.

Given such mismatches between stereotypes and women's actual feelings, it is not surprising that, in some cases, women felt treated according to a misconceived stereotype rather than listened to as an individual:

> 'Again I mention the antipathy to us as 'NCT parents' (because we had an NCT booklet with us).'

In addition, it would seem that some women also approach staff with their own sets of stereotypes. For example, there are assumptions that all older midwives are rigid and authoritarian. Black, Asian and/or overseas midwives and doctors are subject to racist stereotyping. 'Spinster' midwives who are assumed to be without children of their own are disparaged and said not to understand about labour. Such assumptions obstruct the development of a positive relationship between a woman and her caregivers during childbirth.

Systems of care which allow midwives and mothers to get to know each other (preferably before the birth) could do much to reduce reliance on stereotypes, with beneficial results for all concerned. There could be additional benefits if the same midwives were also able to follow through with postnatal care. They would then have the opportunity to discover that their assumptions about who will get depressed, and why, are not always correct.

Midwives (and doctors) are important participants in the experience of childbirth. Their attitudes and the quality of care they provide are central to women's memories of the experience. Some of women's most glowing reflections on their labours centred on staff who treated them as individuals and entered into the experience with warmth and respect. As one woman, who said that the support from the midwife was the best thing about the birth, commented:

> 'The staff at the hospital were marvellous. They treated us as individuals, told us their first names and called us by our first names, asked us what we wanted, and didn't pressure us at all to have things we didn't want. They explained everything they did.'

We end with the words of one happy and fulfilled mother:

> 'I think that in a perfect world every mother should have what I had – a midwife's face that said "Look, we have performed a miracle together" (and there was nothing to it!)'

CHAPTER TEN

Great Expectations Revisited

This chapter was written by Jo Green nine years after the rest of the report. Its purpose is to present some additional analyses, to revisit some of the themes of the study and to look at some more recent research.

The field work for the study was carried out in 1987. The research was done in a climate of protest at the direction that maternity care had taken and a perceived need to put the mother and her feelings back on the map. 'Choice' and 'control' were starting to be buzz words but this was, as much as anything, a general reflection of the consumer culture that 'choice' was desirable in its own right, irrespective of the nature of the choices available. We certainly did not anticipate that within five years of the publication of our study, many of the points that we were making would have been adopted as official policy via *Changing Childbirth* (Department of Health, 1993).

By insisting on the importance of choice and control, *Changing Childbirth* has made people much more aware of these issues. However, by taking them as given, it has not encouraged any questioning of *why* this should be so, and assumptions have been made about how to enhance these aspects of childbearing which do not necessarily take account of the available research evidence. As was the case a decade ago, there is still sometimes the assumption that the provision of 'choice' is a desirable end in itself. This is unlikely to be so unless the options really meet women's needs. From this point of view, *Changing Childbirth*'s other battle cry of 'woman-centred care' is likely to be closer to the mark. This is a phrase which can be interpreted in a variety of ways. However, if what it means is listening to a woman and providing care that fits her needs, then this is likely to enhance her sense of control and her sense of being respected as a person. These are important psychological considerations in any sphere of life. We should also remember that they apply to midwives as well as to the women for whom they care.

Changing Childbirth has been interpreted by many people in many ways. Harmond (1994) quotes one midwife's response to *Changing Childbirth* as:

> 'These days women can do exactly what they want and I have to go along with it and support them as best I can.' (p. 543)

Harmond points out the danger of this interpretation by focusing on hypothetical cases where women have made their choices based on incomplete information and argues that midwives need to be directive as well as supportive.

> 'When I go to the mortgage company for a loan, I do not want my financial adviser to smile and say "It's up to you". I want a considered appraisal of the options which best suit my needs and ability to cope, and some clear recommendations. The birth of a baby is infinitely more important than getting a mortgage but, on rare occasions, midwives give less guidance than the adviser at my local bank.'

This question of which aspects of care contribute to women's satisfaction will be discussed further below.

Further analysis of the Great Expectations data

Women's relationships with their caregiver(s)

It was clear in *Great Expectations* that the relationship between a woman and the people caring for her in labour was of considerable importance. This was revealed in a number of ways, for example:

- ubiquitous importance of feeling in control of what staff were doing
- adjectives to describe staff were related to psychological outcomes
- women were less satisfied if they felt under pressure to have drugs.

While having one midwife throughout the labour was associated with better outcomes, it made no difference whether or not this person had been met antenatally. This is an important finding in view of the current drive to reorganize midwifery services to achieve greater continuity between the antenatal and intrapartum periods. It is indeed a *Changing Childbirth* target that 75 per cent of women should be cared for in labour by someone that they have met antenatally. The findings of a number of other studies (e.g. Walker et al., 1995; Allen et al., 1997) indicate that where women have been delivered by a known midwife they appreciate this, but where they have not been they have not considered this to be important as long as they were still able to establish a good relationship at the time. It is likely that other aspects of the organization of care are more important to women's satisfaction than having a known midwife in labour (Green et al., 1998, in press).

In the study women had circled adjectives to describe the staff who looked after them in labour. We went back to these data to look at the way in which these grouped together. We carried out a factor analysis and found that the adjectives fell into three groups. The first group consisted of the negative adjectives which accounted for 20 per cent of the variance. The second group consisted of 'polite', 'considerate', 'humorous' and 'informative', which accounted for another 12 per cent. The final group was 'supportive', 'sensitive', 'warm' and 'rushed' (negative relationship): 8 per cent of the variance. This last group is a particularly interesting one. Whereas the second group gives an impression of efficiency-with-distance, the third group conveys the idea of a rather more intimate relationship – one that is evidently impaired when staff appear rushed. The distinction between these two groups of (mainly) positive adjectives is particularly interesting in the context of Harmond's comments quoted previously. I will return to the question of how these perceptions contribute to women's satisfaction later in this chapter.

We had conjectured that perceptions of the staff would be independent of the difficulties of the labour. We were able to test this by using regression analysis which seemed to support this assumption. We were also able to test our assumption that a woman's perception of the staff is a major determinant of her feeling of control over and above any contribution made by the difficulties of the labour. This was indeed so. All staff-perception variables were significant predictors of feelings of control even when controlling for length of labour and caesarean section.

Expectations

One of the main aims of *Great Expectations* was to explore the relationships between expectations, events and psychological outcomes. We were keen to do this because of the frequency with which the assumption was made that women have negative outcomes (e.g. postnatal depression) because of a mismatch between expectations and events and that the solution is to give them more realistic expectations. Unfortunately, this stereotype continues to be asserted, despite accumulating evidence of its inaccuracy. *Great Expectations* did not offer any support for this assumption, rather the reverse. However, the issue is a complex one, and so many issues are inter-related that it can be hard to follow the arguments.

There are a number of threads. Firstly, there is the distinction between an 'expectation' and a 'preference'. We postulated in the study that any relationship between expectations and outcomes was likely to be mediated by what a woman wanted to happen. Very few studies have taken account of this point (the study by Slade et al. (1993) (see below) is an exception). Then we need to be aware that experiences are themselves predicted by expectations (Chapter 7), so that separating their effects on psychological outcomes is not easy.

We therefore focused (at the end of Chapter 8) on a composite measure which divided women into three groups: those who wanted something and expected it; those who wanted something but did not expect it; and those who did not have a preference. We constructed this variable for the twelve socio-behavioural aspects of labour. In this study, these were the only areas where we asked parallel questions about both preferences and expectations. However future studies could do the same for other aspects of childbearing, for example regarding the use of different methods of pain relief. By subdividing the sample in this way, we were able to see that the group with the worst outcomes was consistently the group who wanted something but did not expect it to happen. In other words, women with *low* expectations. This has also been demonstrated in a number of other studies as well.

As we also knew that both education and parity were related in various ways to expectations and to outcomes (see, for example, Table 7.14), we went back to these data to try to discover whether the effects that we had found could be explained by these demographic variables. For each of the twelve socio-behavioural events, we carried out factorial analysis of variance (ANOVA) repeating the analysis that was summarized in Table 8.40, but this time adding education and parity. The results broadly confirmed the earlier findings: sometimes education or parity was a significant main effect and sometimes not, but this never overrode the significance of expecting/experiencing an event where it had previously been significant. So, although there is still much to be understood about these relationships, we can feel confident that the results reported in Table 8.40 are not simply a reflection of women with different demographic characteristics having different expectations or experiences.

The Cambridge Prenatal Screening Study (CPSS)

Since *Great Expectations* was first published there have been a number of other studies which have examined some of the same issues. One study that I will draw on heavily is the Cambridge Prenatal Screening Study (CPSS). This study was carried out by Helen Statham, Claire Snowdon and myself between 1989 and 1993. Its purpose was to chart the knowledge, attitudes, anxieties and experiences of pregnant women from before their first hospital appointment through to the postnatal period, with a particular focus on screening for fetal abnormality during routine antenatal care. The emphasis throughout was on normal experience, aiming to understand women's feelings at any given point within the context of the other aspects of their lives. Given this approach, data were collected not only on obstetric and demographic variables but also on a very wide range of other variables such as worries, relationships, attitudes, feelings and personality measures. Its remit and scope, therefore, were much wider than the *Great Expectations* study. However, as with *Great Expectations*, data were collected via postal questionnaires, designed specifically for the study. These were completed on four occasions: at or before 16 weeks, at 22 weeks, at 35 weeks and at 6 weeks after the expected date of delivery. Given the degree of overlap between the studies and the similar methodology, a number of the same questions were asked. It was therefore possible, firstly, to obtain confirmation of some of the *Great Expectations* findings, and secondly to explore some other relationships between variables which had not been part of the *Great Expectations* study.

The Cambridge Prenatal Screening Study: the sample

The women recruited to the study were drawn from nine health districts, all within 60 miles of Cambridge (UK). These included Willowford, Exington and Zedbury, three of the four districts in *Great Expectations*. Women booking between certain dates in the first four months of 1990 were eligible for the study whether they were booking a home, consultant unit or General Practitioner Unit (GPU) delivery. Unlike *Great Expectations* we did not oversample the Exington GPU, so the sample had a slightly lower number of multips. The average age was thus somewhat lower, and there were also proportionately more women under 21 in the CPSS sample. The six additional districts also contained some areas which were quite deprived; one was in an area of heavy industry and one contained within it an area of particularly high unemployment. The result of this was that the women in the CPSS sample were also less well educated than those in *Great Expectations*. Sample characteristics for the two samples are shown in Table 10.1. One thousand, eight hundred and twenty four women returned valid first questionnaires, but most of the findings that I will report here will be restricted to women who completed all four questionnaires, and will exclude those whose babies had died (n = 8) or had a serious health problem or abnormality (n = 26), leaving a total sample of 1285 women.

	Gt Ex n = 825	CPSS n = 1824
Parity 0	39%	44%
Education $\leq$ age 16	51%	57%
Education $>$ age 18	21%	12%
Age $<$ 21years	8%	12%
Age $\geq$ 35 years	9%	8%
Married or living as married	95%	92%
Overjoyed/pleased re discovering pregnancy	73%	70%

Table 10.1: Sample characteristics of the women in *Great Expectations* and in the Cambridge Prenatal Screening Study

Replications of Great Expectations analyses

One finding from *Great Expectations* which attracted a lot of attention was that there were no differences between women with different levels of education in the proportions wanting a drug-free or a pain-free labour. This seemed sufficiently surprising that we deliberately sought to replicate it in The Cambridge Prenatal Screening Study, even though it had little to do with the subject of that study. We found (Table 10.2) that the majority of the CPSS sample agreed with the *Great Expectations* sample in endorsing the use of the minimum quantity of drugs to keep the pain manageable. The same pattern of small differences was also seen between multips and primips: a similar proportion would choose a drug-free labour but more multips than primips would choose a pain-free labour. However, the CPSS sample was somewhat more likely than the *Great Expectations* sample to want a pain-free labour and less likely to want to manage without drugs, although the differences were not significant. This was true for both multips and primips. Could this be because we were sampling a less well-educated population? Apparently not, because, as in *Great Expectations*, there were no significant differences between women with different levels of education.

	Multips		Primips	
	Gt Ex n = 456	CPSS n = 743	Gt Ex n = 292	CPSS n = 610
The most pain-free labour that drugs can give me	11%	16%	6%	13%
The minimum quantity of drugs to keep the pain manageable	65%	65%	70%	69%
To put up with quite a lot of pain in order to have a completely drug-free labour	22%	19%	23%	18%
Other	3%	–	1%	–

Table 10.2: Percentage of women choosing different ideal options for drug use in labour in *Great Expectations* and The Cambridge Prenatal Screening Study

Other aspects of the CPSS data suggest that the differences in preference for drugs may have more to do with the ethos of the hospitals, particularly those hospitals that had not been part of *Great Expectations.* We have shown elsewhere (Green et al., 1994) that women's expectations of their experience on the delivery suite are shaped by this ethos even before they have visited the unit. In general we found that the CPSS sample had worse experiences in labour than the *Great Expectations* sample, and were less satisfied overall. They had more interventions, and circled more negative and fewer positive words to describe themselves in labour. This was true separately for multips and for primips and the pattern of parity differences found in *Great Expectations* was replicated. However, there was one area in which the CPSS sample seemed to diverge from the *Great Expectations* sample and that was involvement in non-emergency decision making. Here the pattern of responses was also particularly interesting when broken down by parity.

	Multips		Primips	
	Great Expects.	CPSS	Great Expects.	CPSS
Staff will make the decisions	6%	4%	2%	3%
Staff will keep me informed	41%	21%	34%	17%
Staff will discuss with me first	32%	44%	37%	44%
I will be in control of decisions	19%	27%	25%	32%
No expectations	3%	4%	2%	5%

Table 10.3: Expectations of involvement in non-emergency decision making

Table 10.3 shows that the CPSS sample expected much more involvement in decision making than did the women in *Great Expectations* (ANOVA, $p < 0.0001$). The vast majority of CPSS women (71% of multips and 76% of primips) expected that staff would at least discuss non-emergency decisions with them, whereas in *Great Expectations* the equivalent figures were 51 per cent and 62 per cent. Why this difference? We can, of course, only speculate, but there is nothing else in the data to suggest that this is a reflection of a particularly woman-centred labour-ward ethos. Rather, I would postulate that we are seeing a reflection of the passage of time between these two studies. In 1987 involving women in decisions about their care in labour was not the norm. *Great Expectations* included two hospitals which were quite forward looking in their woman-centred policies (Willowford and Wychester), but in the other units the modal expectation had been simply to be kept informed. However, by 1990 it was what most women were coming to expect.

So, were these higher expectations matched by more involvement in practice? Table 10.4 shows the reported experiences of the CPSS women alongside those from *Great Expectations.* The answer would seem to be a cautious 'yes': women in the Cambridge Prenatal Screening Study did report significantly more involvement in non-emergency decision-making than women in *Great Expectations,* although not as much as they were expecting. Whereas in *Great Expectations* 51 per cent of multips and 56 per cent of primips said that decisions had at least been discussed with them, in the Cambridge

Prenatal Screening Study the proportions were 65 per cent and 62 per cent. As in *Great Expectations*, differences between multips' and primips' experiences were not significant, although, in both cases, primips had had higher expectations. The difference between expectations and experience was particularly marked for CPSS primips. There were also, as in *Great Expectations*, significant differences between hospitals. Willowford was again amongst those where women felt the most involvement, while Exington women reported the lowest involvement of any of the nine hospitals.

	Multips		Primips	
	Gt Ex	CPSS	Gt Ex	CPSS
Staff made the decisions	13%	8%	10%	8%
Staff kept me informed	37%	27%	35%	30%
Staff discussed with me first	25%	33%	32%	34%
I was in control of decisions	26%	32%	24%	28%

Table 10.4: Involvement in non-emergency decision making

Control and emotional well-being

The predominant message that emerged from *Great Expectations* was that feeling in control is important. Furthermore, it seemed to be important:

- whether we consider 'internal' or 'external' control
- to all women irrespective of social class or education
- for all of the psychological outcomes that we considered
- even to women who, antenatally, said that it was not important.

The data from the Cambridge Prenatal Screening Study gave us some scope for exploring further how and why control is important. As in *Great Expectations*, one of the outcomes of interest to us was emotional well-being. In CPSS this was assessed using the full Edinburgh Postnatal Depression Scale (EPDS) (Cox et al., 1987). We had chosen to use the EPDS, rather than the EWB measure used in *Great Expectations* after a lot of deliberation. The arguments for the EWB measure still seemed valid, but we were conscious of having created a complicated measure that did not allow direct comparison with other studies. Furthermore, as an increasing number of community-based studies reported findings from the EPDS, often treating it as a continuous measure, it began to look as if the EPDS might in fact function as a continuous measure of emotional well-being, even if that was not its original aim or intention (see Green, 1998). We also felt more comfortable with this course of action since we had included additional measures of positive feelings (see below).

One of the issues that arose in *Great Expectations* (see also Green, 1990) was the continuity between antenatal and postnatal emotional well-being. We were able to pursue this more systematically in the Cambridge Prenatal Screening Study because we had data throughout pregnancy, and we also administered the EPDS at 35 weeks of pregnancy as well as six weeks postnatally. We were able to divide women into four groups according to whether they scored above EPDS cut off both antenatally and postnatally (Both n = 66), antenatally only (Ante n = 81), postnatally only (Post n

= 109) or on neither occasion (Neither n = 1016). These analyses are described in Green and Murray (1994) and in Green (1998). The point to be noted here is that various indicators of control in labour were significantly different between the groups, with the 'neither' group always reporting most control, and the 'both' group least. This is shown in Table 10.5

	Neither n = 1016	Ante n = 81	Post n = 109	Both n = 66	p<
Not able to get comfortable in labour	16%	28%	26%	34%	.001
Felt in control of behaviour during labour	52%	37%	48%	36%	.05
Felt in control during contractions	56%	42%	42%	31%	.0001
Felt in control of what staff doing in labour[1]	64%	58%	48%	46%	.0001

Table 10.5: Percentages of women in each EPDS group reporting various feelings of control (see text for definition of groups). Data from the Cambridge Prenatal Screening Study

These data help to suggest at least one piece to fit into the jigsaw created by *Great Expectations.* We appear to see here that low postnatal emotional well-being (as indicated by a high EPDS score) is indeed associated with feeling less in control during labour. It is also clear from these data that not feeling in control may itself be a consequence of low antenatal emotional well-being. A likely model which fits both this and the *Great Expectations* findings on expectations is that shown in Figure 10.1 below.

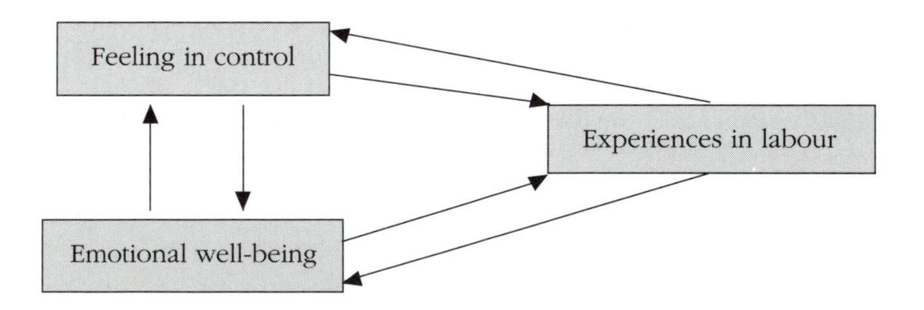

Fig. 10.1: Model of the relationship between control, experiences and well-being

1. We combined the response options 'all of the time' and 'most of the time' in the questionnaire, since we intended to combine them for analysis. The other two options remained as 'some of the time' and 'hardly at all'. This may have been a mistake since it seems to have made people more likely to choose the 'some of the time' option than in *Great Expectations.* This should be a methodological lesson to us all!

POSMO (Positive Experiences of Motherhood)

An additional outcome measure in the Cambridge Prenatal Screening Study was a composite variable called POSMO (Positive experiences of Motherhood) (see Green and Kafetsios, 1997), based on items from Kumar et al.'s (1984) MAMA scale. This was included because one of our concerns in *Great Expectations* about using a depression measure had been that this gave no scope for measuring positive experiences. Using regression techniques we were able to demonstrate that 25 per cent of the variance of POSMO could be accounted for by antenatal variables, principally by expectations of motherhood assessed at 35 weeks. A further 24 per cent of the variance was accounted for by concurrent variables, of which anxiety was the most important. Perceptions of the baby, tiredness and EPDS score also made independently significant contributions. The correlation between POSMO and EPDS was -0.46. Three important points emerge from the POSMO analyses which relate to *Great Expectations.*

Firstly, this confirms the importance of assessing expectations and provides further evidence that *high* expectations lead to better outcomes. EXMO (Expectations of Motherhood), which was the antenatal equivalent of POSMO, was highly correlated with POSMO: the better the experience a woman expected, the more positive her reported experiences. Conversely women with negative expectations of motherhood reported less positive experiences.

Secondly, it tells us that anxiety is an important variable. Anxiety had not been assessed in *Great Expectations* except in the specific context of anxiety about the pain of labour. However, there it proved to be a strong predictor of a number of other measures, and was the only pain-related measure to be strongly related to EWB. The CPSS data would therefore suggest that that question may have been functioning as a surrogate measure of more general anxiety. Certainly we found anxiety, as measured by the State-Trait Anxiety Inventory (Spielberger et al., 1970), to be a ubiquitous variable in the Cambridge Prenatal Screening Study. However, we also found that it was very highly correlated with the EPDS (0.73).

The third finding of importance to *Great Expectations* from the POSMO analysis is that experiences of labour were almost completely uncorrelated with POSMO, and this included the various measures of feeling in control. A likely explanation is that our measure of *positive* experiences of motherhood really is measuring something different from the negatively loaded measures, EWB and EPDS. In other words, it suggests that POSMO is more than just an inversion of measures of negative mood, such as EPDS. The fact that the correlation between POSMO and EPDS was no higher than -0.46 would also support this interpretation. If the two measures were simply inversions of each other, then one would expect a higher correlation. Another way of looking at this is to say that positive and negative feelings can co-exist, and one is not just the opposite of the other. If this is so, and there is evidence from other areas of psychology which would support this, then our attempts in *Great Expectations* to create a single uni-dimensional measure of emotional well-being may have been misguided. It may well be that future studies will gain greater insights by assessing positive and negative feelings separately, as has also been argued by Slade et al. (1993) and Waldenström et al. (1996).

Perceptions of the baby and emotional well-being

POSMO was related to perceptions of the baby, and this is hardly surprising. It faces us with the same dilemma that we had in interpreting the relationship in *Great Expectations* between EWB and perceptions of the baby: which is cause and which effect? Did women perceive their babies negatively because they were unhappy, or were they unhappy because they had difficult babies? When we designed the Cambridge Prenatal Screening Study we had this question in mind and tried to devise a way of answering it. We reasoned that asking women to circle adjectives to describe their baby *before* the baby was born would give us an equivalent measure, relatively untainted by infant behaviour. If negative perceptions of the baby are a consequence of low mood or depression, then women who are depressed antenatally will also be more negative about their babies. If, however, low mood is a response to infant behaviour, we would be less likely to find a relationship between description of the baby and low mood at this time. Women in the Cambridge Prenatal Screening Study were therefore presented with a modified adjective checklist at 35 weeks and asked to circle all of the words that described their baby. We found that just three of the baby adjectives were significantly different between women with high antenatal EPDS scores and those without. Only one of these was highly significant: draining. The other two were 'restless' and 'angry' (both $p < 0.01$), but only six women in the whole sample actually chose the word angry. This would seem to indicate that depressed women were not, on the whole, more likely to describe their babies negatively. Indeed some of the open-ended statements made by women gave an impression more of sorrow than of anger regarding their baby. For example, this poignant comment from a woman with a high antenatal EPDS score:

> 'I have doubts about bringing something so innocent into a world of troubles. It doesn't stand much chance of being happy.'

The list of adjectives that we devised for *Great Expectations* has since been used by a number of other researchers in a variety of contexts. Sikorski et al. (1996) used it in a randomized controlled trial in South East London comparing the normal schedule of antenatal visits with a reduced schedule. There were a number of indications that many women did not like the new schedule. Particularly worrying was that women in the group allocated to the new schedule had less confidence in themselves as mothers and had significantly more negative perceptions of their babies at six weeks postnatally. This was despite the fact that the difference between the groups in the *actual* mean number of antenatal visits was very small and there was no difference in attendance at parentcraft classes. This study is very important for a number of reasons, not least in demonstrating the importance of building women's confidence, not only for coping with labour but for the years to follow.

Other studies

There have, of course, been a large number of studies published since 1988 which touch on some of the same themes as *Great Expectations*. Many suffer from similar problems to those highlighted in Chapter 1, particularly from small samples. Here I shall outline just a few specific studies which have overcome some of these problems and which have a number of points of overlap with *Great Expectations*.

Control and expectations

Amongst the most important contributions on the subject of 'control' has been the work of Ellen Hodnett. Two studies which were being carried out in Canada at much the same time as *Great Expectations* (Hodnett, 1989; Hodnett and Osborn, 1989), looked at predictors of women's sense of control in childbirth. The first compared 80 women who had chosen a homebirth with 80 who had chosen to give birth in hospital. All were interviewed within the last month of pregnancy and again two weeks after the birth. Women completed the Labor Agentry Scale (LAS) (Hodnett and Simmons-Tropea, 1987), which is a 29-item rating scale which measures women's expectations or experiences (depending on wording and timing of administration) of control in labour. Anxiety was also measured using the State Trait Anxiety Inventory (STAI) (Spielberger et al., 1970). Analysis was carried out separately for multips and primips as well as by where the birth took place. No differences were found between the home and hospital groups in third trimester anxiety, but women planning to give birth at home had higher expectations of control, of involvement in decision making and of not using drugs. Broadly speaking, these expectations were realized.

No parity differences were found for women giving birth in hospital, but within the home group, multips had better experiences than primips. Home multips had had the highest expectation of control and actually experienced more control than they had expected. For the other three groups, LAS scores were equivalent antenatally and postnatally (using paired t-tests), i.e. expectation and experience were not significantly different from each other. The author thus concluded that women had realistic expectations of their chosen birth environment, except for the home multips, whose previous hospital experience had led them to underestimate the degree of control that they would have at home. For both multip groups there was a positive correlation between expected and experienced control. Two other studies are cited (both unpublished Masters theses) which also found that high expectations were consistently related to high levels of control and satisfaction. Multivariate analysis explained 33.5 per cent of variance in experienced control with the important determinants being high expectations of control and home environment.

The study by Hodnett and Osborn (1989) was concerned with the effects of continuous intrapartum professional support on childbirth outcomes, and was conducted as a randomized controlled trial. Participants were all attending prenatal classes (Lamaze or General), and were mainly white, middle class and well-educated. Women were recruited in the third trimester. There were 145 women initially, but after the exclusion of those with complications and those who dropped out, 103 were left in the final sample. Measures included anxiety (STAI), expectations of control (LAS) and 'Commitment to Unmedicated Birth' (CUB). The first interview was at 33 weeks, when anxiety and expected control were assessed. Women were randomized after this, either to have continuous support by a known caregiver in labour (the experimental group) or normal care (the control group). Groups were stratified by the type of class that women were attending. Experimental group couples then met their assigned caregiver and established a relationship. Controls also had additional professional contacts at this point but not with someone who would support them in labour. The second interview was at 38–39 weeks. Measures of anxiety and expected control were repeated and commitment to unmedicated birth (CUB) assessed. When labour started, experimental couples contacted their caregiver who provided early labour support at home and continued to be with them until one hour postpartum. All other medical and nursing care was the same for the two groups. Postnatal interviews took place at home two to four weeks after the birth.

Lamaze class attenders were found to have higher expectations of control pre-randomization and higher CUB scores. Women in the experimental group were more likely to have a drug-free labour. CUB, LAS and STAI were all associated with non-significant differences in the use of drugs. Based on the original 145 women, no differences were found between the experimental and control groups in the likelihood of having a caesarean section (18%). Based on the 103 women without complications, the experimental group were found to be less likely to have an episiotomy or to be placed in stirrups for delivery. However, they were *more* likely to have oxytocic induction or augmentation. There were no differences in the number of women who tore, but the experimental group had more intact perineums. There were no differences in the length of labour. Removing from the analysis the 33 women who had oxytocics revealed some significant differences in the remainder – those who had pain relief had longer labours, more experimental than control women had no pain relief and the experimental group had fewer forceps and less electronic fetal monitoring. Within the control group, there were no differences in the LAS scores of women attending Lamaze and General classes, but the experimental group had higher scores and within the experimental group those attending Lamaze classes had higher scores than the General classes. However, repeated measures ANOVA showed only time (i.e. from antenatal to post) as a significant main effect on LAS scores, plus a time x support interaction. Multiple regression showed that expected control at the first interview and being in the experimental group with no pain relief in labour accounted for 30 per cent of the variance in experienced control. In the subgroup of 28 women with unmedicated births, a similar model (adding trait anxiety) accounted for 61 per cent of the variance.

Thus, both of these studies showed, as did *Great Expectations*, that higher expectations predict better experiences. Another study which considered some of these same issues was that by Slade et al. (1993) entitled 'Expectations, experiences and satisfaction with labour'. The focus of this study was in looking at different components of satisfaction and in recognizing that positive and negative emotions can be experienced simultaneously. The participants were 81 primiparous women having antenatal care at a large teaching hospital in the North of England. Expectations of labour were rated at 38 weeks, in the antenatal clinic, and events within 72 hours of birth, on the postnatal ward. Most assessments were made on 10-point rating scales from 'not at all' to 'extremely'. The same items were used antenatally and postnatally with the wording appropriately modified. Questions covered feelings in labour; pain and the use of pain relieving drugs; control (mainly of pain and pain-relief decisions) and, postnatally, whether the experience was as expected and satisfaction with how she had coped. Women who had an elective section were excluded from the analyses.

Mean expectation and experience ratings were found to be the same for: negative emotions (except that women found labour more difficult and less embarrassing than expected) and pain (both overall pain and worst pain). Antenatal ratings were significantly higher than experiences (i.e. optimistic) for: positive emotions (significant for each of the five adjectives and in total); length of labour; use of breathing and relaxation exercises and their effectiveness; use of interventions and degree of control.

Correlations showed that positive emotional expectations correlated well with positive emotional experiences. Negative emotional expectations/experiences were also significantly correlated, but less strongly. Multiple regression was used to predict total positive emotion scores using all emotional, medical and control variables as predictors. The only one found to be significant was expectation of positive emotions. Correlations between expectations and experiences of: worst pain, personal control over duration of labour and staff ability to control the pain were also all highly significant. Correlations for most other expectations/experiences were also significant, although less so.

Women who expected to use medication or epidural generally did, but so did many of those who did not expect to. The relationship between expectation and experience was still significant in most cases, as we had also found in *Great Expectations*. The exception to this pattern was episiotomy: many more women had episiotomies than expected to (60%) and women who expected it were *less* likely to have it. Women who had had unexpected interventions were compared with those who had not in terms of their experience of pain and negative emotions, but no differences were found. Similarly women whose prediction of pain had been an overestimate, underestimate or the same as their experience were found not to differ in terms of their experience of negative emotions.

Personal satisfaction was strongly related to personal control, especially control of panic and the use of breathing and relaxation exercises, but also to the efficacy of exercises, control of pain, duration and position. Personal satisfaction was not predicted by expectations of positive emotions. Comparison between those who attended antenatal classes and those who did not showed few differences.

These findings reinforce *Great Expectations* and Hodnett's studies in showing that positive expectations are associated with positive experiences and that these can co-exist with realistic appraisal of negative aspects. Discrepancies between pain expectations and experiences did not seem to effect emotional experiences or personal satisfaction. The latter was strongly related to control, particularly the ability to control panic. The authors suggest that this is more important than controlling pain and that the efficacy of exercises is in reducing panic and thus increasing tolerance for pain rather than in reducing the pain itself.

Other studies looking at expectations

An earlier study by Knight and Thirkettle (1987) looked at the relationship between expectations of pregnancy and birth and transient depression post-partum ('postnatal blues'). Depression was measured on a visual-analogue scale (respondents marked a point on a line to indicate how depressed they were) because this had been found to be more sensitive than a symptom-based measure in a previous study. Participants were drawn from a group of 180 first-time mothers attending antenatal classes in New Zealand, ninety-eight of whom took part. They completed a questionnaire at 36 weeks consisting of a very large number of 5- or 7-point rating scales. A similar questionnaire was completed at one day postpartum and the depression scale and other mood measures every subsequent day that they were in hospital (an average of seven days). Twelve 7-point scales were used to rate the experience of the birth covering how pleasant, painless, satisfying etc. it was, and on another 7-point scale women rated the extent to which the labour and birth were as expected. This study is thus of interest methodologically because expectations were assessed both antenatally and postnatally.

Few antenatal measures predicted the blues. The most important were trait anxiety (i.e. anxiety as a personality characteristic rather than transient anxiety) and fear of birth. Trait depression and trait anxiety were highly correlated. The correlation between trait depression and the blues 'confirmed several previous findings that level of depression during pregnancy is one of the best predictors of the post-partum adjustment' (p. 356). There was no evidence that the women's evaluation of their birth experience, finding birth to be as expected, or expectations of childbirth were associated with experience of the blues.

No correlation was found between women's ratings ante- and postnatally concerning how pleasant etc. labour would be. However, saying (postnatally) that labour was 'as expected' was the best predictor of a positive rating of the birth experience. The authors translate this as meaning that women who found birth unpleasant report after the event that they were not expecting this to be the case. That is, indeed, consistent with the lack of correlation. What needs to be explained, however, is the opposite, that is that women with positive evaluations of the birth say that this *was* what they were expecting, even though the scales completed antenatally apparently did not indicate this. It could be that the rating scales were not a reliable measure of expectations, or that there was not enough variation in women's responses antenatally to be meaningful. For example if everybody had positive expectations that would explain these findings. Note that the 'expectations' under discussion here are very subjective ones e.g. how pleasant, how satisfying etc. birth would be, in contrast to some other studies which have looked at expectations of rather more objective events such as a drug-free labour or presence of a partner.

A study that went to the opposite extreme in this respect was that by Morcos et al. (1989), which looked at expectations and importance ratings for specific aspects of childbirth. The study was conducted in Alberta (Canada) in the mid-1980s. Only low risk women were included, recruited by their obstetricians during the last six to eight weeks of pregnancy when they were given a questionnaire which was returned at the next visit. Fathers were also included. Out of the 242 couples recruited initially, 95 women volunteered to continue with the study after birth. These were requested to respond to a revised form of the questionnaire in hospital and 90 did. It is not clear why so few were willing to complete a postnatal questionnaire.

As in *Great Expectations*, the authors identified a number of areas of potential importance to parents and asked for each a) how important is it to you? and b) how likely do you think it is to happen? All were answered on a scale from 1 to 5. Topic areas were: prenatal teaching, birth experience, hospital stay, meals, caesarean section and postnatal factors. Items tended to be largely procedural, e.g. prenatal classes should extend over several months; knowing who will be available to attend delivery if own doctor not available; fathers being able to get meals at the hospital. Mean importance ratings given by the mothers were the same (c.3.5) for all the areas. Both mothers and fathers gave higher ratings for importance than for expectations. The wording of the questions did not give respondents scope to say if it was important to them that an event should *not* occur. It is interesting that where there are discrepancies between wants and expectations, the suggested remedy is to give parents information to change one or the other to bring them into line. Nowhere is it suggested that procedural changes might be made so that what parents think is important is more likely to happen.

For the subgroup who returned the postnatal questionnaire, 2-way analysis of variance was carried out with parity as the second variable. For the areas of prenatal teaching, caesarean section and postnatal factors, there were no differences between antenatal and postnatal ratings. For 'birth experience', importance ratings were lower postnatally than antenatally for both multips and primips. For the area of 'hospital stay', primips gave higher importance ratings than multips, and both rated importance lower postnatally than antenatally.

There have also been a number of less informative studies that have considered expectations of childbirth (Crowe and von Baeyer, 1989; Beaton and Gupton, 1990; Fridh and Gaston-Johansson, 1990; Munns and Galsworthy, 1995). The study by Fridh and Gaston-Johansson (1990) is a Swedish study of 50 primips and 88 multips, and is mainly about pain. It starts with the assertion that women with unrealistic expectations of pain experience worse pain, although this is not supported by their data for primips. There are also mismatches between the tables and text which make it difficult to be clear about the study's findings. The main finding was that actual pain was scored higher on a visual analogue scale than expected pain was antenatally, but there was no attempt to discover whether this was simply a measurement issue and whether it mattered to the women, whether they perceived a discrepancy etc. Unfortunately, despite this omission, much of the discussion is taken up with statements about disappointment and lack of satisfaction without assessing either. Little comment is made on aspects other than pain ratings, most of which showed that experience was *better than* expectation.

Satisfaction

A number of other studies have addressed the question of satisfaction with birth experiences. There are, however, problems with the concept of satisfaction and the ways in which we measure it. We had already acknowledged these issues in *Great Expectations*, and this was the rationale for our satisfaction factor analysis. We also argued that our 'marks out of 10' overall satisfaction measure was likely to be more sensitive at the end of a questionnaire when women had already been led through a detailed account of their various potential sources of satisfaction and dissatisfaction, than if it were asked in isolation. However, this has not been tested empirically.

It is quite possible that different measures of satisfaction are actually measuring different things. An interesting paper by Bramadat and Driedger (1993) entitled 'Satisfaction with childbirth: theories and methods of measurement' addresses this issue explicitly. The paper draws on the authors' two PhD/Masters theses, one quantitative and one qualitative, to explore what satisfaction means and how to assess it, and provides a good coverage of the literature. The authors make the important observation that 'satisfaction' is not just *having* a positive experience but a positive evaluation of that experience, in other words it has an affective component. Unfortunately, it does not go on to tackle the question of whether some women may be more easily satisfied than others.

Bramadat and Driedger discuss psychological models of satisfaction, and conclude that they tend to be based on evaluation of the experience relative to expectations. They reject this assumption with examples from Bramadat's study of women with high expectations and bad experiences who said, nonetheless, that they were satisfied. What these women had in common was a very positive perception of the control they experienced during labour and birth. Bramadat did not find that expectations or discrepancy between expectations and events had particularly strong relationships with satisfaction. However, perception of control, measured by the Labor Agentry Scale (Hodnett and Simmons-Tropea, 1987), accounted for 59 per cent of the variance of satisfaction. This emerged as much more important than other perceptions of the event, such as coping with pain and support from partner. Satisfaction ratings seemed to be consistent at different length of follow-up.

A number of small qualitative studies have also made interesting contributions to this area. Bluff and Holloway (1994) carried out interviews with 11 women in the maternity unit of a general hospital. Unfortunately we do not know quite what it was that women were asked, which limits the study's value, but the paper still highlights some interesting issues to do with choice and control. Qualitative analysis of the interviews revealed a 'core construct' which was 'they know best' i.e. midwives are the experts and women therefore trust them. One particular quotation, which says a great deal is:

> 'I hadn't really wanted an epidural, but they said "we feel it might be best", but it was a case of "would you like it?". I did have choice, but I wouldn't have had it if they hadn't said it was best.' (Bluff and Holloway, 1994, p. 160)

This quote highlights the way in which the presentation of an issue is critical to the woman's sense of control. For many women it is likely that the belief that 'they know best', i.e. that one is being cared for by experts, is essential to feeling in control. The alternative feeling – that one is being cared for by people who do not know what they are doing – would almost certainly lead to a feeling of panic and loss of control in all but the most confident woman. Given this need to believe in the staff's expertise, the woman will nearly always follow the staff's advice, but the belief that she *could* have made a different choice enhances her sense of control.

The authors interpret women saying 'they must have had a reason' as evidence of trust in the midwife's knowledge. However, it may be that women *need* to have this belief in order to feel in control. The alternative is to believe that the midwife is acting arbitrarily, which, I have just argued, is likely to lead to panic and loss of control. It was noted that feeling in control did not necessarily mean active participation in decision making, as we also found in *Great Expectations.* In some cases, feeling in control was associated with having an explanation before a procedure was carried out, in others it was feeling *able* to challenge what the midwife suggested, even if this did not happen.

An example given in the paper is of a woman given a third stage injection against her wishes, who felt reassured by someone else taking control when she herself was exhausted, even though the action itself was not what she wanted. The woman's partner did not challenge the injection because 'they know best' and he did not want to argue about it. This example can be taken as supporting the argument above, but we should also remember that to have objected would not only have meant a challenge to the idea that 'they know best', but would also have involved potential conflict, which exhausted parents with their newly delivered baby are unlikely to want. Particularly, given the power imbalance, it is easier to believe that that was the right thing after all. This brings us back to another of *Great Expectations*' key findings: that positive psychological outcomes were associated with the belief that the right thing had happened rather than with the activity itself.

Bluff and Holloway go on to make another very important point:

> 'It is worth noting that while it may appear from the midwife's perspective that the woman lacked sufficient information to make some decisions themselves, the women were unaware of this apparent lack of information. The women perceived that they had received enough information and only wanted more when their wishes had been disregarded.' (ibid., p. 161)

This is a very insightful observation, which probably accounts for the strong contribution of 'information' in the original univariate *Great Expectations* analyses, and its subsequent disappearance from the multivariate analysis. What is probably happening is that those women who say that the information that they were given was in some way unsatisfactory are those who have had some adverse experience that has revealed the inadequacy of their information. Other women, who may have been given exactly the same information (or lack of it), will not report it as unsatisfactory because it will not have been put to the test in the same way. Thus, when we carry out multivariate analysis we discover that reporting unsatisfactory information is just another manifestation of some other unsatisfactory aspect of the birth, rather than an independent source of dissatisfaction.

Another recently published qualitative study is that by Walker et al. (1995). This was based on retrospective interviews with 18 women and three partners on the postnatal ward and another 14 women, three partners and one friend at home three to five months after the birth. This study used purposive sampling, that is to say that women were deliberately chosen to represent the full range of experiences rather than to be typical or randomly chosen. The core category to emerge from this qualitative analysis was the balance between personal control and support. Control came from being able to have support (i.e. the midwife's presence) when it was wanted and not when it was not, and from being able to hand over control or let the midwife take control when appropriate. Thus women are able to make comments like 'it was great, she took control' because the midwife taking control at the appropriate moment was perceived as highly supportive. The key point that these authors make is that staffing levels must be such as to allow parents confidence that the midwife will be there instantly if needed. This study reiterates the point that women need to have confidence in their caregivers.

Two large studies have used multivariate statistical techniques to explore determinants of satisfaction in women giving birth. The first is an Australian study carried out by the Centre for the Study of Mothers' and Children's Health at Monash University (Brown et al., 1994; Brown and Lumley, 1994). All women in Victoria who gave birth in one week in 1989 were sent a questionnaire eight to nine months after the birth. Seven hundred and ninety valid questionnaires were returned (71%). Satisfaction was assessed by one question:

Overall, do you feel your labour and delivery were:

- managed as you liked
- managed as you liked in some ways but not in others
- not managed as you liked?

Women giving the first response were deemed to be satisfied, any other response was considered to be dissatisfied. Thus, 'satisfaction' here has quite a narrow focus on just one aspect of the experience and is much more to do with the activities of the staff than with the contribution of the woman herself. This is in contrast to, for example, Slade et al.'s (1993) concept of personal satisfaction, discussed above, which focuses on women's satisfaction with how they coped. Each of these in turn is probably tapping something different from the global satisfaction measure that we used in *Great Expectations* and which most other studies have also, rightly or wrongly, tended to use.

Brown et al. used logistic regression to model the determinants of satisfaction in their sample. Five factors emerged as significant, although the last two were borderline:

- Having been given an active say in decision making
- Information
- Pain worse than expected/better or same
- Helpfulness of caregivers
- Education

Factors that were not significant in the regression model were:

- Obstetric procedure score
- Held baby soon after birth
- Unwanted people present at the birth
- Length of first stage
- Parity

The other large study that used regression analysis to explore determinants of satisfaction was carried out in Sweden by Waldenström et al. (1996). Thirty-six variables were tested in the model, six of which were significant:

- Support from midwife (sensitivity to needs) (scored 1–7)
- Duration of labour (log hours)
- Pain (scored 1–7)
- General expectations of birth (scored 1–7 from very negative to very positive)
- Involvement and participation in the birth process (scored 1–7)
- Surgical procedures (scored 0/1)

The dependent variable was overall satisfaction with birth on a 7-point scale anchored at very positive and very negative.

These two studies are both valuable additions to the literature. Their lists have some items in common, but as many that are not. Brown et al. found parity differences in their initial analysis, even though these did not contribute to the final model, whereas Waldenström et al. found none. Brown et al. also had education in their model which was not considered in the Waldenström et al. study. Waldenström et al. found obstetric interventions to be significant while Brown et al. did not. Variables that appear more consistently in various guises in both these and other studies are aspects of 'pain' and 'control'. We therefore returned to the original *Great Expectations* data to explore further the contributions of these and other variables to overall satisfaction.

Multiple regression analyses

Pain and satisfaction

We showed in Chapter 8 that many aspects of pain were related to satisfaction (see also Green, 1993). These included the use of Pethidine and epidurals but also antenatal questions such as anxiety about the pain, expected level of pain and preferred level of drug use. However, we also saw (Chapter 5) that drug use was related to many of these antenatal variables (although, interestingly, not to anxiety about the pain). Both drug use and satisfaction were also related to parity. The question that we have since sought to answer is: can differences in satisfaction be explained entirely by drug use, or is there an independent effect of expectations? In other words, for example, is the greater satisfaction of women who preferred a drug-free labour or who expected lower levels of pain attributable just to their lower use of drugs, or is there some additional effect associated with those antenatal attitudes? To answer this question we carried out a hierarchical multiple regression. We entered variables in three groups.

The first group were items from the postnatal questionnaire:

- whether pain was as expected
- use of breathing and relaxation
- use of 'gas and air'
- use of Pethidine or substitute
- use of epidural
- satisfaction with response to pain

The second group were antenatal variables:

- worry about labour pain
- preferred level of drug use
- expected level of pain
- expected usefulness of breathing and relaxation techniques

The final group were the demographic variables parity and education.

All the variables in the first group had been related to satisfaction, and this had been shown to be the case independently for both multips and primips. However, we did not know to what extent they related to each other. For example, it might just be that women who did not use drugs were more satisfied with their response to pain, and that these variables would not both be making independent contributions to satisfaction. This is what the multiple regression technique can tell us.

The findings were that, within the first group of variables,

- whether pain was as expected ($p < 0.001$)
- use of pethidine or substitute ($p < 0.001$)
- use of epidural ($p < 0.05$)
- satisfaction with response to pain ($p < 0.0001$)

were all independent determinants of satisfaction. Use of breathing and relaxation and use of 'gas and air' were not. Thus the apparently strong effect of breathing and relaxation is probably because it is associated with non-use of pethidine or epidural.

When we added in the second group of variables to the regression, we found that just two added significantly to the model: worry about labour pain ($p < 0.01$) and expected usefulness of breathing and relaxation techniques ($p < 0.01$). Preferred level of drug use and expected level of pain were both non-significant. We have, therefore, the curious finding that although the actual use of breathing and relaxation does not contribute independently to satisfaction, their expected usefulness does.

Finally we added parity and education. In the univariate analyses, parity had been very strongly related to satisfaction, but education had not been. Adding them into the multiple regression yielded the opposite result: parity was not significant ($p = 0.75$), but education was ($p < 0.01$). These surprising findings are an excellent demonstration of the value of using multivariate statistical techniques when so many variables are interrelated. What is evidently happening with parity is that the other factors that were significant have accounted for the differences between multips and primips. In other words, the multiple regression allows us to explain the earlier parity difference in terms of differences between multips and primips in their use of drugs, feelings about how they coped, and so on, and there is no additional significant parity effect to be explained. In contrast, a significant education difference is revealed that was masked in the univariate analyses. This shows that women with higher education were less satisfied, and vice versa. However, higher levels of education were also associated with other factors that were associated with *higher* satisfaction such as lower levels of drug use. In the univariate analyses these effects cancelled each other out, but in the multiple regression we are able to see both at work.

In total these factors accounted for 22.7 per cent of the variance in overall satisfaction. The analysis was repeated as a step-wise multiple regression, which means that the computer determines the order of variables to find the best fit, and this yielded the same result.

Control and satisfaction

Three of the control questions:

- feeling in control of the staff
- feeling in control of contractions
- losing control of behaviour

were added to the list of variables in the stepwise regression analysis just described. This increased the variance accounted for to 29 per cent. Feeling in control of the staff made the strongest contribution ($p < 0.0001$), control of contractions was only just significant ($p < 0.05$) and control of behaviour did not contribute significantly to the model. Having an epidural and expected usefulness of breathing and relaxation were no longer significant in this model ($p = 0.06$ and $p = 0.07$) when these control variables were included.

To investigate the relative contributions of different aspects of control further, we took a step back and looked only at control related variables, without the pain-related variables. The first model included only:

- control of behaviour
- being able to get comfortable
- control of staff
- having the right amount of information
- parity
- education

Of these, all except parity were independently significant determinants of satisfaction, and together accounted for 23 per cent of the variance.

We continued generating multiple regressions in this vein: considering groups of variables, such as obstetric interventions and staff perceptions, retaining those that were significant, and at last combining all of these in the final model. This is shown in Table 10.6. This accounted for 37 per cent of the variance

Variable	Beta	significance
Variables in the equation		
Feelings about how well coped with pain	-.204287	.0000
Expectations of usefulness of breathing and relaxation	-.096402	.0074
Being able to get comfortable	.122196	.0017
Feeling in control of what the staff were doing	-.194037	.0000
Having a caesarean section	.165715	.0000
Having an instrumental delivery	.112643	.0040
Education	-.110653	.0020
Perception of staff (Factor 1)*	.093190	.0100
Perception of staff (Factor 2)*	-.090382	.0114
Antenatal worry re labour pain	-.076620	.0291
Episiotomy	.087682	.0290
Having no pain-relieving drugs (or gas & air only)	-.083702	.0260
Variables not in the equation		
Whether pain was as expected	.044634	.2231
Parity	-.025325	.5133
Losing control of behaviour	-.051497	.1797
Feeling in control of contractions	.023831	.5087
Unsatisfactory information	029269	.4316
Having a glucose drip	.001014	.9795
Length of labour	-.028140	.4444
Perception of staff (Factor 3)*	.042780	.2208
Age	-.019998	.5845

* As defined earlier in this chapter:
Factor 1: negative adjectives
Factor 2: polite, considerate, humorous and informative
Factor 3: supportive, sensitive, warm and rushed (negative relationship)

Table 10.6: Final regression model predicting satisfaction (data from *Great Expectations*)

Feeling in control of what the staff were doing was the only one of the control questions to make an independent contribution. As we had postulated, feelings of internal control probably follow from this. However, being able to get comfortable did remain independently significant, even alongside these other variables. It is interesting to see that two of three perceptions of staff factors remained in the model as well. Of particular interest is that the third factor, that associated with intimacy and warmth, was the one that was *not* significant. Rather it was the positive factor represented by polite, considerate, humorous and informative, that was significantly related to women's satisfaction.

Replication of the multiple regression model with CPSS data

The regression model above summarizes the factors that were independently important determinants of satisfaction for the *Great Expectations* sample. The final test that we can apply is to discover whether these same variables also provide a good model for the CPSS sample. Unfortunately, we had not asked all of the relevant questions in CPSS. We therefore had to omit the perceptions of staff and expectations of the efficacy of breathing and relaxation, and questions on information were also not comparable. We were able to add in a couple of other variables that had not been in *Great Expectations*: Trait Anxiety and 'desire for a natural birth', but, in fact, neither made significant contributions. We found that the final model actually accounted for substantially more of the variance than in *Great Expectations* – 52 per cent – as shown in Table 10.7. Having a drug-free labour was inadvertently omitted. However, when it was added in, it was found not to be significant. We therefore present the model without this variable.

Variable	**Beta**	**significance**
Variables in the equation		
Education	-.059231	.0154
Losing control of behaviour	-.067598	.0133
Being able to get comfortable	-.083260	.0026
Feeling in control of what the staff were doing	-.257269	.0000
Having a caesarean section	.229025	.0000
Having a drip	.068804	.0131
Having an instrumental delivery	.072698	.0072
Feelings about how well coped with pain	.359718	.0000
Length of labour	-.105532	.0001
Variables not in the equation		
Parity	-.019524	.4681
Trait anxiety	-.015335	.5406
Having an episiotomy	.005099	8562
Wanting a natural birth (antenatally)	-.041536	.0934
Antenatal worry about labour pain	-.013121	.5978
Age	-.034279	.1749

Table 10.7: Final regression model predicting satisfaction (data from CPSS)

This model is not identical to that for *Great Expectations*, but there is unanimity on the highly significant variables: feeling in control of what the staff were doing; being able to get comfortable; having a caesarean section; having an instrumental delivery; feelings about how well coped with pain and education. We therefore can feel fairly confident that these are indeed independently important contributors to women's satisfaction with birth, or at least for women in the south east of England in the late 1980s and early 1990s.

Conclusion

What can we make of these multivariate analyses? Clearly they do not provide us with a magic wand to wave over the data to tell us 'what really matters', much as I had hoped that they might. They do, however, help us to burrow at least one layer down into the complex inter-relationships. We need to recognize that all the many aspects of giving birth are inter-related. This was especially evident while we were experimenting with different variables to enter into the regression models. The addition or subtraction of just one factor could cause a complete rearrangement of the kaleidoscope. Thus we found, for example, that expectations of the efficacy of breathing and relaxation seemed to be an important predictor of satisfaction, as did antenatal worry about the pain of labour, but these variables tended to wander in and out according to what else had been entered into the model. The explanation, presumably, is that these variables are highly correlated with other variables for which they act as proxies. Clearly there is scope for continuing analyses of these data.

Different studies using regression techniques have not been as consistent as one might like in their findings of what is important. This will be partly a function of the factors that were actually considered. It may also be that no single model fits women in all settings. What should be clear by now is that there is no one 'right' answer to any of the questions in this field. Different studies are all contributing different ways of looking at the picture. The variables identified as important in the original *Great Expectations* study would still seem to be valid. What these additional analyses have done is to help to separate the figure from the background. We may not be able to answer the question 'What *really* matters?', but we can at least reiterate the importance of feeling in control, especially feeling in control of what the staff are doing. That in turn directs our attention to the relationship between a woman and her caregivers, a relationship which may be short-lived but need be none the worse for that. Our factor analysis of adjectives describing the staff gives food for thought here. The factor that did *not* contribute to the satisfaction regression model was that representing the words 'supportive', 'sensitive', 'warm' and 'rushed'. This is a surprising finding which should encourage us to re-examine some of our assumptions about what women value in their relationships with their caregivers. It seems fitting that this new chapter of *Great Expectations* should end as the original study began: challenging assumptions.

Volume II

Volume II of *Great Expectations* presents additional findings from our study of women's expectations and experiences of childbirth. The chapters in this volume cover a number of areas, some of which were not central to the main research questions, but which were worthy of more detailed examination than was possible in Volume I.

CHAPTER ONE

Expectations and Previous Experience

Many studies of childbirth have excluded multips because their previous experiences are a complicating factor. We made a deliberate decision to include multips because it was clearly desirable to attempt to look at the ways in which they felt that their previous experiences were relevant to their current hopes and expectations, even if these could not always be quantified. We therefore included an open-ended question at the end of the booklet which formed part of the main antenatal questionnaire:

> 'If you have had previous experiences that have influenced your hopes and expectations of this labour, please could you tell us about them.'

Two hundred and ninety five women (40%) answered the question, 27 of whom were in fact primips. These mainly described the ways in which their expectations were affected by previous miscarriages or abortions, other hospital experiences (mainly negative), or their own medical/nursing background, 'I feel I am not a pregnant midwife but a pregnant woman'. One woman alluded to her farming background to explain her antipathy to obstetric interventions:

> 'I have spent all my life on a farm rearing and delivering lambs and calves. Most induced calves are dopey and slow to start. It takes 2 to 3 weeks to be 100 per cent the same as the others. (Only noticeable if one is a *very* experienced stockman.) Most labours are left as long as possible unless complications are expected, and if necessary are aided. I would hope to be about the same.'

The 268 multips who answered represent 59 per cent of the multips in the study. The remaining multips presumably did not feel that their previous experiences were relevant or, as one woman actually specified:

> 'Yes I have [had previous experiences], but wish to keep them to myself.'

Well-educated women were considerably more likely to respond than the less well educated.

The range of things that women chose to tell us about in this section was enormous and exceedingly difficult to quantify. The following table shows the number of times particular events were mentioned by the 268 multips who answered the question.

Women could mention any number of these. The percentages represent only the frequency with which the events were identified as being relevant to the question asked. Thus, we find that ARM is mentioned by only four per cent of the multips although the incidence is probably at least ten times higher (see Chapter 6 of Volume 1). Similarly, only 18 per cent mentioned a previous straightforward problem-free birth. Caesarean sections (6%) and forceps (11%) on the other hand are probably mentioned by a much higher proportion of the women who had experienced them.

Obstetric events	n	% of all multips
Straightforward birth	82	18
Induction/acceleration	61	13
Artificial rupture of membranes	19	4
Forceps	48	11
Caesarean section	28	6
Third stage problems	9	2
Suturing	25	5
Postnatal problems	21	5
Other (including episiotomy and epidurals)	120	26
Comments on the experience	n	% of all multips
Staff/environment/management	136	30
Pain	108	24
Self/emotions (e.g. re fulfilment, failure, etc.)	66	15
Control	73	16
n = 455		

Table 1.1: Various aspects of previous births mentioned by women

Overall, 59 per cent of the 331 comments about obstetric procedures were negative,14 per cent were positive and the remaining 27 per cent were either mixed or neutral. The accounts that were most negative typically detailed a succession of interventions, compounded by lack of choice and lack of consideration from staff, as the following detailed quotations show:

> 'My previous pregnancy ended in an induced labour with little choice. I was given an enema (no choice) which left me sore and uncomfortable – waters were broken and labour accelerated by hormone drip. Too much drip led to contractions becoming continuous – Pethidine was given. I insisted on a half dose and came round enough to push at delivery. I had a slight tear. I was not allowed off my bed nor were foam supports available – I was stitched before my local anaesthetic took effect. I saw three doctors and two midwives during labour – my partner was told to stay away until "something was happening" – five hours into labour. He arrived in time to see me sick with Pethidine. Countless strangers wandered in. The baby was removed for bathing etc. and not returned all that night. I developed an infection (contracted *in* hospital) leading to fever and could not breastfeed. Eventually was discharged by my partner after eight days misery.'

> 'Before the birth of my first baby I was told that due to my age (34) I would probably be induced and would need a drip to keep the contractions going. I was taken into hospital when only two days overdue to be induced (I didn't wish this but was told it was for the baby's sake) (no other medical reason B.P. etc.) I was given an enema and then told I could go home as there was no room on the labour ward. After being told to ring every morning to see if there was room, I was taken in four days later and had all induction methods. I was not in control of my body as they kept coming and speeding up my contractions, I ended up with a third degree tear and had to have a general anaesthetic to be stitched. I just wonder if I had been left to "do it myself" I would have been spared all the pain and discomfort this caused. So after the birth I felt far from thrilled at the event and more – that I didn't know "quite what hit me". This time I am trying a different hospital so fingers crossed!'

This comment about trying another hospital was not unique and some women had also evidently been very ambivalent about having another baby at all:

> 'I had to have a forceps lift out last time which I found very traumatic. I have waited six and a half years before finally deciding to go through with having another child.'

> 'All I can say is that I won't let my first experience happen again to me this time, that's why I was put off to have another child for quite a while.'

How previous experience affects hopes and expectations

The expectations of multips who have already experienced a straightforward birth are likely to be high:

> 'My first pregnancy and labour was very healthy and my labour was very quick so as they usually say the second one is easier I expect to go through the labour and birth without any problems.'

The majority of women, however, told us about previous births which had not been as expected, although their reactions to this varied considerably:

> 'Being an "old hand" at this – my second baby means that previous experience tempers former hopes and I am more aware of the realities of giving birth.'

> 'I feel this time I will be more able to cope because I know what to expect... I have higher expectations this time, I think because I'm not so keyed up worrying about the fear of the unknown.'

These two women, both having their second babies after relatively normal previous deliveries, typify the two contrasting reactions which run through multips' accounts. Both women clearly feel that they have learnt something from their experience and are better prepared for their forthcoming labours and both expect to reduce the difference between expectations and events. However, the critical difference is that the first woman sees events as fixed, 'the realities of giving birth', while the second woman identifies aspects of herself ('more able to cope', 'not so keyed up') which will allow events to be different. As a result, while the first woman has lowered expectations, the second actually has higher expectations than she had had as a primip.

A similar polarity of attitudes is to be found among women who had problems with previous births:

> 'Horrific labour last time including acceleration, epidural and eventually caesarean section. Hoping to have another caesarean this time, I've no desire to have a trial labour.'

> 'My first baby was induced against my wishes as the hospital and I disagreed about my dates – result baby distressed, caesarean section... second baby, different hospital, trial labour allowed, much more fulfilling experience, even with forceps delivery. Hopefully I'll get it right this time?'

While for another woman a previous section:

> 'has made me determined to have a *proper* labour and a proper birth that I can experience and remember.'

What is it that leads women to take up such different positions after ostensibly similar experiences? One possibility is that they had approached their first births with differing expectations. If a woman has never felt any commitment to the idea of childbirth as a desirable experience in its own right, she is unlikely to acquire such a stance after a long and painful labour. On the other hand, some women, while not having articulated such a feeling, will feel 'cheated' (a very commonly used word) if they fail to have a normal delivery:

> 'Well you see with my first baby, I hadn't given any thought to my probably having a Caesarean section, I just automatically thought that I was going to experience natural childbirth, so due to complications I had to have an emergency Caesarean section so at the last minute my experiencing Natural Childbirth ended. So really my second time around I would have to fulfil my role as a mother and go through Natural Childbirth.'

On the other hand, other women have evidently worked through such feelings:

> 'The labour was *awful* – persistent posterior position and ketosis and head not engaged resulted in ARM → syntocinon → Pethidine → epidural → forceps → episiotomy that required resuturing some months later – i.e. 36 hours of hell!... I therefore do not have any great expectations about fulfilment, drug free labour, active birth etc. as I had last time – this would leave me too open to feelings of disappointment and failure – far better to be philosophical, accept things as they are and if it does go well then it's a bonus.'

> 'I am under no illusions about the wonders of childbirth this time. I am aiming for a healthy baby by whatever means – the important bit is what happens after the birth – the lifetime to follow. I think many women overestimate the role of the birth and believe it has to be a meaningful experience and failure to achieve this through "natural" birth will severely affect the future... I wasted weeks worrying that I hadn't had a vaginal birth – until I realized that the relationship between me and my baby was no different from other mothers. My baby was alive – without a caesar she would have died, these were the realities.'

Nevertheless, it was clear that women who had had the opportunity to compare birth with and without technology knew which they preferred:

> 'My first labour was under an epidural which although giving me a a pain free labour I was monitored constantly and finally had forceps delivery with my husband out of the room. The whole experience was stressful. There was not an immediate bonding with the baby. The last labour was completely drug free. OK, I felt pain but the satisfaction of having to work for this baby and having done it all on my own was marvellous, and that time there was an immediate bonding. I hope very much that my third labour will be as my second where everything was left up to me with no interference from equipment and technology.'

Treatment by staff

The comments that we have quoted so far have mainly concerned pain and obstetric interventions. Both of these have been identified by previous studies (see Volume 1, Chapter 1) as important determinants of how women evaluate their labours. However, another very noticeable dimension which women identified as being important was the way that they were treated by staff. As Table 1.1 shows, 30 per cent of all multips (51% of those answering the question) commented on the staff/environment/management aspects of their previous labours making this the most frequent class of comment. There were approximately equal numbers of positive and negative comments with a slight preponderance of negative observations, particularly from the least educated women. Complaints were mainly about lack of continuity of care and lack of involvement in decision making:

> 'During the labour of my daughter there seemed to be a rapid change of staff with little consistency in the way I was handled. I therefore feel it best not to have too many expectations, so as not to become angry and frustrated during a time that is already stressful.'

> 'My first son's birth wasn't easy, and the staff totally took over, this I do not agree with, and certainly did not let it happen during my second labour experience which was dealt with by midwives only. Because of the way I was treated by hospital staff, makes me remember my first son's birth as something nobody should go through, and my second labour as one of happiness so I would hope the third will be as fulfilling as the second.'

Apart from lack of continuity and lack of control, three other points kept reappearing in women's complaints about their treatment: husbands being sent away, women being given sleeping pills and being ignored. Women admitted at night who could not convince staff that they were actually in labour were likely to have all three problems. Unlike some of the other negative aspects of previous labours which some women accepted as beyond their control, these experiences were seen as something that they could, and would, resist, even though the benign motivation in giving sleeping pills was acknowledged:

> 'I was given a sleeping tablet to help me get some rest last time as my waters broke late at night and the staff felt it would be a while before the labour got going so they advised me to try and sleep. On reflection I would refuse the tablet next time and in fact the contractions were too strong to allow me to sleep and yet my body was crying out to sleep. In fact, it only made it more difficult for me to concentrate on coping with each contraction. The desperate need to sleep was almost as distressing as the labour pains and I feel this may have contributed to a long labour with very little urge to push.'

> 'I was left alone for three hours. My husband was told to go and get some sleep. I needed a hand to hold. I didn't think I'd be left alone. By the time he came back I was too far gone on pain and drugs. Eventually I was taken to the delivery room because I was making "so much noise I was frightening the other women". I am happy to accept whatever pain relief is on *offer* but I will *not* be left alone in any circumstances this time.'

Another woman summed up her experiences and hopes by saying:

> 'I would like the staff to believe me when I tell them baby's on its way – and not keep telling me what they think should be happening.'

What a number of women felt that they had learnt from previous experience was the need to be assertive:

> 'This time I feel more confident and intend to be more positive and in charge of my labour.'

> 'I expect I shall have to voice my opinions much more strongly – which I find hard.'

> 'I hope I will be able to assert my wishes to the staff, although I expect they will not be granted if they do not suit the staff (i.e. positions for delivery).'

In contrast to the unhappy experiences of these women, others were able to look back on positive experiences that had been enhanced by staff attitudes:

> 'They were supportive and talked to me all the time. It was a wonderful experience. They did everything I asked them to – e.g. putting on my glasses so I could watch my baby being born, and touching her head as it was born. I truly

hope this next labour will be an experience I can remember with pleasure as was the last.'

'First child five weeks early – but still left as naturally as possible and allowed to do own thing. Grateful. Second child four weeks late, monitored closely but allowed to wait and do things naturally. Again, grateful. Both times staff willing to listen to me or offer advice and leave it up to me to decide - good.'

Supportive staff attitudes were particularly valued by those who had expected otherwise:

'Before my previous labours, I anticipated the need to fight to maintain my freedom and thought that the staff would impose themselves on me. This was *not* the case. I was in control (in my second labour, at the GP unit) and my own midwife delivered me. I felt that she was there to help me out when, and only when I needed her. Therefore I feel confident that I will get similar treatment this time.'

There was, however, a small sub-group of women who, appreciating how important the staff had been in making their previous experiences positive, were apprehensive that they would not be so fortunate this time:

'The woman that delivered my child was a coloured woman. If she was worried, so was I. I did as she said, and I came out on top, not a tear or stitches. She inspired me immensely. I would love for her to deliver my baby this time. Unfortunately there's all different people on duty on different days. She told me what to do, when not to, and so-forth, she was caring and approached me at first with reassurance and care. She has really given me my views today. All midwives wouldn't go far wrong if they had the same behaviour as her. I shall be very dubious what happens this time as I probably won't have the same experience again.'

Summary

It will be evident from the range of examples quoted that generalizations about the expectations of multips are impossible. All undoubtedly feel that they have learnt *something* from their previous experience, but what that 'something' is, and what it's implications are for future deliveries is very varied. In some cases it is a very clear idea of what they do and don't want. For example:

'Therefore this time I want:

1. Spontaneous labour.
2. First stage of labour at home.
3. No drugs so that I am alert at birth.
4. Standing or squatting position for birth.
5. No episiotomy.

In short, 'Every mother's dream!'

Such specific wishes, usually based on negative previous experiences, were given by 38 per cent of the multips who answered the question. Table 1.2 shows the number of women expressing particular hopes and expectations. Up to two were coded for each woman.

	n	% of those expressing hopes/expectations
Particular wants	86	38
Feel well prepared	71	31
Expect/hope no problems	64	28
Want to be in control	56	24
Open mind	27	12
Nervous re coping	20	9
No fears: known experience	12	5
Other	40	17

(n = 229. 39 of the 268 women who talked about previous experiences did not express any hopes/expectations)

Percentages add to over 100 per cent because women could be coded in two categories.

Table 1.2: Hopes and expectations expressed by multips

There were no differences between women of different educational levels with respect to these categories. There were also no differences between women booked at different units except that women booked at Little Exington and Exington GP unit were more likely to expect not to have any problems. This is precisely what one would expect since these are 'low risk' units.

CHAPTER TWO

Smoking and Drinking in Pregnancy

Introduction

The association between maternal smoking and adverse outcomes of pregnancy, particularly low birthweight, has been well established over three decades of research (Enkin, 1984). However, the evidence for a causal relationship is not quite so clear cut: smokers and non-smokers may differ in several other environmental, biological and cultural ways.

A similar relationship between alcohol and birth abnormality is also well documented although for healthy women who do not drink heavily there is very little risk.

The connections between smoking, drinking and adverse birth outcomes and later physical and intellectual impairment have led to an enormous amount of antenatal pressure upon women to give up both habits, but particularly smoking, completely. The tone of this pressure is often very authoritarian. For example, Bourne (1975), in his widely read book *Pregnancy,* says smoking 30 cigarettes a day '*almost certainly* causes mental and physical retardation in late childhood' and that 'women *must not* smoke during pregnancy' (our emphasis). Yet women often receive conflicting information from the 'experts'. The Open University/Health Education Council (1985) book *Understanding Pregnancy and Birth* tells women that 'even moderate drinking during pregnancy (two drinks a day) is *known* to result in lower birth weight, lower intelligence and greater risks to the baby' (our emphasis), whilst Huntingford (1985), for example, maintains that drinking in moderation is not dangerous.

While acknowledging that it is better to cut down or preferably give up smoking and drinking in pregnancy, some writers stress that a very heavy propaganda campaign is counter-productive, causing anxiety and guilt in women who are unable to do this (Enkin, 1984; Huntingford, 1985). Clearly, women who smoke and/or drink during pregnancy are under what may amount to strong contradictory pressures both to stop (e.g. advice given by the medical profession at antenatal check-ups and in literature abundantly present in antenatal clinics) and also to carry on (e.g. advertising, social pressure from friends etc.). This is an area of their lives in which they are strongly encouraged to take control. Do they in fact feel able to do so?

Phrasing of the questions

We were interested to know if women did alter their consumption of tobacco and alcohol after they became pregnant, and if so, what led them to make changes. However, we were aware of the sensitive nature of such questions and were concerned not to make women feel guilty if they continued to smoke and/or drink. Nor did we want our questions to be interpreted by respondents as judgemental and answers to be given in a placatory manner i.e. the woman giving a socially acceptable answer. We therefore paid a lot of attention to the phrasing of the questions. There was no compulsion to answer the questions. We explained that what we were interested in were *changes* in smoking and drinking during pregnancy. Women were asked to tell us, *if they had no objection to doing so,* how many cigarettes they smoked a week at the time of the questionnaire (approximately 30 weeks pregnant), and how many they had smoked before they had become pregnant. We then asked an open-ended question to discover what had helped them cut down or stop, or why they had increased (or started). If there was no change in smoking habits, nothing further was asked. The same questions were then asked with regard to the consumption of alcohol. However, with reference to the well-known tendency to under-report tobacco and alcohol consumption (Plant, 1985), it is important to bear in mind that the following results indicate *self-reported* rather than *actual* amounts.

Smoking results

Table 2.1 shows that nearly three quarters of the sample said that they were non-smokers before the pregnancy. Thus, 27 per cent of our sample entered their pregnancy as smokers. This compares to research showing that 30 per cent or more of pregnant women in the UK (and also in the USA and Australia) are smokers at the start of pregnancy (Nowicki et al., 1984; Lumley, 1987), and to a recent British study by Macarthur et al. (1987) in which 29 per cent were regular smokers before pregnancy.

Direction of change	n	%
Never smoked	595	(73)
Decreased (or stopped)	159	(20)
No change in number smoked	46	(6)
Increased	10	(1)
Total	810	(100)

Table 2.1: Changes in smoking habits during pregnancy

Nobody in our study had started smoking during pregnancy but ten women had increased the number of cigarettes they smoked since becoming pregnant. The reasons for this are discussed below. Sixty seven women (31% of smokers and 8% of the sample) had given up completely by 30 weeks pregnant (i.e. at the time of the questionnaire). This is a great deal more than the 15 per cent reported in an unpublished Health Education Council study as giving up smoking on becoming pregnant (quoted in Kitzinger, 1987). A review of the research since the mid 1970s suggests that about 18 per cent of smokers give up by the time of the first antenatal visit, although several more recent studies suggest that the proportion is increasing (Lumley, 1987). In MacArthur et al.'s study (1987), six per cent of women had given up smoking between becoming pregnant and the first antenatal appointment.

There are several possible explanations of why a higher proportion of women in our study had given up smoking compared to other studies.

1. Our women were not telling the truth. We do not find this explanation convincing since it seems more likely that women who smoked would simply say that they had cut down rather than stopped altogether if they wished to disguise the truth. Furthermore, although women frequently under-report the amount they smoke (and drink) during pregnancy, it seems more likely that they would feel able to tell the truth in a questionnaire, where there is no face-to-face confrontation with an interviewer and anonymity is thus ensured, than in an interview situation.

2. We asked our questions at a much more advanced stage of pregnancy – 30 weeks rather than at the time of the first antenatal visit. Consequently, a proportion of women who had not given up at the time of the first visit may well have done so by 30 weeks.

3. Our sample has a middle class bias and middle class women generally are more likely to a) not smoke in the first place (Enkin, 1984), and b) to reduce their intake of tobacco during pregnancy.

4. A fourth possibility is that more women in the late 1980s are giving up smoking as it becomes less socially acceptable and as health education advice takes effect.

In addition to the 67 women in our sample who said that they had given up smoking, a further 92 women (43% of the smokers) said that they had cut down the number of cigarettes they smoked.

Number smoked per week	30 weeks pregnant		Before pregnancy	
	n	%	n	%
1–20 (light smoker)	40	(26)	30	(14)
21–100 (moderate smoker)	80	(51)	100	(45)
101–290 (heavy smoker)	33	(21)	84	(38)
Variable	3	(2)	7	(3)
Total	156	(100)	221	(100)

Percentages are of the number of women who were smokers on each occasion.

Table 2.2: Number of cigarettes smoked at 30 weeks and before pregnancy

Table 2.2 demonstrates the changes in women's smoking habits between becoming pregnant and 30 weeks pregnant, with an increase in the number of women who were 'light' smokers and 'moderate' smokers and a considerable decrease in the number of 'heavy' smokers. Further changes are concealed within each category (i.e. only inter-category changes are shown).

Smoking, education and social class

As expected (Enkin, 1984) there were strong educational differences between smokers and non-smokers ($p < 0.0001$). Women who left school at 16 or younger were the least likely to be non-smokers (64% compared to 91% of the most educated group). Of the women who smoked, it was the most educated women who were most likely to decrease or stop smoking when pregnant and furthermore, none of the ten women who increased the number of cigarettes they smoked fell into the most educated group. However, these differences were not statistically significant.

Social class (by both women's best ever job and by partner's occupation) was significantly related to whether women smoked, with women in classes I and II being least likely to smoke ($p < 0.0001$ in each instance).

Smoking and control

As mentioned in the introduction to this section, women are strongly encouraged to 'take control' over how much they smoke and drink during pregnancy. In general, people (especially women) are exhorted to control their weight, control their appetites and control all the substances that may be taken into their bodies. People who eat, drink or smoke too much are said to have 'lost control' or to lack 'self-control'. This issue of controlling what substances enter the body (and how much of them) takes on particular power for pregnant women. Women who smoke and drink alcohol during pregnancy are often assumed to lack the desire to take any control over their pregnancies, indeed over their lives.

To gain some idea of whether smoking is linked to how 'control-orientated' women are, we examined smoking habits at 30 weeks of pregnancy in terms of whether women antenatally expressed a high or low desire for control over various aspects of labour. (See Volume 1, Chapter 4, for details about 'High' and 'Low Control' women. Only women who were categorized as 'High Control' or 'Low Control' were included in this analysis.) Our hypothesis was that 'High Control' women would be more likely to a) be non-smokers (and non-drinkers) in the first place and b) to cut down/stop smoking (and drinking). In fact, exactly the same proportion of 'High' and 'Low Control' women were non-smokers (74–75%) and 'High/Low Control' scores were not significantly related to changes in smoking habits.

Smoking and birthweight

The mean birthweight of babies born to women who smoked at 30 weeks of pregnancy was significantly lower than that of babies born to non-smokers (3237 gms compared to 3474 gms, t value = 5.01, two-tailed probability < 0.001). Two-way analysis of variance showed that the relationship between smoking and birthweight was still significant when we controlled for the effects of social class (both women's best ever occupation and partners' occupation) and education.

Reasons for changes in smoking

Women's reasons for changing their smoking habits were categorized as in Table 2.3 below. A maximum of two reasons were recorded for each woman. Comments specifying concern for the baby were given priority.

Reason given	n of women giving reason	%*
Being pregnant	35	(21)
Baby-centred	71	(43)
Woman-centred	47	(29)
Pressure or support (external)	13	(8)
Social circumstances	8	(5)
Only a social smoker	5	(3)
Other (e.g. religion, willpower)	31	(19)

n = 165. A total of 210 reasons were given by 165 women.
*Percentage of women who decreased or stopped smoking, and who gave a reason.

Table 2.3: Reasons given for decreasing or stopping smoking

The most frequently given reasons for cutting down or stopping smoking were baby-centred, focusing on the risk to the health of the developing fetus:

> '[I'm] anxious not to hurt my baby. Instead of buying a couple of packets of cigarettes, I buy something for the baby.'

> 'Knowledge of the possible adverse effects smoking could have on the baby was the main motivation for stopping (i.e. guilt!). Financial benefits also a great encouragement to stop.'

> 'The thought of knowing there was another human growing inside me. And the side effects on the baby.'

Sometimes this concern for the baby's well-being took the form of a general comment on what women should do in pregnancy:

> 'I do not believe that pregnant women should smoke.'

It is easier to cut down smoking if it is making you feel ill, and indeed woman-centred reasons such as feeling sick, or not feeling any desire to smoke, were given by over a quarter of the women. The most common combination of reasons was concern for the baby's health followed by a comment on not feeling like smoking anyway, for example:

> 'I wanted to stop due to the baby and also I was sick.'

The third most common reason was 'Being pregnant'. This was coded when no further comments regarding the baby or self were made, although often it was clear by implication that it was the baby's health that the woman was thinking about:

> 'I gave up as soon as I knew I was pregnant.'

Relatively few women said that anything outside these categories had helped them cut down or give up smoking. Sometimes women said that 'external' pressure or support from the family or elsewhere e.g. hospital, was helpful. One women replied that the thing that was of most help was:

> 'My seven year old son saying "it won't do the baby any good".'

Two other categories of reasons are worth elaborating on. A small percentage of women explained that their social and financial circumstances put pressure on them to stop smoking although clearly this is extremely difficult when in the face of severe stress:

> 'I have tried to give up but failed. It was for the baby, my health (I have smoked 11 years) and so expensive. Being unemployed and homeless two plus months does not help the nerves.'

Finally, the 'Only a social smoker' category describes women who wrote that they did not smoke much anyway and so found it no hardship to give up:

> 'I'm only really a "social" smoker and don't enjoy it particularly, so pregnancy was a very good reason to give it up completely.'

Increase in smoking

A small number of women (ten) said that they had increased the number of cigarettes that they smoked per week during pregnancy. Five of them explained that this was due to stress brought on by personal and family difficulties, and another two by the stress associated with pregnancy itself. For some women, cigarettes may be one of the few, or indeed the only comforter in distressing circumstances. One woman increased from 80 to over 140 cigarettes a week during pregnancy, and said:

'I don't really know the reason. Possibly coping with four children and being pregnant, I don't know.'

The judgemental attitudes of the medical profession and society in general towards pregnant women who continue to smoke does contribute, as was mentioned earlier, to feelings of guilt and shame. One woman in our sample, who increased the amount she smoked from a maximum of four packs of cigarettes a week to a maximum of 20 packs a week during pregnancy, wrote at length about the conflicts she experienced:

'If I had not had a cigarette I would have had a hair tearing time, although I disagree enormously on women smoking full stop. If they weren't on the market you couldn't smoke them. The unborn baby would feel better and so would I first thing in the morning. I feel ashamed that I had to smoke so heavy while carrying this baby. I wish cigarettes were never invented, I wish this was a healthy country... The reason for smoking such more cigarettes is it's the only things that kept me sane and in a happy mood.'

Drinking results

Turning now to changes in the amount of alcohol consumed during pregnancy, it is necessary to reiterate the caution about the possible unreliability of self-reported data, although validity varies according to variables recorded and methods used.

Direction of change	n	%
Never drank alcohol	280	(36)
Decreased or stopped	388	(50)
No change in amount of alcohol	111	(14)
Increased	2	(1)
Total	781	(100)

Table 2.4: Changes in alcohol habits during pregnancy

Of the 44 missing cases, only nine were true defaulters. The remaining 35 all gave 'variable' as their response to how much alcohol they drank before and/or during the pregnancy and in addition offered no further information which could help us to deduce any change or the direction of any change.

Only a third (36%) of the respondents said that they had not drunk alcohol either before or during pregnancy. One hundred and ninety eight women (37% of drinkers) had given up alcohol completely by 30 weeks pregnant while another 190 women (35% of alcohol drinkers) had cut down the amount they drank. (These figures are calculated on a number of 536, i.e. the 35 'variables' are included.) Table 2.5 shows the amount of alcohol drunk by women before they became pregnant and at 30 weeks pregnant (i.e. at the time of the questionnaire).

Number of units* of alcohol per week	30 weeks pregnant		Before pregnancy	
	n	%	n	%
Less than 1 a week on average	73	(21)	73	(14)
1 per week	80	(24)	55	(10)
2–12 per week	155	(46)	296	(55)
13–30 per week	0	(0)	35	(7)
Variable or occasional	32	(9)	76	(14)
Total	340	(100)	535	(100)

*One unit = 1 glass of wine, half a pint of beer or 1 measure of spirits.

Percentages are of the number of women who were 'drinkers' on each occasion.

Table 2.5: Number of units of alcohol consumed at 30 weeks and before pregnancy

The maximum amount of alcohol any woman claimed to drink at 30 weeks pregnant (leaving aside the 'variable' group) was 12 units a week, i.e. about two bottles of wine or six pints of beer. The proportion who said they drank only one unit or less a week on average nearly doubled from before pregnancy to 30 weeks pregnant. It is important to remember that only inter-category changes are shown in the table and further changes within categories are concealed.

Drinking habits, education and social class

Whereas the most highly educated women and those in the higher social classes were more likely to be non-smokers, the opposite is true when we look at alcohol consumption. Forty five per cent of the least educated women said that they did not drink alcohol compared to only 18 per cent of the most highly educated women. The same picture emerges by woman's social class and also by husband's occupation. (The relationship between social class and alcohol consumption at 30 weeks is significant at the $p < 0.0001$ level in each case as is the relationship between education and alcohol intake.) Of those women who did drink, the ones who left further education at 19 years or older were the most likely to cut down or stop although the overall pattern is not linear.

Drinking and control

As with smoking, 'High Control' women were no more likely than 'Low Control' women to be non-drinkers: in fact, 27 per cent of 'High Control' women were non-drinkers compared to 31 per cent of 'Low Control' women. Of the women who did drink alcohol at 30 weeks of pregnancy, there were no significant differences in the proportion of 'High' and 'Low Control' women who had changed the amount that they drank.

	Direction of change					
Educational level	No change		Increased drinking		Decreased/stopped drinking	
	n	%	n	%	n	%
16 and under	52	(24)	1	(1)	164	(76)
17–18	43	(28)	1	(1)	111	(72)
19 and over	16	(13)	0	(0)	111	(87)

Percentages are of women of a given educational level.

$p < 0.05$.

Table 2.6: Changes in drinking habits by educational level

(Women coded as 'variable', who also did not give any information from which we could deduce any change or direction of change, were excluded from analysis.)

Drinking and birthweight

Women who said that they did *not* drink alcohol at 30 weeks of pregnancy gave birth to babies whose mean birthweight was significantly *lower* than those born to women who said they did drink some alcohol (3386 gms compared to 3471 gms, t value = 2.12, two-tailed probability < 0.05). However, this difference was no longer significant when we controlled for the effects of either social class (both women's best ever occupation and partner's occupation) or education.

Reasons for changes in drinking habits

Women's reasons for altering the amount they drank were categorized as for smoking and the three most common sets of responses were the same as for smoking.

Reason given	n of women giving reason	%*
Being pregnant	63	(15)
Baby-centred	224	(53)
Woman-centred	125	(29)
External pressure or support	21	(5)
Social circumstances	22	(5)
No problem	27	(6)
Only a social drinker	38	(9)
Other (e.g. religion, willpower)	30	(7)

n = 426. A total of 550 reasons were given by 426 women.

*Percentage of women who cut down or stopped drinking and who gave a reason.

Table 2.7: Reasons given for decreasing or stopping drinking

Women were aware of the effect of alcohol upon the baby's growth and of possible brain damage. Several specifically mentioned Fetal Alcohol Syndrome. Over half of the women mentioned a concern for the baby's health:

> 'I did not want to cause any harm to my unborn child. Forty weeks is a small amount of time to forfeit one's pleasures for a healthy child.'

Some women expressed their concern in terms of a 'moral responsibility to the fetus'.

Over a quarter of the women (29%) mentioned how they themselves felt physically. Frequently this reason appeared in conjunction with concerns for the baby:

> 'Fear of damaging the baby and the fact that morning sickness lasted all day for the first six months.'

The third most common reason was, again, the simple phrase 'being pregnant' although a smaller proportion said this than did for smoking. Again, reasons often appeared in combination:

> 'Being pregnant and also drink seems to send this particular baby potty – i.e. moves around violently.'

It was clear from the responses that the great majority of women were acutely aware of the potential risk to the developing child from maternal use of alcohol and tobacco, and were highly motivated to decrease their consumption of these drugs. Obviously it is easier to cut down when your own body is rejecting alcohol, but some women would very much have liked a drink (or smoke):

> 'I've cut down because it's not good for the baby – willpower is what keeps it down. I often fancy a drink, but resist especially when the baby reminds me with a kick that he/she is there.'

Increase in alcohol consumption

Only two women said that they had increased their intake of alcohol after they became pregnant. However, five women made comments which implied that they had increased the amount they drank, albeit very slightly. Two said that this was for so-called medicinal reasons e.g. drinking a small amount of Guinness a week for its iron content. Three women explained that they were under a great deal of personal stress. The explanation for this small imbalance in numbers lies in the fact that several women felt they had cut down overall, but that occasionally they did have a drink. For example, one unhappy single parent with two toddlers said she had stopped drinking but occasionally did drink 'a half of a Carlsberg Special to reduce sadness and to help me sleep'.

Conclusion

Smoking and drinking alcohol were both related to women's educational level and social class, although in opposite directions: the least educated and lower social class women were the most likely to smoke while alcohol was more of a well-educated, middle class habit. There was a tendency for well-educated and higher class women to be more likely to take control of their smoking/drinking habits by cutting down or stopping. Even so, our hypothesis that it was 'High Control' women (i.e. women who expressed a strong desire antenatally for control over particular aspects of labour) who would be the most likely to cut down/stop smoking and drinking during pregnancy was not supported.

Smoking was significantly related to birthweight with women who smoked giving birth to smaller babies. This relationship was independent of social class and education effects. There was also a weaker, but still significant relationship between alcohol and birthweight where it was the non-drinkers who primarily gave birth to smaller babies. This finding is a function of the fact that it was the less educated, lower social class women who were most likely not to drink alcohol, and when class and education were controlled, it was no longer significant.

Women were well aware of the potential risk to the developing child from their intake of tobacco and alcohol and made it clear that they often put great effort and willpower into reducing their intake of these substances. Where they had difficulties in doing so and had occasionally even increased their smoking and drinking, they described sometimes quite overwhelming feelings of guilt and distress. However, cigarettes and alcohol often act as comforters and relaxants for women undergoing sometimes great personal stress.

CHAPTER THREE

Birth Plans

Introduction

The questionnaire introduced the 'birth plan' section with the following statement:

> 'Some women make sure that their wishes about the birth are put down in writing. This is sometimes called a 'birth plan' – the hospital may provide a standard form and/or you might write down some of your feelings yourself to be kept with your notes.'

Our definition was deliberately vague so as to tap the variety of ways in which women might have had their wishes recorded. We were also aware that the number of women who actually wrote their own birth plans without guidance from a midwife was so small that we would be unlikely to be able to say much about them. Throughout this section it is important to remember that 'birth plans' refer to a variety of ways in which women's wishes may be recorded.

Antenatal data

Knowledge of unit practice and intentions re birth plans

We first asked women if they knew whether birth plans were usual practice in their hospital: 57 per cent said they did not know, 15 per cent said yes, they were, and 28 per cent said no. We also asked women whether they intended to have their wishes written down. Only 16 per cent of the sample had already written, or said they were intending to write, a birth plan, 7 per cent were undecided, 8 per cent had considered but rejected the idea and the majority, 69 per cent, had never thought about writing down their wishes. For ease of reference we will refer to these groups as 'pro birth plan', 'undecided', 'anti birth plan' and 'never considered' respectively.

Not surprisingly, women's responses varied depending on which unit they were talking about. Willowford and Zedbury were the only places where more than a handful of women said that birth plans *were* the usual practice in their hospital.

	Yes		No		Don't Know	
	n	%	n	%	n	%
Exington consultant	3	(4)	30	(40)	43	(57)
Exington GP unit	5	(7)	20	(26)	52	(68)
Little Exington	1	(2)	24	(51)	22	(47)
Willowford	43	(23)	25	(14)	116	(63)
Wychester	7	(4)	67	(36)	112	(60)
Zedbury	50	(30)	40	(24)	77	(46)

Percentages are of women in a given unit.

$p < 0.0001$

Table 3.1: Whether women thought birth plans were usual in their unit (by unit)

It was also at Zedbury and Willowford that women were most likely to be pro birth plan. A third of the women at Zedbury had completed (or were about to complete) a birth plan as were a fifth of those at Willowford.

	Pro birth plan		Undecided		Anti birth plan		Never considered a birth plan	
	n	%	n	%	n	%	n	%
Exington consultant	9	(12)	4	(5)	3	(4)	58	(78)
Exington GP unit	8	(11)	0	(0)	8	(11)	60	(79)
Little Exington	1	(2)	3	(6)	3	(6)	40	(85)
Willowford	34	(19)	22	(12)	15	(8)	112	(61)
Wychester	9	(5)	14	(8)	22	(12)	139	(76)
Zedbury	52	(3)	6	(4)	8	(5)	101	(61)

Percentages are of women in a given hospital unit.

$p < 0.0001$

Table 3.2: Intentions re birth plans by unit

In fact, according to the Directors of Midwifery, midwives record women's wishes antenatally in all six units. However, only at Zedbury was this a matter of written policy and here they had developed a 'Maternity Care Plan'. This plan is part of the Maternity Notes which women carry throughout their pregnancy and the women's wishes are recorded by the midwife at booking. The care plan is updated throughout pregnancy and wishes confirmed with the woman when she is in labour.

The Zedbury 'Guidelines for Midwives' suggest that the plan should cover the woman's relationship with her partner (if any), 'language problems', 'dietary, spiritual and cultural needs', social circumstances and support as well as the woman and her partner's wishes during labour. It is also used as an opportunity to discuss with the woman options about parentcraft classes, infant feeding and entitlements to maternity benefits. The Maternity Care Plan then potentially provides a structure for comprehensive discussion; however, it is very much under the control of the staff and is very different from the kind of woman-initiated birth plan envisaged by some childbirth activists (Kitzinger, 1987).

We are not able to say how the care plans were completed in practice. However, it is interesting to note that despite the unit policy being for every woman to have such a plan, 24 per cent of the women booked at Zedbury said that having their wishes about labour recorded was *not* usual in Zedbury (and 61% had 'never thought' about having their wishes recorded: see Table 3.2). This discrepancy could be because, i) midwives were not actually implementing the policy or ii) women's wishes about labour were not recorded as they had not at that point thought much about it. The unit policy did clearly state that 'in many cases it may be necessary to complete this section ['Interests and needs for care in labour'] at a later date when they have formulated their ideas'. However, it should be noted that women answered our question about birth plans within four weeks of their expected date of delivery. Also, none of the women mentioned an updating of their plan and indeed one described the Zedbury Maternity Care Plan as 'a standard form (do you want painkillers etc.) provided by the hospital and signed at 12 weeks'.

A third reason for the discrepancy between the hospital policy and the women's reports might be that women do not equate the process of the midwife completing the Maternity Care Plan with a recording of their own feelings. The Director of Midwifery at Zedbury said that only a 'small unknown number' of women write down their wishes for themselves. There is some evidence that women may sometimes have felt actively discouraged from recording their wishes. As one woman at Zedbury volunteered:

> 'I asked the hospital if I could have things written down. They told me just to wait until labour and tell the midwife what I want.'

A fourth possibility is that despite our explicit attempt to define birth plans as something that a woman could write herself or which could be written on her behalf, women may have assumed that a birth plan only referred to the former.

Finally, women may have had the opportunity to record their wishes but did not feel they had anything in particular to say. They therefore perhaps neither noticed that they had an opportunity to have their wishes written down (only 30% knew it was usual practice) nor had they thought about it (61%).

	Women often write their own wishes	Midwives record women's requests automatically	There is a written policy relating to birth plans
Willowford	No	Yes	No
Exington consultant unit	No	Yes	No
Exington GP unit	No	Yes	No
Little Exington*	No	Yes	No
Wychester	No	Yes	No
Zedbury	No	Yes	Yes

*Little Exington is in the process of having new forms printed incorporating a standard form and developing a written policy.

Table 3.3: Approaches to recording women's wishes in writing in the six units

On paper Willowford appeared similar to the other units which, unlike Zedbury, had no written policy on birth plans and where women rarely wrote their own. However, about a quarter of the women in Willowford said that it was usual practice to record their wishes, as compared to just a handful of women at all the other units except for Zedbury (see Table 3.1). Almost a third of the women at Willowford said that they already had completed, or were about to complete, birth plans (as compared to between 9% and 18% of women at the other units). We would suggest that this reflects Willowford's emphasis on women's choice and control in childbirth and the attitude of the staff (see Chapter 5 on unit ethos, in Green et al., 1986). However, it should also be noted that, on the other hand, it was precisely the staff's positive approach to women having choice and control that was given by some women as reason for not having a birth plan. They felt confident that the staff would respect their wishes and therefore decided that a birth plan was redundant. As one woman commented:

> 'There is no point writing a birth plan because Willowford has a super attitude towards mum. You can do as you like.'

Whether or not women feel that they have been offered the opportunity to have their wishes written down (and whether or not they feel they have done so) is clearly influenced by unit policy and staff attitude. It also depends on women's perceptions of birth plans or 'care records' and how they perceive their own wishes about labour (e.g. whether they feel their wishes are 'unusual'). We would suggest that there is a distinction between writing down your own wishes and having them written down for you. This issue will be explored in the section on postnatal data.

Social class and education

Women of higher social class (as defined by their own best ever occupation) were more likely to say whether or not birth plans were the normal practice at their hospital (although they were not always right), and more likely to have completed a birth plan or at least to have considered the possibility. (84% of women in classes IV and V had never considered writing a birth plan as opposed to 52% in classes I and II.) A similar pattern was found for education.

Parity

Women who had had previous experiences of childbirth were more likely to claim that they knew their unit's usual practice re birth plans but there was very little difference between the intentions of multips and primips.

	Primips		Multips	
Birth plan intention	n	%	n	%
Never considered	190	(66)	326	(72)
Pro birth plan	43	(15)	64	(16)
Undecided	27	(9)	25	(6)
Anti birth plan	30	(10)	29	(6)
Total	290	(100)	444	(100)

Table 3.4: Birth plan intentions by parity

Perceptions of the pros and cons of birth plans

We asked all women what they thought were the advantages and disadvantages of 'writing things down' as well as reasons for thinking there might be 'no point' in doing so. They were offered 16 pre-set options drawn from views about birth plans recorded in the literature and expressed by women in the pilot study. There was also space for women to add their own statements. In designing this part of the questionnaire we were very aware that what one woman might see as an advantage of birth plans, another woman might perceive as a disadvantage. We therefore included similar statements under different headings. Thus, 'I want to help myself stick to whatever I decided before I went into labour' was included under the list of possible advantages of birth plans, while the statement 'If I write things down it might stop me changing my mind during labour' was one of the options offered as a *disadvantage* of birth plans. Tables 3.5 to 3.7 show how many women agreed with statements describing the advantages, disadvantages and pointlessness of birth plans.

	Number of women agreeing	% of total sample
The advantages of writing down what you want are:		
Even if I don't know the staff who attend me in labour they'll be able to know what I want by reading what I've written	416	(55)
When I'm actually in labour I won't be in such a good position to tell staff what I want	393	(53)
If it's in writing the staff are less likely to do things to me that I don't want	260	(35)
Writing things down helps me to sort things out in my head	253	(34)
I want to help myself stick to whatever I decided before I went into labour	42	(6)
Other (please say what)	23	(3)
n = 751		

For Tables 3.5 to 3.7, women could tick as many statements as they wished. Women who did not tick these statements were not necessarily indicating disagreement. Statements are given in the order of popularity, not in the order that they appeared in the questionnaire (see Appendix for questionnaire).

Table 3.5: Advantages of writing things down

	Number of women agreeing	% of total sample
The disadvantages of writing things down are:		
If I write things down it might stop me changing my mind during labour	346	(46)
Writing things down can get you labelled as a trouble maker	102	(14)
It might upset the staff	85	(11)
It seems a bit of a cheek	77	(10)
The decisions should rightly be taken by the staff, it's not up to me to decide what I want	75	(10)
Other (please say what)	52	(7)
n = 751		

Table 3.6: Disadvantages of writing things down

	Number of women agreeing	% of total sample
There is no point in writing down what you want because:		
It's not possible to know what you are going to want during labour in advance	504	(67)
I'm sure I can say what I want at the time	335	(45)
I think the staff understand what I want anyway	129	(17)
There is no need, I don't want anything out of the ordinary	122	(16)
I don't suppose anyone will take much notice of it anyway	62	(8)
I don't like the standard form they gave me to fill in	4	(1)
Other	37	(5)
n = 751		

Table 3.7. Reasons why there is no point in writing things down

As Table 3.5 shows, the main advantage seen for birth plans was that they aided communication. On the whole, women perceived more advantages than disadvantages, the main disadvantage being restriction of the woman's flexibility in labour. Related to this is the fact that two thirds of the sample agreed with the statement that there was no point in writing down your wishes because 'it's not possible to know what you are going to want during labour in advance'.

Perceptions of birth plans by parity

Having or not having had prior experience of birth was cited by women as influencing their response to the birth plan questions – in particular, their sense of being able to predict some of the events of labour. Primips were particularly likely to stress that it was hard to plan in advance:

> 'Not having experienced labour before how on earth can one tell what will actually be needed?'
>
> 'How can you make any decisions when you don't know what being in labour is like?'

This was reflected in the large proportion of primips (72%) who ticked the statement 'It's not possible to know what you are going to want during labour in advance'. Nevertheless, 64 per cent of multips also ticked this statement and stressed the unknown quality of the experience with comments such as 'Experience has taught me all labours are potentially different' or 'In my last labour all my ideas went out of the window!'.

There were, however, no differences between primips' and multips' assessment of the need for flexibility as reflected in the statement that birth plans help you stick to whatever you decided before you went into labour, and the statement that birth plans might stop you from changing your mind.

The only other significant difference between multips and primips perceptions of birth plans was, sadly, that more women with previous experience of labour felt that there was no point in writing down their wishes as 'I don't suppose anyone will take much notice of it anyway' (11% of multips compared to 4% of primips). As one woman said 'You don't get a choice anyway, the doctors don't give you a choice' and another woman, commenting on how her birth plan had been ignored last time, stated:

> 'Therefore this time (I shall go to the same Maternity Hospital) I shall be more wary of the staff handling my labour – and certainly less trusting that they will *all* automatically read and observe the guidelines of my birthplan.'

Perceptions of birth plans by social class and education

There were only five significant social class differences in perceptions of the pros and cons of birth plans. Women in the lower social classes were more likely to tick three statements concerned with the idea of birth plans impinging on the professionals domain: 'It might upset the staff', 'The decisions should rightly be taken by the staff, it's not up to me to decide what I want', and 'It seems a bit of a cheek'. (It is possible that working class women may get a more negative reaction to their birth plans than middle class women.)

The fourth difference was that lower class women were more likely to agree that an advantage of writing things down was 'to help myself stick to whatever I decided before I went into labour'. Contrary to the stereotype of the inflexible middle class woman with her long lists (see Volume 1, Chapter 1), this statement was *not* more favoured by middle class women. Finally, lower class women were also more likely to say that there was no point in writing their wishes down because the staff understood what they wanted anyway.

	Social class grouping						
Statement	I + II		IIIn + IIIm		IV + V		p <
	n	%	n	%	n	%	
Writing things down helps me stick to decisions	9	(3)	22	(6)	8	(10)	0.01
Might upset staff	19	(7)	46	(12)	18	(22)	0.01
Staff should make decisions	9	(3)	48	(13)	15	(18)	0.001
Seems a bit of a cheek	13	(5)	42	(11)	18	(22)	0.001
Sure staff understand my wishes anyway	36	(13)	62	(17)	25	(31)	0.01

Percentages are of women in a given social class.

Table 3.8: View of birth plans by social class

A similar relationship to that with class existed between education and attitude to birth plans. The only differences were that i) there was no relationship between education and whether women thought birth plans might upset the staff, and ii) more educated women were more likely than the least educated to say that writing things down helped to sort things out in their heads ($p < 0.01$). Only 29 per cent of those who left school at 16 or under agreed that 'writing things down helps to sort things out in my head', as opposed to 33 per cent of those who left at 17 or 18 and 45 per cent of those who were still in full-time education at 19 or over.

Perceptions of birth plans by unit

Women's anticipation of staff reaction to birth plans varied widely between units. For instance, 20–28 per cent of those booked in the Exington units thought that writing things down could lead to them being labelled as a 'trouble maker' as opposed to 8–13 per cent of women booked elsewhere. Similarly, 22 per cent of the women booked at Exington consultant unit thought no-one would take much notice of a birth plan even if they wrote one, whereas only four per cent of those at Willowford felt this would be the case. Further analysis could be carried out to explore these differences and their interrelationship with parity and social class. Preliminary investigations suggest, however, that population variations do not explain women's different assessments of the staff. We would also note that women's assessments of staff reactions in different units are consistent with our own observations of 'unit ethos' from our earlier research (Green et al., 1986), and are related to the units own official position on birth plans (see also Green et al., 1994).

Women's intentions to use birth plans and their perceptions of the advantages and disadvantages of them

(To simplify the presentation of this section the small group of women who were 'undecided' about birth plans have been excluded from the analysis.)

Pro birth plan women: those who intended to use birth plans

The women who intended to use birth plans were, not surprisingly, more positive about plans than other women. Women intending to use birth plans focused on the birth plan as a tool for ensuring that their wishes were understood and respected. Women who were pro birth plans were twice as likely as those who had rejected the idea to say that 'If it's in writing the staff are less likely to do things to me that I don't want' (50% compared to 22% of anti birth plan women), and 'Even if I don't know the staff who attend me in labour they'll be able to know what I want by reading what I have written' (76% compared to 36%). They were less than half as likely to feel that birth plans were unnecessary because they were sure they could say what they wanted at the time (22% compared to 58%), or they thought the staff understood what they wanted anyway (8% compared to 22%). (NB. This does not mean that they necessarily felt that the staff did not understand what they wanted but simply that they did not feel birth plans were made redundant if the staff did understand what they wanted.)

Most of the pro birth plan group, unlike the women who had rejected birth plans, felt that it was useful to consider what they might want during childbirth before going into labour, or at least they did not feel that the uncertainty of how the labour might go made a birth plan redundant. Only 39 per cent of the pro birth plan group agreed that there was no point writing down what they wanted because 'it's not possible to know what you are going to want during labour in advance' as opposed to 73 per cent of the anti birth plan group.

It would appear that women who decide to use birth plans more often believe in thinking in advance about what they want in labour and that they wish to communicate their wishes to the staff.

Anti birth plan women: those who have considered but rejected birth plans

Women who rejected the idea of birth plans tended to agree that 'It's not possible to know what you are going to want during labour in advance'. They were also more likely to think that the staff understood what they wanted and said that they didn't want anything unusual. They did, however, see some advantages of birth plans: notably that when they were in labour they would not be in a good position to tell staff about their wishes and that written requests would help different staff (who may have never met them before) realize what they wanted. However, given that staff sometimes see the writing of a birth plan as an expression of lack of faith in the staff's good will (Green et al., 1986: Chapter 5), it is ironic that, in some ways, the women who rejected birth plans expressed *less* faith in the staff's responses than did the pro birth plan group. Twenty five per cent of the anti birth plan women said that a disadvantage of a plan would be that it could 'get you labelled a trouble maker' (compared to 14% of the pro birth plan group) and 10 per cent thought that it 'might upset the staff' (compared to 4% of the pro birth plan group). Fear of staff reaction was, therefore, presumably one of the factors influencing these women against writing a plan which, in some other respects, they might have found useful. The women who did write plans had, in some way, more faith in the staff's cooperation and support.

The anticipation of staff reaction was one of the factors influencing women's perceptions of birth plans: women who anticipated staff cooperation saw birth plans as facilitators of good communication, whereas those who expected adverse staff response saw birth plans as inhibiting good communication. Women also differed in their perceptions of what counted as a 'real' birth plan. Some women who rejected birth plans obviously saw them as lists of demands drawn up by women without consultation with the staff. Thus, one woman (who had decided against a birth plan) commented that birth plans were a bad idea because:

> 'I would write it down for my own purposes, to discuss with the midwife. But I'm not happy with giving a written list. I feel it's a better approach to talk together.'

A pro birth plan woman, on the other hand, commented that plans were a good idea precisely because 'It gives staff a chance to discuss my wishes with me'.

Women who had never considered birth plans

The majority of women (69%) had never considered writing a birth plan. They were distinguished from both of the other groups by their greater acceptance of the professionals' control over childbirth. They were more likely than any of the other women to agree 'decisions should be taken by the staff, it's not up to me to decide what I want' and that writing down one's wishes seemed to be 'a bit of a cheek'. Eleven per cent of this group also indicated that they did not suppose anyone would take much notice of a birth plan anyway – the experts would just get on with it. They were more likely to think that childbirth *should* be left to the experts as well as believing that the experts would not listen to women anyway. It was, however, even within this group, only a minority of women who were so fatalistic.

Are women who write birth plans inflexible?

Are women who write birth plans saying that they want to stick to the plan come what may? From our earlier hospital based research we were very aware of some staff's view of women who write birth plans as inflexible and antagonistic:

> 'NCT people who come in with long lists [and] put people's backs up' (Green et al., 1986, Chapter 5).
>
> 'They read all the books and try to take over.' (ibid.)

However, our data suggested that this is not the intention of most women who write plans. Women who intended to use birth plans were just as likely as anyone else to emphasize flexibility. Out of the 117 women intending to use a birth plan, just five said that they wanted it to 'Help myself stick to whatever I decided before I went into labour'. In fact, only six per cent of the whole sample ticked this statement and there was no significant difference in response to this item between women in each of the three groups (pro plan, anti plan, never considered a plan).

However, there were some differences in the responses to the statement that birth plans might stop women changing their minds during labour. Women who had rejected the idea of a birth plan were almost twice as likely to tick this statement as those who were intending to use birth plans (63% compared to 33%).

Many of the anti birth plan women thought that writing things down reflected a certain rigidity:

> 'Every labour is different and you should go in with an open mind.'
>
> 'Why write things down... things don't always go according to plan (Nature might not read your notes!).'

Or as a third woman wrote:

> 'I feel a birth plan is too rigid. I want to approach my third labour with an open mind – to be flexible.'

These women feared that birth plans encouraged unrealistic expectations and therefore might lead to a sense of failure and disappointment:

> 'Strong pre-conceived ideas about labour can cause great disappointment if not lived up to.'
>
> 'It's better to take things as they come instead of trying to plan ahead and possibly getting let down because what you want is not possible for whatever reason.'
>
> 'I may feel I have failed, if for whatever reason I have to have some sort of intervention I had previously decided against.'

This view of birth plans as rigid documents encouraging and reflecting high expectations and employed in an adversarial manner against staff contradicts the image of birth plans promoted by those activists campaigning in favour of such plans (e.g. Simpkin, 1984; Kitzinger, 1987). For instance, in the three page discussion of birth plans in the Health Education Council/Open University handbook for expectant parents, *Understanding Pregnancy and Birth*, there are more than a dozen reminders to women to discuss their plans with staff and not to approach them with distrust or antagonism: 'It is important to remember that an agreed "agenda" does not take the place of a relationship in which you feel able to trust your care givers. Any birth plan works best as part of a relationship of understanding and trust between you and those caring for you' (HEC, 1985, p. 111).

Flexibility is also encouraged in the discussions of birth plans that we found in the literature (Snell, 1983; Evans and Durward, 1984; Flint, 1986; Kitzinger, 1987). The Health Education Council/Open University book, for instance, includes a section called 'When the Unexpected Happens' which reminds women that, however carefully they plan ahead, labour is bound to bring some surprises and also has another section, 'Changing Plans', which starts by advising women that 'sometimes your birth plan has to change in these last weeks (of pregnancy)' (HEC, 1975). It was this understanding of birth plans that was reflected by the women who intended to use them. The pro birth plan women in our sample emphasized the need for both trust and flexibility. As one woman who intended to use a birth plan commented:

> 'Childbirth is not a predictable situation. Therefore I would only want to list preferences and want to be as adaptable to the situation as possible.'

Postnatal data

In the event, 84 women had their wishes written down by the time they went into labour. (This was rather fewer than expected given that 117 women said that they already had written down their wishes or were intending to do so 'soon' when they responded to the antenatal questionnaire.) Of these, 35 women (i.e. less than half) found the birth plan helpful, three found it actually unhelpful and 44 felt it was not particularly helpful or unhelpful (two women did not answer). We then asked an open-ended question about what, in practice, they had found to be the advantages or disadvantages of birth plans.

Advantages of the plan (volunteered postnatally)

The women who found the plan helpful volunteered that it helped communication, helped them to get what they wanted and was useful over shift changes. They also said that it helped to sort things out in their own heads and yet still allowed them to be flexible:

> 'It was invaluable as most of the time I was not in a state of mind to insist on what I wanted.'

> 'The advantage I found was that my wishes were respected, and having them written down meant very little decision making whilst in labour.'

> 'It made me think, in advance, of all the options that might be available so I might consider whether these options were/were not what I might wish for if the labour was straight forward.'

Disadvantages or pointlessness of birth plans

Of the 47 women who did not say that their plan had been helpful, ten (12% of the women who used plans) felt that the plan had been completely ignored by the staff:

> 'Didn't make any difference the midwife wouldn't and didn't do anything I had asked for.'

Another nine women felt the plan was made redundant by the turn of events – the labour was too fast for the plan to be followed, emergencies arose which meant the plan did not apply or they simply changed their mind:

> 'Advantage was psychological only. I felt prior to labour that my wishes would be taken into account. But when labour commenced my wishes differed dramatically from those expressed on my birth plan.'

Seven women felt the plan was unnecessary as, in the event, the situation to which it applied did not arise (e.g. wishes regarding a caesarean section); three women felt happy to look to staff for guidance at the time and chose not to refer to the plan.

Intentions to use birth plans in a future birth

Most women still did not feel that they would use a birth plan next time but 131 women were unsure and 95 definitely would use one. This represents a shift towards being more pro birth plans from women's antenatal feelings. Only 16 women who had used a birth plan this time would not use one in the future.

Why did women change their attitude to birth plans?

Finally, we were interested in what influenced women to consider a birth plan for their next labour although they did not use one this time? Were these women different from those who did not use a birth plan this time and still would not next time round? Women who did not use a birth plan for this labour but would use one in the future found birth a less satisfactory experience ($p < 0.05$) and felt less in control of what staff did to them than women who did not use a birth plan this time and would not in the future. They were also more likely to be dissatisfied with the amount of information they had received ($p < 0.01$), less likely to describe the staff as 'informative' ($p < 0.05$) or 'considerate' ($p < 0.01$), and more likely to describe them as 'bossy' ($p < 0.01$). These results echo some of the statements multips made antenatally, i.e. a previous unsatisfactory experience can lead women to consider the use of a birth plan next time around. In exactly the same way, women who had used a birth plan this time but had found the experience unsatisfactory would not use one for a future birth.

It is thus clear that dissatisfaction with care does not in itself lead women to be pro or anti birth plans – it makes them want to try an alternative approach next time.

Summary

Most women in our sample did not wish to, and did not, have a birth plan. Birth plans were used mainly at the two units which encouraged women to have their wishes written down and where women were less likely to anticipate negative staff reactions. Birth plans were also more popular with the more educated and higher class women. However, they were not an exclusively middle class phenomenon.

Women's attitudes towards birth plans were also related to their previous experiences of staff (and of birth plans) and more generally to their attitude towards the role of professionals in childbirth. Above all, they reflected women's understanding of the role of birth plans themselves. All the women, for instance, wanted good communication with staff and subscribed to the need to have a flexible approach to labour. The difference was that the anti birth plan women believed birth plans would obstruct both these things whereas the pro birth plan group believe that birth plans do not pre-empt changes of mind and positively facilitate good communication.

In practice, however, less than half of those using birth plans said that they had been helpful and 12 per cent felt that the plan had been completely ignored by the staff. It is clear that birth plan campaigners have a long way to go if they are to convince many women and staff.

CHAPTER FOUR

Women's Views of Pain Relieving Drugs

Antenatal data

We were interested in women's attitudes towards and knowledge about the major forms of obstetric analgesia. We therefore included a series of questions asking women about what they saw as the advantages and disadvantages of epidurals, Pethidine (or alternative such as Meptid) and gas and air. The responses to these open-ended questions gave us a general picture not only of what women knew but also of how they felt about different drugs and of their priorities regarding pain relief. The results are discussed below.

Gas and air

Over a fifth of the total sample (22%) did not feel able to offer any comment on the advantages and disadvantages of gas and air.

Perceived advantages of gas and air

The most commonly cited advantage (given by 29% of the sample) was that it 'helps the pain' and 'Immediate good pain relief – I wouldn't have a baby without it!'. This was closely followed by the statement that the intake of gas and air is under the control of the woman herself (mentioned by 25% of the sample).

> 'It's totally self service. You get total control over how much you want and when you want it.'

> 'This is my favourite drug as I can have as much or as little as I require.'

Fourteen per cent of the total sample also mentioned that it had little effect on the baby and another 14 per cent said that it was a fast acting and convenient drug. Eight per cent of the sample emphasized that gas and air did not deprive the woman of being involved in the birth so implying that they thought other drugs did:

> 'You don't lose control or feelings so you can take an active part in the birth.'

> 'Gas and air is least damaging to the birth experience.'

Other women (7% of sample) specified that gas and air was useful at some time (e.g. just in the first stage of labour), six per cent said there were very few side effects and another six per cent said it 'distracts you' or 'gives you something to hold':

> 'A psychological prop, it stops one cutting off the blood supply to partner's hand by providing an alternative thing to hold!'

Some women said it helped their breathing and pushing rhythm and a few commented positively on its effects on the brain:

> 'You can legally get high on it (only joking!). It's marvellous stuff!'

> 'Wonderful stuff, I am thinking of having it plumbed in.'

Six women also commented on how gas and air leaves one mobile:

> 'Using gas and air doesn't restrict your movements – not like an epidural or the Pethidine which made me so woosy I couldn't stand up.'

The remaining comments were coded under 'Other' – this category included such miscellaneous statements as 'Gas and air is natural, it's not really a drug'.

Perceived disadvantages of gas and air

The most commonly cited disadvantage of gas and air (mentioned by 14% of the sample) was that it could result in a loss of involvement or control:

> 'I definitely do not want this. I have had gas and air and it makes you feel in a different world.'

> 'If you take too much it makes you sleepy. I slept for a minute and dreamt I had had the baby. It was a shock to realize I still had a lot to do.'

The next most commonly mentioned disadvantage (mentioned by 11% of the sample) focused on the physical side effects on the woman – sore throats and numbness – and another 11 per cent commented on the problems of using the mask correctly and the necessity of adequate instruction antenatally. Eight per cent felt it was quite useless as a pain relieving drug:

> 'This is the only *so called* pain relief I have had and I do not consider it to be effective.'

Six per cent mentioned their fear of the mask:

> 'I hate the thought of placing a black mask over my nose and mouth (memories of childhood visits to the dentist!).'

> 'Gas and air has no advantage to me personally as I would fight off having to wear the mask.'

A scattering of women made comments about the side effects of gas and air, its effects on pushing or other problems.

	n	% of sample
Helps with pain	214	29
In control of it yourself	186	25
Little/no effect on baby	106	14
Quick and easy to use	104	14
Can still feel and be aware	56	8
Good at times	51	7
Little/no side effects on woman	45	6
Distracts you/something to hold	41	6
Helps breathing/pushing	20	3
Makes you high	16	2
Still mobile	6	<1
Other	56	8
n = 744		

Table 4.1: Perceived advantages of gas and air

	n	% of sample
Loss of control/awareness	101	14
Side effects on woman (physical)	83	11
Self-administration difficult sometimes	79	11
Ineffective	61	8
Dislike mask	42	6
Side effects on baby	9	1
Dulls the experience	7	< 1
Inhibits pushing	7	< 1
Makes you behave badly	3	< 1
Timing problems	2	< 1
Other negative	21	3
n = 744		

Table 4.2: Perceived disadvantages of gas and air

Pethidine (or alternative such as Meptid)

Over a quarter of the total sample (28%) did not feel they knew enough about Pethidine to be able to list a single advantage or disadvantage. In practice very few women seemed to have heard of Meptid, though one woman who was in our sample (who had trained as a nurse) did comment:

> 'Pethidine makes both baby and mother drowsy and is an unnecessary risk. Meptid is a better form of pain relief as it has no effect on baby, can be given at any time during labour and doesn't knock you senseless!'

Perceived advantages of Pethidine

Almost half the sample commented positively on the pain relieving properties of Pethidine. Thirty eight women (5% of the total sample) made the rather surprising comment that Pethidine left you alert and aware, did not dull your mind or stop you being in control:

> 'This is quite a good form of pain relief because it still allows you to know about the labour you are going through.'

There was an implicit comparison with the effects of other drugs in such comments. Some emphasized that Pethidine was a positive help because it:

> 'Gives the patient a rest and a chance to get back in control.'

Or

> 'Takes the edge off the pain and relaxes you so you are more in control.'

Twenty eight women (4% of the whole sample) emphasized that Pethidine (unlike an epidural) did not dull the *physical* sensation so they could still feel the birth.

> 'Helps keep the pain to a small amount but still enough for you to experience childbirth.'

	n	% of all women
Helps with the pain	341	46
In control, alert and aware	38	5
Can still feel sensations	28	4
Easy to administer	19	3
Generally safe	7	<1
Little/no side effects on baby	7	<1
Still mobile	7	<1
Little/no side effects on woman	5	<1
Other	44	6

n = 744

Table 4.3: Perceived advantages of Pethidine

Perceived disadvantages of Pethidine

The most commonly cited disadvantages of Pethidine were the side effects on themselves and their babies. Side effects on the woman were mentioned by 28 per cent of the sample. Specific side effects ranged from 'It can give you a numb leg for a few days' to 'It made me feel that I was too drugged and when my baby was born I felt almost too tired to hold him'. One hundred women (13% of the sample) specifically commented on the loss of control that could result from the use of Pethidine.

> 'Makes you drowsy, not in control of yourself. I prefer to suffer and experience all the pain, so I know what I'm doing.'

> 'You may be too drowsy to react to contractions/focus on what is happening, essentially have to rely on outside help, midwife etc.'

A quarter of the sample also expressed concern about the effects of Pethidine on the baby. In particular, they were concerned that it could affect the baby's breathing or sucking responses and 'interfere with bonding'. Some were particularly concerned about events during previous labours in which they had been given Pethidine.

> 'Pethidine nearly stopped my first baby's heart – I wouldn't like to put this one in danger.'

> 'I had an induced birth last time and had Pethidine which I think is a good analgesia. But my baby took 8 minutes to breath spontaneously, was this due to Pethidine?'

The other two most commonly mentioned problems were the difficulties of getting the timing of drug administration right (mentioned by 11% of the sample) and the ineffectiveness of Pethidine as a pain relieving drug (7% of the sample).

	n	% of sample
Side effects on woman	210	28
Side effects on baby	186	25
Loss control/awareness	100	13
Timing/administration problems	83	11
Ineffective pain relief	51	7
Slows/stops labour	18	2
Uncomfortable with method	6	<1
Other negative comment	41	6

n = 744

Table 4.4: Perceived disadvantages of Pethidine

Epidurals

Almost a quarter of the total sample (22%) did not feel they knew enough about epidurals to note down even one advantage or disadvantage.

Perceived advantages of epidurals

Almost a third of the sample (32%) volunteered that they thought that having an epidural would guarantee a pain free labour, another 13 per cent made vague or qualified statements saying it was a 'good' pain relief or 'almost always' provided a completely pain free labour. Another way of looking at the responses is to note that of the 332 women who mentioned the pain relieving qualities of epidurals, over two thirds of them (233) thought that epidurals guaranteed a complete absence of pain. (However in practice about 1 in 20 epidurals are not successful or only partially successful in this sense (Huntingford, 1985, p. 85).

Eighty nine women (12%) volunteered positive comments about the function of epidurals for caesarean sections:

> 'It does allow the mother to at least be a part of the birth which must be better than a GA.'

A further five per cent of the women wrote that an epidural was useful in a vaginal delivery to enable a woman to be involved and in control. Other drugs and pain itself were seen to cause loss of control and an epidural was therefore welcomed:

> '[An epidural means I'm] totally conscious and aware of what is happening without the pain to blur the experience. Also to be able to communicate with my husband and hospital without feeling drugged.'

> 'Complete pain free - able to take active part in birth.'

> 'With my first child I had an epidural and I'm going to ask this time for one. It made things very calm and I didn't shout out. I was in full control of my feelings and that is very important to me.'

	n	% of sample
Guarantees complete pain relief	238	32
Helps pain, often complete pain relief	99	13
Good for Caesarean section	89	12
Gives you control	40	5
Good for long labours	27	4
Good for the baby	17	2
Good for the woman	13	2
Allows birth to be fulfilling	8	1
Easy to administer	4	<1
Less distressing for birth companion	2	<1
Other advantages	19	3
n = 744		

Table 4.5: Perceived advantage of epidurals

Perceived disadvantage of epidural

The most commonly mentioned disadvantage of an epidural was the loss of sensation it entails. This disadvantage was volunteered by almost a third of the total sample (31%). Women talked about feeling 'robbed' and 'cheated' of previous experiences of birth under epidurals and were concerned about feeling they had not 'participated in' or 'contributed anything much to labour'. Women felt they would miss out on the birth:

> 'For me it would take away the excitement of birth. To carry the baby for nine months and then not to feel it coming into the world must be awful.'

> 'No pain at all but your childbirth seems to have happened to someone else and it takes a while to believe that it is actually you that has given birth.'

Nineteen per cent said that epidurals led to a loss of control over your body. (Control as a theme in women's attitudes towards pain relief is discussed in Volume 1, Chapter 5). A further 16 per cent of the sample commented that epidurals could lead to further interventions. However, even among these women, although many mentioned things like catheters, few showed any awareness of the association of epidurals with, for instance, forceps deliveries. The incidence of forceps delivery among women having epidurals is 70 per cent for primips and 40 per cent for multips (Hoult et al., 1977). Concern was also expressed by 13 per cent of women about postnatal side effects ranging from 'lingering numbness' to 'it leaves a mark on your back like a pimple'. In addition 13 per cent of women commented on the slight risk of long term injury.

> 'Although the midwife has assured me there is no danger of spinal injuries I am a bit reluctant to have an injection in this area of my body.'

A further 12 per cent commented on the loss of mobility during labour itself and another seven per cent of the sample disliked the method of administration: 'The thought of a needle in my back makes me sick'. Only 24 women (3% of the sample) volunteered the information that epidurals do not always work.

	n	% of sample
Loss of sensation/miss out on birth	230	31
Loss of control	140	19
Leads to medical interference	117	16
Side effects on woman (postnatally)	94	13
Risk of paralysis	94	13
Loss of mobility	89	12
Uncomfortable re method of admin.	52	7
It might not work	24	3
Side effects on baby	19	3
Timing problems	15	2
'Not right'	9	1
Other negative	41	6
n = 744		

Table 4.6: Perceived disadvantages of epidurals

Women's attitudes towards pain relief clearly reflect their views of how birth should be – their 'philosophy' of childbirth. In some cases this was explicitly stated, as in this comment about epidural analgesia:

> 'Ideal for the people that want it, but personal view is that pain draws you closer to your unborn and suffering makes you feel proud and deserving at the first glimpse at the trouble that caused it.'

Relative views of different drugs

In general women listed more positive comments about gas and air than negative ones, but the reverse was true for Pethidine and epidurals. This is, however, a very crude measurement as the disadvantages listed ranged from the very minor to the very severe (as perceived by the woman herself).

	Gas and air	Pethidine	Epidural
Mean no. of advantages per woman	1.2	0.7	0.8
Mean no. of disadvantages per woman	0.6	0.9	1.2

Table 4.7: Advantages/disadvantages per woman of pain-relieving drugs

Women's attitudes towards epidurals for caesarean section

Women were asked:

'If you were to have a caesarean section, would you prefer a general anaesthetic (completely unconscious) or an epidural (numb from the waist down, but fully conscious)?'

Responses were:

Epidural	42%
General anaesthetic	38%
Don't know	20%

Although most women were not keen on epidurals during labour, there was more enthusiasm for epidurals in the event of a caesarean section. Thus, although only 8 per cent of the sample wanted an epidural for pain relief during labour, 42 per cent would want one for a caesarean section in preference to a general anaesthetic.

Attitudes towards epidurals for caesarean section and women's educational level

There was a clear relationship between women's attitudes towards epidurals for caesarean sections and their educational level. The longer a woman had stayed in full time education, the more likely she was to prefer an epidural.

Age of leaving education	Would prefer epidural		Would prefer general anaesthetic		Don't know	
	n	%	n	%	n	%
16 or less	114	(31)	170	(46)	85	(23)
17 or 18	98	(46)	78	(37)	36	(17)
19 or more	97	(61)	37	(23)	26	(16)

Percentages are of women of a given level of education

$p < 0.001$

Table 4.8: Choice of anaesthesia for caesarean section by education

A similar relationship exists between women's attitudes and social class as defined by their best ever job (but not partner's class). Only 17 per cent of women in social class V would prefer an epidural for a caesarean section, whereas the vast majority (83%) in social class I would prefer an epidural.

Relationship between attitude towards drugs and perceived familiarity with or knowledge about each drug

Women sometimes explicitly drew attention to their familiarity with a drug as a factor which predisposed them towards it – knowing something about the drug in itself made it more acceptable.

> '..(Pethidine) is the sort I would have, as the others are unknown to me.'

> 'I think this (an epidural) is what I might go for if labour pain gets unbearable because I know more about it.'

The degree to which women felt the staff had explained things to them openly and thoroughly was also important. Thus, one woman who felt the staff had explained epidurals had great confidence in this method:

> 'Made an appointment to see an anaesthetist at the hospital to ask about epidurals. He spent an hour explaining certain worries we had, with my husband and I. We feel this is a safe and effective way of pain relief, and feel confident in our hospital and anaesthetist.'

While another commented:

> '... I have been offered this but I do not feel they are familiar enough with it yet. They really do not explain anything about how it works, what it entails. Therefore you have no confidence in it.'

Knowledge of advantages/disadvantages of drugs and preferences about use of drugs

Women who did not list any advantages or disadvantages for each pain relieving drug (indicating instead that they 'didn't know or weren't sure') were likely to go on to say that they 'didn't know enough to make a choice' or 'didn't mind' whether they used that drug. By contrast, women who wrote down at least one comment about the particular drug were more likely to indicate a definite preference about it. This in itself is not surprising. However, it is worth noting that the majority (63%) of women who did not feel able to write down any 'advantages' or 'disadvantages' of epidurals still expressed a preference – they still had feelings about them even if they felt unable to respond to the invitation for comments.

If women felt able to write comments, what were their preferences?

Women who wrote comments about gas and air were as likely to reject it as those who did not, but were also much more likely to actively want gas and air.

Women who wrote comments about Pethidine were both more likely to want and to reject Pethidine than women who did not. However, women who wrote about the pros and cons of epidurals were more likely to reject epidurals than those who felt unable to make any comment.

It would seem therefore that feeling able to comment on the pros and cons of gas and air is associated with wanting to use it, whereas feeling able to comment on the pros and cons of an epidural is associated with rejecting it.

Knowledge about pros and cons	Indicated no preference/ choice	Rejected drug	Wanted drug
Women who said they didn't know about the pros and cons of gas and air	59%	23%	18%
Women who wrote down at least one comment about gas and air	24%	20%	57%
Women who said they didn't know about the pros and cons of Pethidine	52%	38%	9%
Women who wrote at least one comment about Pethidine	24%	52%	25%
Women who said they didn't know about the pros and cons of epidurals	37%	56%	7%
Women who wrote at least one comment about epidurals	5%	86%	9%

Table 4.9: Knowledge about drugs and preference for use

Prior experience of and current attitude towards particular forms of pain relief

Women who had previously used gas and air, Pethidine or an epidural were more likely to want to use it this time around than those who had not. There are three obvious explanations for this:

1. Women who have experienced these forms of pain relief realize how genuinely good they are.

2. Women who have experienced these forms of pain relief cannot imagine giving birth without them.

3. Women who have not experienced these drugs have, at least in the case of multips, positively resisted having them. They were predisposed against them in the first place in contrast to women who have experienced them.

Women with previous experience of gas and air were twice as likely as women who had not used it to 'definitely want it'. Women who had not used gas and air were more likely to feel that they did not know enough to make a choice (Table 4.10).

	Previous experience		No previous experience	
	n	%	n	%
Don't know enough to make choice	4	(1)	26	(7)
Prefer not/definitely don't want	68	(18)	85	(23)
Don't mind	95	(26)	107	(29)
Quite like	94	(25)	101	(27)
Definitely want	110	(30)	57	(15)

Percentages are of women in a given column.

Table 4.10: Previous experience of gas and air by current attitude towards using it

Although some of the multips without experience of gas and air may have had elective caesareans, most will have had a previous labour in which the option of gas and air was available and therefore have probably actively chosen to avoid it. In fact, 27 per cent of the multips had never used gas and air and they were much less positive about gas and air than the other multips (see Table 4.11). However, if we compare these women with primips who also have no experience of gas and air, we see again that they are much more negative about using it. Differences in attitudes are not, therefore, simply a consequence of experience.

	Multips with prior experience		Primips without prior experience		Multips without prior experience	
	n	%	n	%	n	%
Don't know enough to make a choice	2	(1)	12	(5)	14	(12)
Definitely don't want/prefer not to have	60	(18)	31	(12)	54	(45)
Don't mind	86	(26)	75	(29)	32	(26)
Definitely want or quite like	186	(56)	137	(54)	21	(17)
Total	334		255		121	

Percentages are of women in a given column.

Table 4.11: Current attitude towards gas and air by previous experience of it and parity

Similar associations were found for Pethidine and epidurals. More of the women who had experienced these methods of pain relief in a previous birth wanted them this time round than those who had not. However, any effect of previous experience seemed to disappear once the data were broken down by parity because the multips without prior experience were a distinct minority with very different views from the majority of primips.

	Multips with prior experience		Primips without prior experience		Multips without prior experience	
	n	%	n	%	n	%
Don't know enough to make a choice	3	(1)	31	(12)	16	(11)
Definitely don't want/prefer not to have	123	(40)	131	(49)	93	(63)
Don't mind	87	(28)	65	(24)	27	(18)
Definitely want or quite like	94	(31)	41	(15)	12	(8)
Total	307		268		148	

Percentages are of women in a given column

Table 4.12: Current attitudes towards Pethidine by previous experience of it and parity

	Multips with prior experience		Primips without prior experience		Multips without prior experience	
	n	%	n	%	n	%
Don't know enough to make a choice	1	(1)	21	(7)	27	(8)
Definitely don't want/prefer not to have	52	(55)	235	(81)	303	(84)
Don't mind	18	(19)	12	(4)	10	(3)
Definitely want or quite like	24	(25)	21	(7)	19	(5)
Total	95		289		359	

Percentages are of women in a given column

Table 4.13: Current attitude towards epidurals by previous experience of them and parity

Postnatal data

General comments about pain relieving drugs

Postnatally, women were asked to respond to two open-ended questions: 'Please add any other comments that you wish to about pain relieving drugs' and 'If there is anything else you'd like to say about (the way you responded to the pain of labour) please tell us about it in your own words'. Over half the sample responded to this question. We coded up to four responses for each woman. The responses discussed below are therefore based on post hoc codings.

	n	% of women who made comments
Side effects of Pethidine/(or alternative e.g. Meptid)	69	(19)
Positive comments about drugs	67	(19)
Felt in control	60	(17)
Side effects of gas and air	53	(15)
Bad timing of drug administration	47	(15)
Positive comments on how dealt with pain herself	44	(12)
Would have liked more pain relief	25	(7)
Felt out of control	23	(6)
Negative comments on staff support	22	(6)
Pragmatic acceptance	21	(6)
Mixed comments on control	19	(5)
Would have liked less pain relief	18	(5)
Positive comments on staff support	17	(5)
Side effects of epidural	14	(4)
Unprepared/false expectations re coping with pain	12	(3)
Ashamed/disappointed	12	(3)
Wanted pain relief at time but now happy didn't	11	(3)
Proud of self	8	(2)
Other positive	60	(17)
Other negative	34	(9)
349 women made no comment		
636 comments were coded		
n = 362		

Table 4.14: Comment about the pain and pain relief

Comments about drugs and side effects

About a fifth of the women who wrote something volunteered positive comments about pain relieving drugs:

> 'I'm pleased I had an injection of Pethidine – it made me relaxed and certainly worked for me.'

> 'I found the gas and air a marvellous help.'

> 'Epidural was excellent and I was very glad to have one.'

However, these positive comments were outweighed by the negative comments about side effects – 19 per cent of the respondents to this question made negative comments about Pethidine, 15 per cent made negative comments about side effects of gas and air and 14 women (20% of those who had one) complained on the side effects of Epidurals. The criticisms of Pethidine were of it making women feel sick and/or out of control. Similar criticisms were made of gas and air:

> '...did not relieve the pain but made me feel very sick and faint. Also made me lose control – I didn't know where I was.'

Sometimes the combined effects of Pethidine and gas and air could make women feel very 'out of it':

> 'I felt totally out of control. I did not realize when my baby was born. I feel an epidural would have helped.'

Some complaints about epidurals concerned the pain of administering them. One woman who said the epidural was the worst thing about the birth commented:

> 'It was extremely painful and I would not recommend it to anyone.'

Or the pain of disconnecting it:

> '...the agonising part of the epidural was taking off the sticking plaster from my back when it was all over – I felt I was being skinned alive!'

However, the main complaint about epidurals were about postnatal problems:

> 'The pain due to the injection lasted about five weeks after. If I had been told I would have refused it point blank.'

> 'I have still got numbness in my right foot and a clot in my blood vessel has come up due to the needles from the epidurals and drips.'

Women who would have liked more pain relief

Twenty five women volunteered that they would have liked more or earlier pain relief:

> 'Now that the birth is over I can see that I should have asked for pain relief sooner, but didn't want to be a bother, and just kept holding out thinking that the pain couldn't get any worse.'

In particular, some of them expressed the desire for an epidural (or at least a more effective epidural):

> 'I only wish the epidural could have been topped up right until he popped out – coward aren't I!'

Another woman was very distressed by the pain of a rotational forceps with only gas and air to relieve the pain:

> 'I was unprepared for the pain of a rotational forceps delivery under gas and air. I feel the birth was a very frightening procedure and I now find it upsetting to think about. I am very envious of mothers who had a straightforward time or had an epidural as I think this would have helped a great deal, but realize in my case the medical staff could not have foreseen the need for one.'

On the whole, these women saw the lack of pain relief as due to their own refusal to take drugs only to find themselves overwhelmed by the pain, or as a failure in the timing or administration of the drugs. However, two women, both from Willowford, commented:

> 'It is obvious the midwives would prefer you not to have pain killers, so often they are administered later than you'd wish, by which time you may panic.'

> 'It seems as though the doctors and midwives would prefer to have you have your baby as natural as possible. So now in the 80s you have to almost demand an epidural for total pain relief.'

Only 18 women said they wished they had had less pain relief.

Changing and mixed feelings about pain relief

A few women expressed mixed feelings such as one woman whose first labour was under epidural but whose second was so well advanced when she was admitted that staff thought there was no time. Her labour however slowed down and:

> 'I had three hours with no pain relief. I found this very hard as I had not experienced that before and wished I'd had another epidural at the time. However I recovered so quickly after this labour compared with the after effects of an epidural I was finally glad that I managed without one.'

Eleven women specified that they were now glad that they had not had as much pain relief as they wanted at the time:

> 'I got annoyed when she didn't want to give me extremely strong pain killers – she gave me gas and air, and now I am very glad she did what she did.'

> 'My midwife belonged to the NCT and massaged a lot, if she had offered pain relief I probably would have accepted at the time, but glad she didn't.'

Pain relief and staff support

Some of the negative comments about staff centred around staff failure to consult or involve women in decisions about pain relief:

> 'I was not asked I was just injected.'

> 'Some midwives made me feel I ought to "do as I was told" and made me feel under pressure to have pain relief I never really wanted by telling me how awful it would get and how long I would be there.'

> 'I wasn't asked about having Pethidine and felt unable to control my own body.'

Other comments were about staff's failure to support women (e.g. 'no-one helped me to breathe correctly').

Positive comments about the staff, on the other hand, described support, negotiation and consultation. As one woman commented:

> 'From previous pregnancies I knew I didn't like the gas and air. I told my midwife this during the 1st stage of labour and she respected my wishes. Unlike the midwife I had while delivering my second child, here I was very pressurized. Also because of having a bad time with the second labour I was petrified of my third and consequently, was very frightened of having injections of Pethidine but my midwife handled me very well and offered me only half a dose when I wished, which I eventually took.'

And this woman went on to write:

> 'I feel the relationship you have with the staff with you during the labour plays a very important part in how you deal with pain etc... This being my third child I have had experience of three different midwives. The one delivering my first did not force me to do anything or take anything. I was happy with how I coped with the pain. But with my second baby the midwife was very forceful but at the same time she seemed to be panicking. Due to this I was not at all confident. I was not happy about this labour. With my third baby I had a very good relationship with my midwife and we worked together. I was very happy with the way things went.'

How women felt they coped with the pain

Many of women's postnatal comments about the pain centred around the issue of control. Sixteen per cent of all comments made in response to the open-ended question about drugs and dealing with pain focused on control. Nine per cent referred to a positive sense of having control, four per cent to a negative sense of loss of control and three per cent to a 'mixed' experience of control.

> 'I felt in control to begin with, but they put me on a drip as things were only moving slowly. After this I felt out of control and only half there. I think I panicked and left the midwives to get on with it. I just tried to do what they asked me to do. I feel disappointed.'

Women who were pleased with the way they coped with the pain were often pleased to have coped without drugs:

> 'I was very pleased that I was able to go through this stage of labour naturally without any interference from drugs etc.'

> 'I feel very proud to have coped with such pain without any form of pain relief. It gave me a sense of inner strength. Now I feel I can cope with almost any pain.'

For some women, going without drugs or managing with only a few drugs was a source of tremendous satisfaction and pride:

> 'Even though labour is painful, the less painkillers I could use made me feel more satisfied, feminine and pleased with myself.'

Other women, however, were not convinced. As one woman who had a very fast labour and arrived too late to have anything but gas and air wrote:

> 'It is nice to know I did it without – although I wouldn't again if I could have pain relief. Maybe I'm just a coward – but I don't think natural childbirth is all it's cracked up to be.'

Women who were not pleased with the way they coped with the pain wrote of their shame and disappointment:

> 'I felt I was rather a handful for the poor midwives as I'm not very brave when it comes to pain and I am quite ashamed.'

CHAPTER FIVE

Alternative Ways of Dealing with Pain

Breathing and relaxation exercises

The majority of our sample intended to use breathing and relaxation exercises during labour.

	n	%
Yes, definitely	316	(42)
Yes, probably	274	(37)
Don't know	91	(12)
Probably not	58	(8)
Definitely not	8	(1)
Total	747	(100)

Table 5.1: 'Do you intend to use breathing and relaxation exercises during labour?'

Most women (91%) thought that such natural methods of pain relief would be 'very' or 'a bit' helpful in controlling the pain. However, only 13 women (2% of the sample) thought that they would allow them to control the pain completely. Interestingly, more women thought breathing and relaxation exercises would be helpful than in fact intended to use them.

	n	%
I am sure that they would allow me to control the pain completely	13	(2)
I think that they would be very helpful in controlling the pain	307	(41)
I think that they would probably help a bit	373	(50)
I wouldn't expect them to help at all	26	(3)
I have no expectations	28	(4)
Total	747	(100)

Table 5.2: 'How useful would you expect breathing and relaxation exercises to be?'

Actual use of breathing and relaxation exercises

Sixty three per cent of women used breathing and relaxation exercises 'all' or 'most of the time', 27 per cent used them 'for a bit' and only 10 per cent of women who went into labour did not use them at all.

Some women who had intended to use breathing and relaxation exercises found in practice that they soon gave up. One woman felt too much emphasis was placed on the exercises because:

> 'By the time you give birth the last thing you can remember is the breathing exercises.'

And another felt she had not practised enough:

> 'I wish I'd practised breathing and relaxation exercises so that they'd been more useful. For three hours I found the pain pretty terrible and kept wondering why I'd let myself in for this pain the second time around.'

Several women commented on the importance of staff support at the time:

> 'Staff should encourage patients to use the breathing exercises by breathing with the patient. I was told to remember my breathing and left to get on with it.'

When staff did help women to use their breathing exercises this sometimes made all the difference:

> 'I'm afraid I wasn't prepared. I didn't feel I had been taught to breath properly. It was only when the midwife got me to breath more deeply that I could cope.'

> 'I never realized that blowing out with pain made you dilate quicker. I started breathing as the midwife told me to at nine o'clock at which time I was 3 centimetres dilated, and by 10.19 she was born. I always believed breathing classes were silly until now and this is after having two children.'

Overall, women found the exercises more useful than they had expected. Of the women who used breathing and relaxation exercises, only five per cent found that they did not help at all.

	n	% of women who used breathing and relaxation
They allowed me to control the pain completely	30	(5)
They were very helpful in controlling the pain	299	(49)
They only helped a bit	249	(41)
They did not help at all	27	(4)
Total	605	(100)

Table 5.3: 'How useful did you find breathing and relaxation exercises?'

Women who antenatally said they expected labour to be only moderately uncomfortable were the most likely to use breathing and relaxation exercises and to find that they were very helpful.

Relationship between breathing and relaxation exercises and the independent variables

The more educated and/or middle class women were more likely to intend to use breathing and relaxation exercises. However, social class and education made no difference to reported use of breathing and relaxation exercises postnatally.

Primips were more likely than multips to intend to use breathing and relaxation exercises during labour (85% compared to 75%). In the event, more primips tried breathing and relaxation exercises during labour at least for a bit (92% compared to 79%, $p < 0.05$) but multips and primips were equally likely to use these exercises throughout labour. It is interesting to note that when multips did use breathing and relaxation exercises they were more positive about them than primips ($p < 0.05$). Fifty eight per cent of multips found that they were very helpful or even allowed them to control the pain completely, as opposed to 48 per cent of primips.

There were also some interesting unit differences. Surprisingly, 20 per cent of the women booked at the (low risk) Exington GP unit did not intend to use breathing and relaxation exercises during labour as opposed to 6–11 per cent at the other units, and this was reflected in their actual use as reported postnatally.

Alternative methods of pain relief

Just over one fifth of our sample were thinking about using alternative methods of pain relief (other than breathing and relaxation exercises). The most popular option was Trans Electronic Neural Stimulation (TENS) closely followed by massage. These methods of pain relief were being considered by 86 and 83 women respectively (i.e. approximately 11% of the whole sample). (Each woman could have up to two responses coded, so there is some overlap between women who indicated one method and another.)

Fifteen women mentioned their intentions to use ice packs or hot waterbottles, twelve mentioned yoga and a similar number mentioned movement and/or position. Only seven women mentioned using a bath to help with the pain and one or two mentioned things such as prayer or hypnosis:

> 'Prayer, we asked for a more relaxed labour, about two hours notice before birth and not much pain – extremely helpful before and during.'

Most women (four fifths of the sample), however, were not considering alternatives.

Alternative methods of pain relief: postnatal data

In the event, 154 women (i.e. about a fifth of the women who experienced labour) used alternative methods of pain relief. In fact, probably more women tried different methods than this but did not perceive them as 'alternative methods of pain relief'. It seems unlikely, for instance, that only six women moved about to relieve pain.

Alternative method	n	% of women experiencing labour who used this method
Massage	85	(13)
TENS	36	(5)
Bath	22	(3)
Hot water bottles/ice pack	12	(2)
Movement	6	(<1)
Prayer	5	(<1)
Yoga	4	(<1)
Other	4	(<1)
n = 675		

Table 5.4: Use of alternative methods of pain relief

Massage was enjoyed because of the physical contact and comfort as well as the pain relief it afforded. TENS was also popular with the 36 women who used it. Being able to adjust the intensity and push the button during contractions was a distraction in itself and women also liked it because:

> '... it put me in control of relieving the pain.'

> 'TENS was wonderful: it gave pain relief without the side effects of drugs.'

However, some women who wanted TENS were, in the event, unable to have it – either because the staff on duty did not know how to use it, or because TENS was not available:

> 'I was disappointed – I had to have an injection of Pethidine instead of using TENS as I had wanted because the midwives on duty were unfamiliar with TENS.'

'I originally requested the use of a TENS machine when I went into the labour ward but there is only one available and this was in use.'

Antenatally, 86 women had said they were thinking of using TENS but less than half of those actually used TENS during labour. On the other hand, there were a few women who may have used TENS without knowing what it was. One woman, for instance, said she did not use any alternative form of pain relief such as TENS but said:

'I had this thing strapped to my back and every time I had a pain I had to press this button and it sent like electric shocks up my back. It helped the pain quite a lot.'

Relationships between alternative methods of pain relief and the independent variables

The more educated and/or middle class women were both more likely to intend to use alternative methods of pain relief and to report doing so postnatally. Also, primips were more likely than multips to intend to use, and to actually use, alternatives. There were some surprising unit differences concerning the use of alternative pain relief. Few of the low risk women in Exington GP unit and Little Exington intended to use alternative methods of pain relief – only nine per cent and 11 per cent respectively compared to 18 per cent to 27 per cent at the other units ($p < 0.05$). This result might reflect parity differences in the sample, given that most of the women at Exington GP unit and Little Exington were multips and multips were less likely to intend to use alternative methods. Further analysis would need to be carried out to explain these differences.

Movement and position

We asked women: 'Were you able to get into the positions that were most comfortable for you during labour and delivery?'. If there were times when they were unable to get into the most comfortable position, they were asked why this was so.

	n	%
No, hardly ever	100	(15)
Yes, some of the time	258	(38)
Yes, all of the time	315	(47)
Total	673	(100)

Table 5.5: 'Were you able to get into the most comfortable positions?'

Less than half the sample were always able to get into the position they found most comfortable (a recent survey by *Mother and Baby* (1988) found that a third of women would have liked more freedom of movement). When women were encouraged to be mobile they were sometimes surprised by how much it helped the progress of the labour:

> 'It was much easier once I turned over on to my hands and knees.'

> 'The second midwife encouraged me to get off the bed and walk around, which I did and labour sped along.'

Some women expressed great satisfaction with active birth:

> '[The best thing about the birth was] the satisfaction of delivering my third child in an "active" position after an active birth, having had two previously "orthodox" labours and forceps deliveries.'

Some women were convinced that changing their position had made all the difference. One woman, for instance, who was being prepared for a forceps delivery, wrote:

> 'It was thought necessary as baby was distressed [But] as soon as I changed position on the bed, and episiotomy was done, the baby came out unaided by forceps.'

Another woman who had a positive experience of an active labour wrote:

> 'Last time everything slowed down when I arrived at hospital which I put down to immobility.'

Mobility was also seen to help control the pain:

> 'Being allowed to be in the position I chose helped enormously in controlling the pain.'

> 'I was able to keep on top of the pain by walking about and swaying whilst standing. If I lay down the pain would engulf me.'

> 'I had an "active" labour and at no time was confined to a reclining position on the bed. I felt that being able to do exactly what came naturally and what I found to be most comfortable was probably the reason for the relatively small amount of severe pain that I had.'

It should not be assumed that women who were mobile and who were always able to get into the most comfortable position necessarily had staff support for this. For example, one woman described how she was only able to get into the most comfortable position:

> 'At my insistence. I was *told* to get into a certain position that was *not* comfortable at all – I refused.'

Moving around and getting comfortable: women who were not successful

Just over half of the sample (53%) felt that they were not always able to get into the most comfortable position during labour and delivery. Usually this was because of some kind of physical constraint such as the monitoring equipment (12%) or drip (6%).

	n	% of women who experienced labour
Fetal heart monitor limited movement	82	(12)
Staff influence/control	55	(8)
Couldn't find any comfortable positions	50	(7)
Drip limited movement	43	(6)
Too painful to move	30	(4)
No time, labour too fast	20	(3)
Too tired/no inclination to move	18	(3)
Miscellaneous physical constraints (e.g. stirrups)	18	(3)
Epidural limited movement	17	(3)
Gas and air, or Pethidine made woman too woozy	10	(1)
Other	23	(3)

n = 675

(Up to two reasons were coded for each woman)

Table 5.6: Reasons why women could not get as comfortable as possible

Thirteen per cent of the sample indicated two reasons for their discomfort. The raw data show that more than 16 per cent of the women specifically felt unable to get comfortable at times because of the mechanics of interventions:

> '[The worst thing about the birth was] being unable to change position or get off the bed because of the monitor.'

> 'I could hardly move because if I did the scalp monitor played up.'

The women who were connected to more than one piece of apparatus gave graphic descriptions of their discomfort:

> 'I had an epidural, a drip, a monitor which was attached to the baby's head and then the actual delivery – a consultant standing between my legs (stirruped) pulling on a suction unit which was on the baby's head. "Comfortable" was a word of the past.'

Quite apart from the arguments about the physiological benefits of being able to move around, there are also psychological aspects:

> 'I was surprised just how painful the first stage was – I feel that had I been able to walk around (I was attached to a continuous fetal monitor) I would have been able to manage with just gas and air – it is very different when you cannot move – at 3 a.m. – you have nothing else to do but feel the contraction and breathe through it as best you can.'

The second most common reason given by women for why they were unable to get comfortable was because of staff control: 'I was made to lie on my back', 'The midwife kept telling me what to do', 'She wouldn't allow me to "wriggle around"'.

> 'The midwife was rather unenlightened and wanted me to lie down for delivery. I would really have preferred to sit up, but she was adamant.'

Sometimes staff used physical manipulation or force to place women into the position they wished:

> 'The sister forcibly pulled me on to my side.'

> 'The midwife insisted on turning me on to my back, which I was in no state to argue with, having had two sleeping tablets before going into labour, and having gas and air.'

At other times women were advised to move into the position that was 'easiest for the staff' or 'best for the baby':

> 'Most comfortable for me isn't always easiest for staff to see what's going on.'

> 'For the delivery I was told to lie on my side and when I questioned this, they said the baby preferred it that way.'

Sometimes women were unable to get comfortable because the staff did not believe they were in labour and tucked them up in bed:

> 'They told me to lie down and go to sleep, couldn't really convince them I was in labour.'

> 'Put into general ward "for a sleep" after waters broke and kept there until contractions quite strong. As others in ward were asleep discouraged to get out of bed.'

'Internal' reasons for being unable to get as comfortable as possible

Seven per cent of the women quite simply could not find a 'most comfortable' position:

> 'There weren't any! – The hospital provided all manner of options – bean bags, mattress, bed, birthing stool etc. – but I couldn't face leaving the bed!'

Four per cent of the sample said it was 'too painful' to move, three per cent that labour was too fast, they had no time to get comfortable, and three per cent that they were too tired or could not get up the enthusiasm to shift their position:

> 'I was too tense, I was frightened to move most of the time.'

> 'I was so tired by that stage that the effort seemed too much. I got as far as *thinking* about changing position!'

The women who described feeling 'too tired' or had no inclination to move had often also had Pethidine or sleeping tablets (the numbers, however, are too small for statistical analysis).

> 'During the latter part of labour I was given some sleeping tablets and when a strong contraction woke me up I felt too dopey to do anything other than to lie down.'

> 'I had been given sleeping tablets and I did not really know what I was doing as I felt drunk.'

> 'The pain was quite intense at times and the Pethidine made me very drowsy and made me sleep at times. Therefore I "forgot" to be bothered about or consider comfortable positions.'

However, only ten women specifically identified 'wooziness' induced by drugs as the reason for their inability to get into the most comfortable position. Seventeen women identified the physical constraints of having an epidural as an inhibitor to getting comfortable. This represents 26 per cent of all of those who had an epidural.

Women were also prevented from getting comfortable by inadequate provisions:

> 'I am very sad I had to give birth on my back – but the staff couldn't find any more pillows and the bed didn't adjust.'

Some women found the hospital beds narrow and uncomfortable:

> 'The design of the beds are made to suit doctors and not patients. i.e. the mattress is divided across in the middle into which I kept sinking having to ask to be helped up at regular intervals.'

One woman discovered after the event that what she had really wanted was a birthing chair:

> 'I felt best able to cope with the pain when sitting on the toilet as this was a very comfortable position and felt I would like to give birth in such a position. I discussed this later with the district midwife and was told that a birthing chair had been available at the hospital for a trial period but was sent back due to lack of interest. I feel I would have benefited from such a chair.'

A rather sad case was the woman who was offered the special option of the pool, the pride and joy of Willowford, but wrote:

> 'The put me in a "pool" which I didn't find at all comfortable probably because it only had six inches of water in it!'

Relationship between 'getting comfortable' and the independent variables

There were no education or social class differences with regard to finding comfortable positions, but multips were more likely to be able to get comfortable than primips.

	No, hardly ever		Yes, some of the time		Yes, all of the time	
	n	%	n	%	n	%
Primip	48	(18)	116	(43)	104	(39)
Multip	51	(13)	142	(35)	212	(52)

Percentages are of women in given row.

$p < 0.005$

Table 5.7: Ability to get comfortable by parity

There were striking differences between units. Women at the Exington GP unit were the most likely to have been able to get comfortable all the time, while women at Exington consultant unit and Zedbury were the least likely. In part, this is a factor of the higher intervention rates at the Exington consultant unit (and the concentration there of 'high risk' women). However, it also reflects both different staff attitudes and the design of the consultant unit, which requires women to be transferred during labour:

> 'Transferring from the bed to the labour room couch was difficult and I felt so much pressure from the baby and with the pain I didn't seem to have the strength. The sister present, I felt, did not seem to realize this and her attitude was upsetting.'

	No, hardly ever		Yes, some of the time		Yes, all of the time	
	n	%	n	%	n	%
Willowford	17	(11)	53	(33)	91	(57)
Exington consultant	17	(19)	40	(44)	34	(37)
Exington GP unit	8	(16)	12	(24)	31	(61)
Little Exington	7	(16)	13	(30)	24	(55)
Wychester	16	(10)	71	(43)	78	(47)
Zedbury	28	(20)	61	(43)	54	(38)

Percentages are of women in a given unit.

$p < 0.01$

Table 5.8: Ability to get comfortable by unit

There are clear differences between units concerning staff attitude to movement and position. Although the women in Exington consultant unit often mentioned interventions such as monitoring and drips as the cause of their discomfort, 15 per cent of all the women who gave birth there (and 14% of women at the GP unit) said they were (at least sometimes) prevented from getting comfortable by the staff (lack of support, physical manipulation or prohibitions). In contrast, no-one at Little Exington gave this as a reason for not being able to get comfortable.

Provisions for movement and supporting 'unconventional' positions also vary between units. Willowford, in particular, has a reputation for encouraging 'active birth' and provides a pool, bean bags and cushions to help women:

> 'I must give credit to the sympathetic atmosphere at the hospital, and their pool and active birth room, both of which I was lucky enough to use. I was able to move around as I liked, coped with most of the pain by rocking on all fours and gave birth kneeling upright leaning forward over bean bags on the floor.'

(Twenty eight per cent of women giving birth at Willowford in 1987 gave birth in non-conventional positions.)

The high rates of discomfort at Exington consultant unit cannot be explained away by reference to the higher risk population in this unit. To pursue the comparison between units we also looked at the figures in terms of parity. It is clear that Exington consultant unit and Zedbury come out particularly badly both for multips and primips. (In contrast to Exington consultant unit, low risk multips are not filtered away from Zedbury.) This may reflect some aspects of the unit ethos as well as of provisions (see Green et al., 1986).

	No, hardly ever		Yes, some of the time		Yes, all the time	
	n	%	n	%	n	%
Willowford	8	(9)	30	(32)	55	(59)
Exington consultant	9	(18)	21	(43)	19	(39)
Exington GP unit	7	(15)	10	(21)	31	(65)
Little Exington	4	(12)	11	(33)	18	(55)
Wychester	7	(8)	32	(38)	45	(54)
Zedbury	13	(15)	32	(38)	40	(47)

Percentages are of multips in any given unit.

$p < 0.05$

Table 5.9: 'Were you able to get comfortable?' by unit, multips only

	No, hardly ever		Yes, some of the time		Yes, all the time	
	n	%	n	%	n	%
Willowford	9	(13)	23	(34)	36	(53)
Exington consultant	8	(19)	19	(45)	15	(36)
Wychester	9	(11)	39	(48)	33	(41)
Zedbury	15	(26)	29	(50)	14	(24)

Percentages are of primips in any given unit.

$p < 0.05$

Table 5.10: 'Were you able to get comfortable?' by unit, primips only

Little Exington and Exington GP unit have been omitted from analysis because of the very small numbers of primips at these units. Wychester and Willowford, with their mixed 'risk' population, came out relatively well in this analysis. A higher proportion of women in these units are able to get comfortable all of the time than at the comparable unit of Zedbury and more were able to get comfortable for some of the time than at the 'low risk' GP and satellite unit at Exington.

As was shown in Volume 1, Chapter 8, being unable to move into the most comfortable position possible was significantly associated with negative psychological outcomes. Freedom of movement was also closely tied in with women's sense of 'external' control (see Volume 1, Chapter 7).

Perhaps the clearest implications for service provisions from this section of the study is that, in some units, provisions for non-drug pain relief such as TENS need to be improved and staff could develop greater understanding of, and support for, women's desires to move about and get comfortable during labour.

CHAPTER SIX

The Third Stage of Labour

Introduction

The third stage of labour is defined as the time between the delivery of the baby and the completion of the delivery of the placenta (Clinch, 1985). However, in clinical practice the limits of the third stage have been extended so that active management of the third stage with the injection of an oxytocic drug begins before the baby is fully delivered, in what is still technically the second stage of labour (ibid). Shortly after the delivery of the baby, the uterus naturally begins to contract strongly again, causing the placenta to separate and descend into the vagina. The classic signs of descent are a show of blood, a lengthening of the cord and a rising up of the contracted uterus in the abdomen. The placenta may then be delivered by the mother pushing out the placenta with the aid of gravity ('maternal effort') or by the staff pushing ('fundal pressure') or by pulling on the cord ('controlled cord traction'). Manual removal of the placenta under general anaesthetic is necessitated if the placenta or fragments of it are retained in the uterus, as the uterus will then be unable to contract properly, possibly resulting in postpartum haemorrhage (Clayton et al., 1975; Inch, 1982).

Active management of the third stage

With the isolation of ergometrine as the active principle of ergot in 1935, oxytocic drugs were introduced into obstetrics for the treatment and control of postpartum haemorrhage, previously a major cause of maternal mortality and morbidity (Inch, 1982). The administration of first ergometrine and then, in the 1950s, Syntometrine (a combination of 0.5 mg Ergometrine and 5 units of Syntocinon) for prophylactic purposes became common practice in the United Kingdom, although other oxytocic drugs are used in different countries (Elbourne et al., 1988). The routine administration of Syntometrine with the birth of the anterior shoulder in association with early cord clamping and cord traction is standard policy in nearly every maternity unit in the country (see the results of a survey of policies for the care of low risk women in maternity units cited by Prendiville et al., 1988). In practice, there may be variations in the management of the third stage, such as in the timing of the injection of syntometrine, or when the woman requests a natural childbirth.

Whilst the therapeutic value of oxytocic preparations in the control of postpartum haemorrhage has been widely acknowledged and praised, the preventative value of such preparations has been questioned by a minority which includes doctors (see Dunn, 1985, cited by Prendiville et al., 1988), midwives (see Inch, 1982; Ward, 1983) and women (e.g. Stewart, 1982). Ergometrine in particular, especially when given intravenously, can have severe side effects, most notably causing a sharp rise in blood pressure, but also resulting in headaches, dizziness, nausea and vomiting and an increased incidence of retained placentas. Inch (1985) has argued that routine management of the third stage with oxytocics results in a 'cascade of intervention' i.e. early clamping and cord traction with negative consequences for both the mother and baby.

In a thorough review of thc research, Inch concludes that the existing evidence throws doubt on the scientific basis for the routine management of the third stage with oxytocics. Prendiville et al. (1988) analysed data derived from nine published reports of randomized controlled trials of routine oxytocics. They concluded that the use of routine oxytocics significantly reduces the risk of postpartum haemorrhage by about 40 per cent. However, other aspects of third stage management (position of mother, early cord clamping and controlled cord traction) were not recorded in the trials and Prendiville et al. point out that such aspects 'may predispose to the problems which routine oxytocic administration would otherwise prevent' (p. 14).

In a further analysis on the benefits and disadvantages of different oxytocic preparations, Elbourne et al. (1988) concluded that Syntometrine appeared to be the safest and most effective preparation but that the quality of the data was poor.

Information about what is involved in the third stage of labour tends not to be readily available to the pregnant woman. Very little space, if any, is allocated to discussion of the third stage in most of the books and pamphlets aimed at educating and informing the pregnant woman, although much attention has been paid to other aspects of labour such as the advantages and disadvantages of the various forms of pain relief, and interventions such as induction. For example, the generally informative and well thought out Open University/Health Education Book 'Understanding Pregnancy and Birth' describes the delivery of the placenta and what the placenta is. However, it says absolutely nothing about the drug syntometrine which is routinely used throughout Britain to hasten the delivery of the placenta and to control bleeding. The word 'syntometrine' does not even appear in the index of the book yet it is probably the most common intervention of them all. The only aspect of third stage management that the book does mention is clamping and cutting the cord, which for some reason appears under the sub-heading 'The Second Stage': 'The midwife may clamp and cut the umbilical cord immediately or wait until blood stops pulsating through the cord from the placenta'.

Other books aimed at pregnant women do devote more room to discussion of the third stage (see Bourne, 1975; Huntingford, 1985; Kitzinger, 1983, 1987; and Inch's excellent book (1982) which explores the whole issue of the third stage and its management in depth). However, these books are probably only read by a minority of motivated women who are likely to be already relatively well-informed and who are aware that the issue, and options around it, exists. The material which is most likely to reach the least informed people, i.e. is provided free at antenatal clinics, does not provide this information. It is actually possible to go through the entire pregnancy, attend antenatal appointments and give birth and still be unaware i) that there is a third stage, i.e. that anything else happens after the delivery of the baby, and ii) that it is routinely managed by the midwifery staff. (In fact, 13 of the multips in our study did say they knew 'nothing' about the third stage, as did 9 primips, and 33% of multips only knew 'very little'.) This state of general ignorance is in sharp contrast to knowledge about the first and second stages, especially about 'minor' interventions and pain relief. (For example, only one per cent of multips said they did not know enough to make a choice about fetal heart monitoring, four per cent did not know enough to make a choice about Pethidine and six per cent did not know enough to make a choice about epidurals. However, ignorance about 'major' interventions was as widespread among multips as about the third stage.)

One section of the main antenatal questionnaire was designed to discover what women knew about the third stage of labour and how they felt about routine management. Postnatally, we looked at whether women got what they said they wanted regarding the third stage and at how women remained unaware of the routines of third stage labour. We hypothesized that, antenatally, relatively few women are aware of the options for third stage of labour. Also a significant proportion of women do not realize that the third stage is routinely managed with an injection of Syntometrine followed by cord clamping and controlled cord traction. Furthermore, we hypothesized that some women are unaware that the delivery of the placenta follows the birth of the baby.

Third stage of labour: antenatal results

How much knowledge do women have?

We defined the third stage as 'The time between the delivery of the baby and the completion of delivery of the afterbirth (the placenta)'. We did not give any information about how the third stage is normally managed. In the pilot version of the questionnaire we had included specific questions about whether women wanted an injection of Syntometrine, when the cord should be clamped and about controlled cord traction. We abandoned these questions in the main survey in favour of a much vaguer format (see Appendix A4), partly for ethical reasons (women might be frightened by references to syntometrine and its use to stop uncontrolled postpartum bleeding) and partly to avoid any possibility of leading questions. Thus we first asked women 'How much do you know about how the third stage of labour is managed?'.

Over half the sample (53%) felt they knew 'quite a bit' and 11 per cent said they knew 'a great deal'. This leaves a third (33%) who only knew 'very little' and three per cent who felt they knew 'nothing'. It is probably fair to say that many of the women who said they knew quite a bit or a great deal were, in reality, not nearly so well-informed as they believed, as we shall see overleaf.

Parity, education and knowledge of the third stage

Multips were nearly twice as likely as primips to say that they knew 'a great deal' (13% compared to 8%). An equal proportion of primips and multips said that they knew 'nothing' or 'very little' (35–36%). However, the relationship between parity and perceived knowledge did not reach significance ($p = 0.06$). Perceived knowledge of the third stage and women's educational level were significantly related.

Educational level	Know nothing		Know very little		Know quite a bit		Know great deal	
	n	%	n	%	n	%	n	%
16 and under	14	(4)	145	(39)	180	(47)	31	(8)
17–18	4	(2)	61	(29)	119	(56)	28	(13)
19 and over	2	(1)	35	(22)	99	(62)	24	(15)

Percentages are of women of a given educational level.

$p < 0.0001$

Table 6.1: Knowledge of the third stage of labour by education

Women who left full-time education at 19 years or older were twice as likely to say they knew 'a great deal' as women who left at 16 years or younger (15% compared to 8%). Conversely the least educated women were twice as likely to say that they knew 'nothing' or only a 'very little': 43 per cent compared to 23 per cent of the most highly educated women.

This association between knowledge and education is to be expected. Educated women are probably more likely to read about or to discuss issues with staff than less educated women who may more often feel intimidated by staff (Hubert, 1974). Staff may make more effort to explain and discuss issues with educated women, believing they are more rational and able to understand. Or, quite simply, educated women may be more likely to perceive themselves as knowledgeable regardless of 'actual' knowledge.

There is also a highly significant association between perceived knowledge of the third stage and social class as defined by the woman's best ever job, but no significant relationship with partner's occupation.

Discussion of the third stage with the staff

We then asked women whether a doctor or midwife had discussed the management of the third stage with them. Only 23 per cent said yes and a further 15 per cent had discussed it during a previous pregnancy but not during this one. Three per cent were not sure, which leaves over half of the sample (59%) who had never discussed the third stage with a doctor or midwife. Thus, it seems that the majority of women do not get information about the third stage from staff and have no opportunity to discuss it. It would appear that professionals do not believe women need to be well-informed about the third stage. This may be because they accept the management of the third stage as commonplace and/or just noncontroversial.

Parity, education and discussion with staff

There was a highly significant relationship ($p < 0.0001$) between parity and whether women had discussed the third stage with staff. Twenty four per cent of multips had discussed the third stage with staff in a previous pregnancy, but primips were much more likely to have discussed it with staff in this pregnancy (46% compared to 8% of multips). Staff may assume that multips already know a lot about the third stage, although, as we have seen, this is not necessarily true. Half the primips (49%) and 65 per cent of the multips had never discussed the third stage of labour with staff.

We expected to find that well-educated women would be the most likely to have discussed the third stage with staff. However, although there was a relationship between educational level and discussion with staff in the expected direction, it was not statistically significant.

Decision making in the third stage

Women were asked:

> Are you happy to leave matters to staff once the baby is actually born, or do you wish to make the decisions yourself about how the third stage of labour is managed?
>
> I will leave it totally up to the staff to make the right decision
>
> I would like the staff to advise me and I will probably take their advice
>
> I would like the staff to advise me but I will still make up my own mind even if my decision is different from their advice
>
> Other – please say what

Most women were happy to leave the decisions to the staff (29%) or were predisposed to take the staff's advice (56%). Only 14 per cent were inclined to assert their own wishes, but, as we shall see, only 13 per cent had any views to express.

Views on third stage decision making were significantly related to parity ($p = 0.001$). Interestingly, it was primips who were more likely to say they would make up their own mind whatever the staff said. The women who had already been through childbirth were more likely to say they would depend on the staff.

	Parity			
	Primips		Multips	
	n	%	n	%
Totally depend on staff	60	(21)	154	(34)
Take staff's advice	181	(62)	236	(53)
Still make up own mind	51	(18)	54	(12)
Other	0	(0)	4	(<1)

Percentages are of women of a given parity.

p < 0.001

Table 6.2: Decision-making in the third stage by parity

Decision making by education

Once again we see a significant relationship with education ($p < 0.001$) with the least educated women being more likely to leave decisions entirely up to staff (33% compared to 17% of the most educated group). Conversely, 22 per cent of the highly educated women would assert their own wishes compared to only 11 per cent of the least educated.

Decision making was also significantly related to woman's best ever job ($p < 0.0001$) in the expected direction.

Expressed wishes about the third stage

Women were asked 'Do you have any particular feelings or wishes about what you do and don't want to happen in the third stage?' and, if so, what these wishes were. We were especially interested in discovering how knowledgeable women were about third stage management, and having already asked them directly how much they knew, these questions were, in part, included to test their perceived knowledge. The question was designed so that women could interpret it in whatever way seemed most meaningful to them. We would thus pick up all those who had strong views on the medical management of the third stage (whether for or against) as well as misconceptions about what the third stage involves.

Only 13 per cent of the sample (n = 99) said that they did have particular wishes for the third stage. Two thirds (64%) said that they had no wishes and 22 per cent said that they were not sure or did not know enough about it.

It is important to bear in mind throughout the following cross-tabulations that the results refer to a small minority (13%) of women who did have specific wishes for the third stage.

Parity, education and expressed wishes

Parity was significantly related to whether women had any particular wishes for the third stage ($p < 0.01$). Primips were less likely than multips to say they had no particular wish concerning the third stage, and more likely to be undecided. There was, however, no effect of parity among women who did specify a wish.

There was a highly significant relationship ($p < 0.001$) between women's educational level and the specification of wishes about the third stage. Educated women were much more likely to express a wish: 27 per cent of women who left full-time education at 19 years or older, compared to 14 per cent who left at 17 or 18 years, and 7 per cent at 16 years or younger.

	Had particular wish(es)?					
Educational level	Yes, wishes		No, wishes		Don't know	
	n	%	n	%	n	%
16 and under	27	(7)	245	(66)	97	(26)
17–18	29	(14)	138	(65)	45	(21)
19 and over	43	(27)	94	(60)	21	(13)

Percentages are of women of a given educational level.

$p < 0.001$

Table 6.3: Expressed wishes about the third stage by education

A similar pattern was evident between third stage wishes and women's own best ever occupation ($p < 0.001$) and partner's occupation ($p < 0.001$).

Perceived knowledge and expressed wishes

Expressing particular wishes for the third stage was also, as one might expect, related to the amount that women said that they knew about the third stage. Over half of the less well-informed women answered 'Don't know' to the question about specific wishes. However, it was still only a fifth of the more knowledgeable women who expressed particular wishes (compared to 4% of less well-informed women).

Perceived knowledge	Yes, wishes		No, wishes		Don't know	
	n	%	n	%	n	%
Know nothing	2	(9)	7	(32)	13	(59)
Very little	8	(3)	104	(43)	129	(54)
Quite a bit	70	(18)	305	(77)	22	(6)
A great deal	18	(22)	63	(76)	2	(2)

Percentages are of women in a given row.

$p < 0.0001$

Table 6.4: Expressed wishes about the third stage by perceived knowledge

There was also a significant relationship ($p < 0.0001$) between expressed wishes and discussion of the third stage with staff. Over half of those who had not discussed the third stage said they did not have any wish and another third were unsure – it seems that for these women there was no basis on which to make a decision. Women who had talked about the third stage with staff were more likely to express a particular wish.

What were women's feelings/wishes about the third stage?

Table 6.5 shows post-hoc categorizations of the third stage wishes which were expressed. Up to three responses were recorded for each women, giving a total of 146 different responses from 95 women (13%) of the total sample).

	n	% of women stated a wish (n = 95)	% of total sample (n = 751)
Response: stated wish for third stage			
A. Natural third stage	29	(31)	(4)
B. Delay cord cutting till no pulsation	16	(17)	(2)
C. Delay syntometrine	5	(5)	(<1)
D. Delay cord cutting (no mention of pulsation)	10	(11)	(1)
E. Placental comments and stories	6	(6)	(1)
F. Contact with baby/peaceful atmosphere	43	(45)	(6)
G. Involvement of husband/partner	5	(5)	(1)
H. Medically managed third stage	7	(7)	(1)
J. Stitches	3	(3)	(1)
K. Other	22	(23)	(3)

Table 6.5: Feelings about/wishes for the third stage

We can see that within the small proportion of women who did specify a particular wish concerning the third stage, just under half of their comments concerned its management (medical or physiological, see responses A, B, C, D and H in Table 6.5). Over a third (41%) of the wishes were for a natural third stage, specifically no syntometrine, and/or delayed cord clamping and cutting:

> 'I want to be able to sit quietly with my baby whilst still attached to the placenta. I would like the placenta to be delivered without injection if possible, but I have no real objection to the injection if it is necessary.'

> 'I do not want an injection automatically to hurry up the placenta removal. I do not want the cord cut automatically. I would use acupuncture as a first choice to hurry the process up if there is a problem.'

(This woman had discussed third stage with the staff, the previous one had not.)

Several women made it clear that they had thought out carefully the procedure they wanted and had taken into account potential problems:

> 'I would like things taken as slowly as possible. Assuming there are no complications (i.e. cord damaged/twisted; baby not breathing at all), I would prefer the cord was left attached until it stops pulsating. (See Leboyer *Birth without Violence*)'.

Five women said that they would accept a compromise of delaying the injection of syntometrine until after the baby was born:

> 'I'd rather not have syntometrine but I've struck a compromise – the midwife will delay clamping and cutting the cord till it's stopped pulsating and baby is at the breast, then she'll give the syntometrine if that's how she feels happiest.'

Nearly a third of the comments (30%) concerned either the desire to have contact with the baby as soon as possible (e.g. for the baby to be delivered onto the stomach) or the desire for a peaceful atmosphere:

> 'I want the baby to be handed to me immediately and to be left to discover its sex for myself. Otherwise I don't have any particular wishes.'

> 'I would like to hold and breastfeed my baby right away.'

The category 'placental comments' included several women anxious about the delivery of the placenta, often as a result of a previous bad experience:

> 'I want to make sure that the placenta has been properly removed this time.'

> 'I had trouble with the afterbirth with the first child – would not like to have to go to be operated on for it to be removed.'

One woman wrote about a very unhappy experience of a late abortion of a handicapped baby:

> 'I would like, if possible, for the afterbirth to be delivered naturally. When having Sam a particular doctor decided to deliver it manually. He failed to get it out in one go and therefore "lost" part of the cord. This resulted in me haemorrhaging and needing an ERPC. The stupid thing was my body delivered the remainder of the placenta several minutes later.'

She said no-one had discussed the third stage with her, although she was very happy with the way the hospital had helped her deal with the traumatic abortion. (Although only six women wrote about feelings and past experiences regarding the delivery of the placenta in response to this question, others described their own experiences at other points during the antenatal and postnatal questionnaires.)

Seven women specified that they wanted medical management and explained they thought it was too risky to do otherwise:

> 'I would hope to have an injection because I think this reduces the risk of parts of the placenta remaining and therefore reducing risk of infection.'

Five women requested the involvement of their partner in the third stage:

> 'I want the cord to stop pulsating before it is cut – and by my husband – and therefore to allow the baby to breathe first... and my husband to bath the baby.'

Three women expressed anxiety about stitches, although suturing would not normally be seen as part of the third stage as defined at the beginning of this section.

Finally, there is a larger 'ragbag' category of comments that did not fit into the previous groups. One woman simply remarked:

> 'I do not want to see it!'

Presumably she meant the placenta, not the baby. There were several women who seemed rather confused about the third stage, although both women quoted below said they knew 'quite a bit' about it.

> 'Yes, there is one particular wish about my third stage of labour and that is that I have a normal delivery, everything to go smoothly and to use as little pethidine as possible (I don't want an epidural).'

> 'I feel I need advice about methods/positions in how to give birth but may not want to be tied to any one position until the time comes.'

One woman summed up her attitude which is probably representative of that of many other women and also of many staff:

> 'I have understood that the delivery of the placenta (third stage) was relatively uncontroversial and apart from deciding whether to see the placenta or not, there wasn't much to it.'

Hospital policy

Given that over a third of the sample knew 'very little' or 'nothing' about the third stage and that over half had not discussed it with the staff, we expected that many women would not be aware of the routines of third stage management even after the event. Secondly, we did not expect more than a small minority of women to have strong feelings on the subject as a result both of lack of awareness of the procedures antenatally and lack of awareness of them *as* they are being performed. Indeed, women's responses to the questions about the third stage of labour were often confused. As we shall see, sixteen per cent of the sample were unsure whether they had had an injection of syntometrine and even some of those who thought that they were sure, later made comments which cast some doubt on this. As the data on the third stage of labour seemed so confused and therefore unreliable, we asked each unit to clarify its policy on the following:

a) Is syntometrine given routinely? Under what circumstances would it not be given? When is it administered? (e.g. with the anterior shoulder, crowning or after delivery, etc.)
b) What is the policy as regards controlled cord traction? Is CCT routine even if syntometrine is not administered?
c) What is the policy as regards cutting and clamping the cord? (e.g. before/after pulsation ceases)
d) Are babies routinely aspirated? If not, under what circumstances would they be aspirated?

The hospitals responses are recorded in Table 6.6.

Willowford is the only unit in our study where syntometrine is *not* administered routinely to manage the third stage of labour. As described in the introduction, it is extremely unusual for maternity units not to administer oxytocics routinely in the third stage, and Willowford may possibly be the only unit in the country which does not adopt such a policy. Nevertheless, it is still a minority of women who do not receive syntometrine at Willowford (personal communication). At all the other five units syntometrine is routine, excepting certain situations, usually when the woman actively objects.

In five units, controlled cord traction is routine if syntometrine has been administered. In Exington GP unit, it depends on the situation. When the cord is clamped and cut is more variable – only in Exington consultant unit was it specified that the policy is to clamp and cut the cord before pulsation has stopped (see Inch, 1985, for a discussion on advantages and disadvantages of different times of clamping and cutting). Babies were not routinely aspirated in any of the units.

The third stage of labour: postnatal results

Perception of receiving an injection (of syntometrine)

Women who had a caesarean section or forceps delivery under general anaesthetic were not included in this section. We asked women: 'Did you have an injection as the baby was born (to speed up the third stage and stop bleeding)?'. (A few women said they had received the injection *after* the baby was born. This may also have been true for other women who did not volunteer the information.) We did not specify an injection of syntometrine as we thought it unlikely that many women would have heard of syntometrine and also we wished to allow for the possibility of other ocytocic drugs being used on occasion. However, we do sometimes ourselves refer to syntometrine in the following account as it was the preparation of choice in all the units studied. Fifty five per cent of the sample said that they had had an injection, 29 per cent said that they had not and 16 per cent were unsure (total n = 638).

Hospital	Policy as regards Syntometrine	Policy as regards cutting and clamping of cord	Policy as regards controlled cord traction	Policy as regards aspiration of baby
Willowford	Not routine. Not given at woman's request, or in natural labours where there has been no intervention, or in very fast labours. Given with the anterior shoulder, or after delivery if the midwife is on her own.	Depends on woman's request and if Syntometrine was given.	Only if Syntometrine is given. Otherwise maternal effort to deliver the placenta.	Not routine. Only if much mucus or if meconium is present.
Wychester	Routine. Not given at woman's request or if medically contraindicated. May not be given if woman is on a syntocinon drip. Given with the anterior shoulder.	Cord cut and clamped after baby is placed on mother's stomach and covered with a warm towel. The cord has normally stopped pulsating.	Routine, unless Syntometrine not given. However, is at the midwife's discretion.	Not routine. Only if much mucus or meconium present.
Exington consultant unit	Routine, except for medical contraindications or after oxytocin infusion. Given with anterior shoulder.	The cord is cut and clamped before pulsation ceases.	Routine, unless no oxytocin of any kind has been given.	Not routine.
Exington GP unit	Routine. Not given 'if the mother refuses'.	No written policy – very variable	No written policy, depends on situation.	Not routine
Little Exington	Routine. Not given 'at patient's request and after counselling patient'. Given with anterior shoulder or after delivery. Very unusual not to be given.	Varies with midwife and the woman's request, type of delivery and condition of baby.		Not routine. Only if meconium present or low Apgar score.
Zedbury	Routine. Not given at woman's request or if medically contraindicated. Given with the anterior shoulder.	Cutting and clamping of the cord occurs after pulsation has stopped.	Routine, unless Syntometrine is not given.	Not routine.

Table 6.6: Hospital policy on third stage of labour

Thus, only just over half of the sample thought that they had had syntometrine when it is likely that a much higher proportion in reality received the injection as it is routine in all but one of our hospitals. In a small number of cases confusion may have been caused by our explanation that the injection was 'to speed up the third stage and stop bleeding', while not mentioning the placenta. One woman denied having such an injection but later said:

> 'The only injection I can remember was to help the placenta/or afterbirth be removed after the birth of my son.'

Our assumption is that women have under-reported the management of the third stage and that the figures presented are not accurate but represent women's perceptions rather than the actual state of affairs. This assumption will be tested in a further piece of analysis with data taken from the hospital records.

Hospital unit and perception of injection

Perception of receiving an injection is related to hospital unit.

	Yes		No		Unsure	
	n	%	n	%	n	%
Willowford	85	(54)	59	(37)	15	(9)
Exington Consultant	36	(46)	23	(29)	20	(25)
Exington GP	25	(49)	18	(35)	8	(16)
Little Exington	28	(64)	7	(16)	9	(21)
Wychester	91	(59)	33	(21)	31	(20)
Zedbury	73	(55)	41	(31)	20	(15)

Percentages are of women in a given unit.

$P < 0.05$

Table 6.7: Perception of receiving syntometrine by hospital unit

The figures given above would seem to confirm the hypothesis that women's perception of the administration of syntometrine differs markedly from the actual course of events. The highest percentage of women saying they had been given an injection gave birth in Little Exington where there are no sophisticated emergency facilities on hand. However, the smallest percentages of women replying 'yes' gave birth in the Exington consultant and GP units, where policy on management of the third stage is also strict (see Table 6.6). Women at Exington consultant unit were the most likely to be 'unsure', suggesting that the figures from there are the least accurate. However, in all the units, except Willowford, between 15 per cent and 25 per cent of women were 'unsure' of what happened. This suggests that many women are not informed about how the third stage is usually managed in hospitals, and further that the injection of syntometrine is being given without their knowledge or informed consent. The lack of communication between staff and women about the injection of syntometrine was quite apparent. For example, one woman commented:

> 'Although I know I had an injection for the third stage the only reason is that I was expecting it and my husband told me they gave me it.'

Others reported:

> 'There was a needle given to me in the top of the thigh – nothing was mentioned before or after it was given.'

> 'They did it without even telling me until I had the needle in my thigh.'

> 'No mention was made of an injection at this stage as far as I can recollect.'

Lack of communication may have even more significance in emergency situations:

> 'I had to have an injection of something as I lost a lot of blood. Everything happened so quickly, doctors rushing about, but nobody really told me what was going on and that scared me.'

The much smaller percentage of women who were 'unsure' at Willowford seems to indicate superior communication and sharing of information about this issue there. However, staff at Willowford were by no means exempt from criticism about how they managed the third stage:

> 'I was just given the injection while [baby] was being seen to. I don't know what I was being given or why... they stuck it in before I even knew it was coming.'

Parity, education and social class

There was no significant difference related to parity in the numbers of women who said that they received an injection (60% of primips compared to 51% of multips).

Educational level, though, was strongly related to the women's perception of receiving syntometrine. The most educated women were the most likely to say they had had an injection, and the least educated where the most likely to feel sure they had not. A higher percentage of the two least educated groups were also more likely to be unsure. Since the chances of receiving and being physically aware of the injection are probably about the same for all women (other things being equal), we would hypothesize that these differences may arise from the fact that well educated women are more likely to know that the injection is normal practice (see antenatal results). It may also be that staff are less likely to explain things to the less educated women.

Educational level	Yes		No		Unsure	
	n	%	n	%	n	%
16 and under	149	(48)	99	(32)	60	(20)
17–18	101	(56)	52	(29)	28	(16)
19 and over	99	(68)	31	(21)	15	(10)
Total	349	(55)	182	(29)	103	(16)

Percentages are of women of a given level of education.

$p < 0.01$

Table 6.8: Perception of receiving syntometrine by educational level

Social class (as represented by women's best ever occupation) was also very strongly related to perception of administration of syntometrine, as would be expected from the relationship with education ($p < 0.0001$).

Reasons for women's uncertainty

Women who said they were 'unsure' about having had an injection of syntometrine were asked: 'What do you think are the reason(s) for your uncertainty about whether or not you had an injection in the third stage?'.

One hundred and five women were eligible to respond to this question. Out of this, 102 did so, with 17 women giving two reasons for their uncertainty. Their responses are shown below (pre-coded statements had been derived from pilot questionnaires).

A	The staff made the decision and didn't tell me what it was	9	(9%)
B	I was confused as such a lot of things were happening all at the same time	20	(20%)
C	I was in a lot of pain at the time and didn't notice what was happening	19	(19%)
D	I was very involved with my newborn baby and didn't notice what was happening	40	(39%)
E	I was still affected by the drug(s) I'd had so I didn't notice, or feel an injection	17	(17%)
F	I was not aware that anything else might happen after the birth of the baby, so I didn't notice	8	(8%)
G	Other, please say what:	6	(6%)

n = 102

- Numbers/percentages are of women giving each reason. Percentages add up to more than 100 per cent because 17 women gave two reasons.

Table 6.9: Reasons for uncertainty about having had an injection

Obviously, several of these reasons, which are themselves interrelated, might explain why any one woman could be unsure about having received syntometrine. However, they were not explicitly told they could tick more than one category, and only a minority did so. The most commonly given reason was the arrival of the baby involving and distracting the woman to the exclusion of all the events going on around her. Nevertheless, the general confusion and disorientation (reasons B, C and E) and complete lack of knowledge (as indicated by reasons A and F) on the part of a sizeable minority of women, is also evident.

The 'other' category, while only ticked by six per cent of responders, is interesting in that women explained in their own words why they did not know if they received an injection in the third stage. Several women explained that the staff had broached the subject but that they cannot now remember.

> 'I was being talked to throughout all stages however I can't really remember the details now.'

> 'The midwife suggested the injection, and I asked her to wait to see how things went without it, but neither my husband nor I remember whether I got the injection in fact.'

Another woman could not tell what was happening because of the effect of her episiotomy:

> 'Hospital practice is to inject as the baby is delivered (so I was told beforehand) so, as I had had an episiotomy, I wasn't aware of anything else much down there. (My husband tells me that I *did* have the injection).'

Several women said they were totally exhausted after the birth and did not take in what was going on:

> 'I was too exhausted and was relieved to lie down relaxed and wait to be stitched up.' (also ticked E and F)

> 'Totally exhausted, so half asleep.' (also ticked B, C, E and F)

Ninety four women answered the question on what they thought accounted for their uncertainty in having had syntometrine despite the fact that they were ineligible to do so. Two thirds of them had previously said that they had received an injection of syntometrine while one third had said they had not. The responses they gave are shown overleaf:

A	The staff made the decision and didn't tell me what it was	16	(17%)
B	I was confused as such a lot of things were happening all at the same time	7	(7%)
C	I was in a lot of pain at the time and didn't notice what was happening	8	(9%)
D	I was very involved with my newborn baby and I didn't notice what was happening	36	(38%)
E	I was still affected by the drug(s) I'd had so I didn't notice, or feel an injection	14	(15%)
F	I was not aware that anything else might happen after the birth of the baby, so I didn't notice	12	(13%)
G	Other, please say what:	4	(4%)

n = 94

- Numbers/percentages are of women giving each reason. Percentages add up to more than 100 per cent because three women gave two reasons.

Table 6.10: Reasons for uncertainty about having had an injection: 'ineligible' women

These women (18% of all the women who said 'yes' or 'no' to having had an injection) may be indicating that there is, after all, some doubt in their minds. However, it should be remembered that their knowledge of whether or not they had the injection need not have come from their own direct perception. As we saw above, for example, they may know because the staff or their partner told them about the injection afterwards. Their answers are not, therefore, necessarily contradictory. Whatever the degree of their uncertainty now, their identification with the options given is a valid statement about factors which mitigated against them knowing whether or not they had had an injection. The particular reasons given indicate a lack of information about third stage rather than confusion about events at the time.

Decision making

We asked women who had answered 'yes' or 'no' to the injection question how the decision had been made. The responses are shown below:

	n	%
The staff were insistent that I take their advice and I didn't feel that I could refuse	6	(1)
I was happy to follow the staff's advice on the matter	134	(26)
I made my own decision with the staff's approval	28	(5)
I made my own decision against the staff's advice	0	(0)
It all just happened and so there wasn't a decision made as such	311	(61)
Other (please say what)	35	(7)
Total	514	(100)

Table 6.11: How decisions about the third stage were made

Nearly two thirds of the women said a decision as such had not been made (or at least not one which involved negotiation beforehand with them). Instead, everything 'just happened' at the time. This goes some way towards explaining why 18 per cent of this group of women may have been in doubt about whether they had had an injection or not. Another quarter of this group were happy to follow the staff's advice, i.e. to leave the decision about the third stage procedures up to them. Only five per cent reported that the decision had been their own. This compares to 14 per cent of the sample at the stage of the second antenatal questionnaire who had said that while they would take into account the staff's advice, they would still want to make their own decision even if it differed from that advice. A few women explained that the situation had been discussed with them antenatally, and that a plan for the management of the third stage had been made at that time:

> 'I had discussed the matter fully with the GP and midwife in advance. It was decided that since I had no strong feelings either way, we would leave it to the midwife, depending on circumstances. This decision was confirmed when the birth was imminent.'

> 'I bled badly after my previous two babies, so it was decided beforehand to have the injection to prevent this.'

(Both these women gave birth at Wychester.)

However, more typically, women just went along with whatever happened at the time, in which case they ticked '...there wasn't a decision made as such', or if they were aware of what the midwife was doing and there had been some communication on the issue, 'I was happy to follow the staff's advice'.

Several women who gave birth at Willowford where syntometrine is not administered routinely gave examples of how the third stage had been managed according to their personal circumstances:

> 'Everything was normal and the midwife felt that nature was doing its job.'

> 'My midwife gave me the injection 20 minutes after my daughter was born as she and I hoped I would not need it. But as I lost a bit of blood I think it worried my midwife and she decided on the injection. I was happy to follow her decision.'

However, another woman at Willowford said:

> 'The staff told me what they were going to do and I accepted it. I wasn't asked if I wanted the injection.'

It seems clear from the way women described what had happened in the third stage that a lot depends not only on hospital policy, but also on what one hospital described in their policy statement (see Table 6.6) as 'the midwives' discretion'. Thus, the midwife may or may not discuss the management of the placenta with the woman, she may or may not favour waiting to see if the placenta delivers naturally, she may go by the woman's own wishes or follow her own routines.

Unit differences

The most notable difference between the hospital units in how the decision was made is that women were more likely to make the decision themselves at Willowford: 17 out of the 28 women who decided for themselves about the administration of syntometrine gave birth at Willowford. No woman who gave birth at the Exington GP unit or Little Exington made the decision and women at these units were the most likely to say 'it all just happened'.

Education and social class differences

Women's educational level was related to how the decision about the injection was made ($p = 0.05$). Twelve per cent of those who left school after the age of 18 years made the decision themselves compared to four per cent of the intermediate group and three per cent of the least educated group. Correspondingly, the more educated women were least likely to say 'it all just happened'. Women's social class was also related to how the decision was made but the relationship is not linear and no clear pattern is discernable. Parity was not related to the decision making process.

Feelings about what happened

Women were asked six weeks retrospectively 'How did you feel about having had, or not having had, the injection?'.

	n	%
I was very pleased about it	151	(29)
I was fairly happy about it	66	(13)
I was quite unhappy about it	8	(2)
I was very unhappy about it	2	(1)
I had no particular feelings about it	278	(53)
Other (please say what)	22	(4)
Total	527	(100)

Table 6.12: Feelings about what happened re the injection

Over half of the women asked said that they had no particular feelings about the injection (or lack of it). This indifference is reflected in the lack of awareness that we have documented about the administration of syntometrine and the overwhelming lack of involvement on the part of women in decisions about the management of the third stage. Only ten women in the sample reported that they felt unhappy at all with what happened, and it is interesting that seven out of this ten gave birth at Willowford, where we found the greatest communication about the third stage between staff and labouring women.

In at least one of these cases the woman's unhappiness does not relate to the staff: she had not wanted the injection but asked for it after attempting to push the placenta out herself and not succeeding. She explained that her unhappiness was due to disappointment in having to have syntometrine after a drug free birth. Unit was not related to women's feelings about having or not having the injection, but it is interesting to note that women at Willowford had a tendency to express stronger feelings than other women and were the least likely to say they had no particular feelings (women at Little Exington were the least likely to say they were 'very pleased' and the most likely to have no particular feelings). Parity, education and woman's social class were not related to feelings about the injection.

We next looked to see if women's feelings varied according to their perceptions of having received an injection and found that indeed they did. The main differences were that women who said they had not received an injection were more likely to feel 'very pleased' than those who thought they had (38% compared to 24%), and less likely to say they were only 'fairly happy' (9% compared to 15%).

As the number of women who expressed any unhappiness is so small, conclusions regarding them cannot be drawn. Nevertheless, the words they used very clearly illustrate just how powerless and vulnerable they may feel:

> 'Under the circumstances I felt I was in no position to reject [it], as I had already been pumped full of every other drug available.'

However, other women who were not asked by staff if they wanted the injection were pleased that they had had it. For example:

> 'If I had been consulted I would have insisted on having the injection as I am certain it reduces the risk of haemorrhage. I know a member of the Radical Midwives Association who refused this drug and haemorrhaged (I know you can't draw conclusions from a sample of one...)'

The management of the cord and the placenta

All the women were then asked if the cord was clamped and cut before it finished pulsating and whether the placenta was delivered by controlled cord traction (explained by us as 'gently pulling on the cord'). Both these procedures are the usual practice in most British hospitals, particularly if an oxytocic drug has been administered, although there is variation, for example, in when the cord is clamped and cut. Table 6.6 shows the policy as regards these procedures in the study hospitals.

Clearly, the question of when the cord was cut is extremely specific and we did not expect to find that women were aware of the timing, or perhaps even aware of the cord at all. This is borne out by the results: 77 per cent were unsure when the cord was clamped and cut, 14 per cent said it was done before the cord had finished pulsating and 9 per cent said the cord had stopped pulsating.

However, women were more aware about the delivery of the placenta by controlled cord traction: 58 per cent asserted that it had occurred and 13 per cent that it had not. Nevertheless, this still leaves nearly a third of the women who did not know – despite the fact that a midwife pulling on the cord is something that one might well expect a woman to notice even though she has just given birth.

As information about management of the cord and delivery of the placenta is not recorded in the labour ward records, we were not able to check how accurate women were in their perceptions.

Perception of when the cord was clamped and cut varied by unit ($p = 0.05$) as did perception about controlled cord traction ($p < 0.001$). Women at Little Exington were the least likely to say the cord was clamped and cut before pulsation had ceased, and to say controlled cord traction had taken place. Women at Willowford were the most likely to be able to answer 'yes' or 'no' to these questions i.e. they were more sure about what happened one way or the other. Education was not significantly related to perception of when the cord was clamped and cut, although the least educated women were more unsure about it. Education and perception of cord traction having taken place were related ($p = 0.05$), with the most educated women being more sure about what happened.

Comments about the cord and delivery of the placenta

THE CORD

The vast majority of women did not make any further comment specifically about the cord. Several comments were made by women at Willowford regarding the husband taking part at this point of the birth. It seems that staff sometimes offer partners the opportunity to clamp and cut the cord at Willowford. The comments on this were generally favourable. One woman said humorously:

> 'They asked my husband if he would like to cut it, he refused – I'm glad he did, the thought of him wielding a pair of scissors would have had me on valium straight away.'

Other women explained the cord had been cut immediately because of complications, loosely describing the act as one of 'medical necessity' – for example, situations where the cord was round the baby's neck. Naturally, they appreciated the necessity of swift action. One woman said she had not known that the cord would pulsate anyway and it seems most likely that this is the case for many other women. Another woman who had strong wishes about clamping and cutting the cord was unhappy when the midwife did not observe these wishes:

> 'Midwife apologized for having done this against my wishes immediately she had done it – she said it came to her so automatically that she had forgotten my request.'

THE PLACENTA

However, although women said little about the cord, rather more was said about problems with the delivery of the placenta. Several women described it as the worst part of the whole birth (In answer to the question: What was the worst thing about the birth?)

> 'The pain, then when the placenta wouldn't release and the midwife was pushing and pulling.' (Willowford)

> 'When I couldn't stop bleeding and was taken down to the theatre for a D & C which showed nothing was wrong – it frightened me a bit.' (Willowford)

> 'Having the retained placenta. Not only was it most distressing but it was the worst thing I've ever experienced.'

(This woman gave birth at Little Exington but then had to be transferred to Exington consultant unit to have a manual removal of the placenta which obviously contributed to the unpleasantness of the situation.)

Other women described elsewhere in the questionnaire how unpleasant and painful it was when the placenta did not deliver easily:

> 'I was not very happy at all. They eventually manually removed it after much tugging.' (Willowford)

'[The third stage] along with the delivery of the baby was not at all pleasant. The placenta broke up as they tried to pull it out and so they were pummelling my stomach for ages to help get it all out.' (Willowford)

'Painful. The afterbirth wouldn't come away for some time. The midwife was rubbing my stomach which left bruises.' (Wychester)

Despite the fact that we were not selecting quotations by unit, it is noticeable that many of the most negative experiences were at Willowford, the only unit not to administer syntometrine routinely. One woman associated this directly with the third stage and postpartum problems she experienced:

'I was not given an injection for the third stage after the baby was born. At the time I didn't mind either way but I had excessive bleeding after the delivery of the placenta and had to have the injection anyway. The blood loss left me weak and anaemic and I feel I should have had the injection in the first place. I also had excessive bleeding during my first period after the birth and this could have been due to retained membranes because the placental delivery was not as efficient.'

Clearly, it is impossible to do more than draw attention to a possible association between placental problems and unit procedure since we have selected the quotes in a non-random fashion to illustrate certain observations we wish to make.

On a more positive note there were several comments from women in all units describing the delivery of the placenta as interesting and well managed:

'I wanted to see and know about the placenta so the midwife inspected it in front of us and told us all about it.' (Exington consultant unit)

'The midwife waited until the contraction expelled the placenta but then gently helped pull it out. Third stage lasted 8 minutes, placenta weighed 450 gms, the whole thing was managed very sympathetically, I was allowed to cut the cord myself after it had stopped pulsating.' (Willowford)

'Delivery of the placenta was fascinating and the midwife showed me all the bits – which side was attached and the membranes.' (Exington GP unit)

'Found it useful to see the placenta before it was removed.' (Little Exington)

'I think the third stage of labour is the most exciting.' (Willowford)

'It was interesting to see the placenta after it had done such an amazing function over the past nine months, keeping baby alive.' (Zedbury)

ASPIRATION OF THE BABY

Women were asked: 'Was the baby aspirated (mouth, throat and nasal passage gently sucked out to remove any liquid)?'

Fifty per cent of the sample (320 women) answered yes, 36 per cent (230 women) answered no and 14 per cent (88) women said they were not sure.

There were highly significant differences by hospital unit, in perception of whether babies were aspirated ($p < 0.0001$). The lowest figures were for Willowford (one third of babies) and the highest at Wychester (two thirds of babies). Women were most unsure of what had happened at Little Exington (21%) and Exington GP unit (18%). Wychester and Willowford had exactly the same policy regarding the aspiration of the baby (see Table 6.6).

Parity, educational level and woman's social class were not related to perception of aspiration of the baby.

Few women commented on aspiration – where they did so, it was usually to explain the necessity for it:

> 'Extremely happy [about aspiration]. I know of two babies who *nearly* died because they were not aspirated at birth, and one baby who did die.'

> 'I was happy about this as it was a necessity with me having genital herpes.'

Only half a dozen women voiced disquiet over aspiration. One said:

> 'I know they have to do this but I don't feel comfortable about how they do. I have mixed feelings.'

We looked to see how many of the mothers of babies who had been aspirated had reported that their child had had any problems at birth, to try and get an idea of whether there may have been a medical reason for this procedure. In fact, only 30 per cent of the babies who were aspirated were reported by their mothers to have had a problem at birth. (Seven per cent of babies who were not apparently aspirated also had at least one problem at birth.) Fifteen per cent of babies that were aspirated were also admitted to a special care baby unit (compared to 10% of those who were apparently not aspirated).

Postnatal wishes

Finally we asked women 'Was there anything in particular that you wanted immediately after delivery, such as having the baby delivered onto your stomach, putting your baby straight to the breast, or being left alone with your partner and child?'. This question was included to enable a check back to the same antenatal question which had asked women if they wanted anything specific to happen (or not happen) in the third stage. Fifty one per cent (328 women) said that they had had particular wishes, compared to 13 per cent (97 women) at the antenatal stage. This big difference is largely accounted for by the fact that we specified possibilities in the postnatal question (derived from the most common antenatal responses), whereas the antenatal equivalent was left open. Nineteen women specified two wishes.

	n	% of women who stated a wish (n = 328)	% of total sample (n = 710)
Any/all of the above (i.e. possibilities mentioned in the question)	29	(89)	(41)
Involvement of husband/partner	5	(2)	(1)
Placental comments	5	(2)	(1)
Natural third stage	2	(1)	(1)
Cup of tea/cigarette/gin and tonic etc.	18	(5)	(1)
Other	15	(5)	(2)

11 women did not specify their wishes

N.B. Numbers are of women giving each reason.

Table 6.13: Women's wishes for the third stage

A comparison of antenatal and postnatal wishes for what should happen in the third stage showed no consistency at all. Although, for example, 29 women said antenatally they would like a natural third stage (i.e. they did not want syntometrine) and others made specifications about the management of the cord, only one of these said postnatally that she had wanted a natural third stage. None of the seven women who said antenatally they wanted a medically managed third stage reiterated this postnatally. The only area of consistency was with respect to women who had said that they wanted contact with the baby: 91 per cent of these women confirmed postnatally that they had wanted this.

The majority of women (79%) who did specify postnatally that they had particular desires for the third stage, got what they wanted, while 19 per cent did not. The remaining eight women had specified two wishes and only one was realized. One woman who had wanted 'my baby immediately on my stomach, and I wanted to put her on my breast to feed' and did not get this, said: 'I was bloody annoyed at the staff for not doing this when I asked them to'. Several women said they had wanted contact with the baby immediately and were pleased to get this even though they had not expressed their desire:

> 'I was very pleased how they dealt with the third stage. I wanted all the things in the above question but I did not ask for them. So I was very pleased when I got them all, as I did not get all of them with my previous children.'

Other women said they had not been able to hold the baby immediately because it was cold or they were told the baby had to be kept warm:

> 'The baby was wrapped when I had wanted as much skin contact as possible but I understand it was important to keep the baby warm so this was necessary.' (Wychester)

> '[I wanted] the baby delivered onto my stomach and [to hold] her wet and naked body next to mine. [But] She was given to me wrapped in a blanket.' (Wychester)

> 'The reason the cord was clamped and cut early and that I could not have her on my stomach or at the breast straight away was that the room was too cold and she had to be wrapped up. We *were* left alone however.' (Exington consultant unit)

There was no relationship between postnatal desires for the third stage and either unit or parity. However, there were significant differences by education ($p < 0.0001$) with the most educated women being more likely to have specific wishes (62% compared to 42% of the least educated women). Woman's social class was also associated with wishes ($p < 0.05$).

Control over the staff and women's psychological outcome

There were several significant, though hardly surprising, relationships between certain aspects of the third stage and control over what the staff did. The less in control the women were, the more likely they were to be unsure about whether they had been given an injection ($p < 0.05$), and the more likely they were to say everything had 'just happened' instead of a decision being made ($p < 0.05$).

There was little relationship between any aspect of the third stage and the four psychological outcome variables. Women who thought they had not been given an injection were the most satisfied with birth ($p < 0.05$), and women who had particular wishes for the third stage which were realized were both more satisfied ($p < 0.0001$) and more likely to be fulfilled ($p < 0.05$).

Conclusion

Our hypothesis that a significant proportion of women do not realize that the third stage of labour is routinely managed by the staff is confirmed. A large minority of women knew very little or nothing about the third stage of labour, including many women who had given birth previously. Furthermore, the majority of the women had had no opportunity to discuss the third stage with health professionals during the antenatal period or in any previous pregnancy. These results would seem to confirm that staff accord a low priority to the concept of the third stage as a major part of the childbirth process which women need to be well-informed about. Women tended to be correspondingly confused or indifferent about the third stage, desiring little part in decision making and having few, if any, opinions about how it should be managed. They were particularly unclear about when the cord had been clamped and cut (i.e. before or after it had finished pulsating) and whether the placenta was delivered by controlled cord traction.

CHAPTER SEVEN

Suturing

The pain of suturing and postnatal problems

The pain of suturing

The whole process of suturing and the later consequences were discussed by women as a matter of great concern. Although often seen as a minor operation by staff, it is, as the discussion below will show, of major importance to women. The pain of suturing was a particular issue for two thirds of the sample.

One in three women experienced no pain at all during suturing but almost one in five experienced 'a lot of pain' during the procedure.

	n	%
Felt a lot of pain	88	(19)
Felt a bit of pain	227	(49)
Felt no pain at all	150	(32)
Total	465	(100)

Table 7.1: Pain during stitching

The NCT episiotomy study found similar rates: 40 per cent of women felt no pain at all during suturing and 23 per cent found it painful or very painful (Fox, 1979).

The high proportion of women experiencing pain seems surprising given the fact that 76 per cent of the women were given local anaesthesia for the procedure and a further seven per cent were already anaesthetized (e.g. with an epidural). In some cases, it was clear that staff were not waiting for the local anaesthetic to take effect. Some women said that the pain of suturing was worse than the pain of delivery:

> 'The anaesthetic was painful and pointless as it was not given time to work. The stitching was far more painful than the actual delivery.'

In fact, 12 per cent of the women who answered the question 'What would you say was the worst thing about the birth?' said that it was the suturing afterwards:

> 'Without doubt [the worst thing was] when they cut you and the stitches afterwards. I would rather give birth again than be cut and have the stitches – awful!'

> 'The pain of stitching was far more painful than the birth.'

Others felt that the suturing had spoilt their memories of the birth experience:

> 'The SHO who gave me my sutures was off-hand and sarcastic. After administering the lignocaine he asked if I could feel the needle prick, I said yes and he said "Oh well, just hang on to the gas and air!". After my delivery being handled so well by the midwife it was a shame for it to be spoilt by a half awake doctor who was more interested in talking to the auxiliary about the weather!'

It was not just the pain of being stitched that was the problem but, for instance, having the baby taken away:

> 'The worst thing was having to be stitched, because the baby was taken away during this period.'

Women also complained about the lack of information. Over a third did not know what degree of tear they had had and one woman commented:

> 'The nursing sister who was in charge at night and who stitched me up seemed loth to tell me how many stitches I had. I don't think knowing that was going to worry me after managing to give birth I was just interested to know as it is my body.'

Over and above this, however, the complaint that came up time and again was of the delay in being stitched. We do not have information on how long each woman waited to be sutured, but the NCT survey found that although 61 per cent of women were sutured within half an hour of delivery, 13 per cent had to wait for over an hour (Fox, 1979). A few women in our study mentioned a wait of up to two hours:

> 'The only thing wrong with the birth is that the doctor took more than one and half hours to turn up to stitch me up.'

Such delays mean that numbness from the actual delivery may have worn off and hence a local anaesthetic may be needed. In addition, delays could be anxiety producing and meant that women could not relax, put the birth behind them and focus on their new baby:

> 'I would rather had my stitches more or less straight away rather than waiting two hours because it was worrying me and I couldn't concentrate fully on the baby.'

When women were left up in stirrups the delay was particularly distressing:

> 'The stitches were humiliating because I had to wait a long time with my legs strapped up before they stitched me.'

Having the process of stitching interrupted also caused distress:

> 'The doctor started to stitch me and then had to leave and do an emergency caesarean and he returned later to finish stitching. I realize he had to go but it was horrible having to be put back in the stirrups and given more local anaesthetic and the whole thing started again.'

On the other hand, where women did receive prompt attention they were often very grateful:

> 'I think one of the nicest things was that the Doctor came into the delivery room and waited until after my baby was born, to see if I needed stitches. So it meant I was stitched straight away after the birth. When I had my little girl at Exington consultant unit I was left with my husband for two hours before someone came to stitch me.'

Postnatal problems with the stitches

Women were also asked an open-ended question as to whether they had experienced problems with the stitches in the postnatal period. Ninety nine women, 21 per cent of the women who were sutured, had problems later on. We coded a maximum of two problems for each woman.

	n	% of women who were sutured
Sore/stinging	43	(9)
Stitches gaping/came undone	24	(5)
Too tight	22	(5)
Infection	12	(3)
Stitches not dissolving	8	(2)
Had to be unstitched and redone	4	(1)
Other	13	(3)
n = 465		

Table 7.2: Type of problem with stitches

The most common complaint about the stitches was soreness and stinging. Five per cent of women had stitches that 'gaped' or came undone and another five per cent had stitches that were too tight:

> 'I only wish I'd had to have had no stitches or at least they weren't put in so tight then I wouldn't be having the problems I am now – so much for a sex life!'

Infection was also a problem for 12 women (3% of those who had stitches):

> 'I had my six-week check (at seven weeks) only to find I was septic inside. I feel I should have had a check earlier, perhaps a swab on leaving hospital. Intercourse is still off. First stitches then discharge now septic. I should have been checked earlier, and treated.'

Four women had to have their stitches taken out and redone. A few women had severe and/or multiple problems:

> 'Two days after, they started to make me swell and I had to be cut with scissors four times to release the blood pressure. Also one week later they came undone and left a gap about 2 cm long which became infected. I still haven't healed and am very sore. It's up to me if I need to be cut and stitched again.'

> 'I thought I must just be making a fuss as I was in agony with my stitches and I felt very weak and dizzy. It was only after speaking to other Mums and my community midwife (who was great) that I became aware that not everyone (in fact no-one else on my ward) had stitches and that I had lost a pint of blood.'

Some women, however, specifically praised the person who did their suturing. One woman, for instance, who complained about the way the midwife did the episiotomy ('hacking my tail end') was grateful to the doctor for the skill with which he repaired the damage:

> 'I would like to say also that the doctor (Registrar) who sutured me made a very good job as the bruising and swelling were quite bad, he did comment as to what the midwife had done.'

Another woman felt that the skill, care and consideration of the SHO actually resulted in an improvement:

> 'I feel he took time and care, as with my first baby after my episiotomy my vagina was I can only describe as 'lop sided'. Now after the SHO stitched me my 'shape' has returned to 'near normal' and is no longer uncomfortable.'

Postnatal problems with the stitches and parity

Multips and primips were equally likely to have some kind of problem with the stitches postnatally. However, interestingly, primips were more likely to complain of stitches being too tight (29% compared to 14% of multips), while multips complained of stitches being too loose (32% compared to 18% of primips).

Who sutured – and with what result?

It has been suggested that the pain of stitching and later problems may be related to who did the suturing. In particular, queries have been raised about the skill of medical students. As Flint writes:

> 'I often think of my 20 year old son when I see medical students suturing women... To my knowledge he has never sewn a button on... If he were a medical student, he could be sewing a woman's perineum – learning how to sew on the most sensitive part of a woman's anatomy!' (1986, p. 102)

Women themselves also suggested that it is preferable to be sutured by experienced staff (as opposed to medical students), or by midwives rather than doctors. One woman, for instance, who was sutured by a midwife without pain or problems, compared this to her previous experience:

> 'I felt very uncomfortable with my first child, and was stitched by a doctor.'

Researchers have also suggested that midwifery suturing may be associated with a lower infection rate and less pain (Greenshields, 1987) but there is little empirical evidence. We therefore analysed our data on stitching by who sutured. In the first place we found that, as expected, women who had episiotomies were more likely to be stitched by a doctor than women who had tears. Eighty two per cent of the women who had episiotomies were stitched by a doctor as opposed to 54 per cent of those who had tears only.

Who sutured?	Episiotomy		Tear	
	n	%	n	%
Doctor	152	(83)	133	(55)
Midwife	26	(14)	104	(43)
Medical student	5	(3)	6	(2)

Percentages are of women in a given column.

Table 7.3: Type of perineal damage by who sutured

Again, as expected, doctors were more likely to suture third degree tears. Women tended to be less likely to know what kind of tear they had if stitched by a doctor.

Who sutured?	Don't know		1st Degree		2nd Degree		3rd Degree	
	n	%	n	%	n	%	n	%
Doctor	63	(40)	47	(30)	39	(25)	7	(5)
Midwife	36	(33)	46	(43)	25	(23)	1	(<1)
Medical student	2	(27)	2	(29	3	(43)	0	(0)

Percentages are of women in a given row.

Table 7.4: Knowledge of type of tear by who sutured

Women who were sutured by doctors were more likely to have some kind of pain relief – 79 per cent were given local anaesthetic, 8 per cent were already anaesthetized and 2 per cent used gas and air. Only eight per cent had no pain relief at all. However, 19 per cent of those sutured by midwives had no pain relief at all. This finding probably reflects the fact that midwives were more likely to deliver women and do the suturing before the numbness in the perineum due to the birth had worn off.

There was no difference in the experience of pain of women stitched by a doctor or by a midwife. There were, however, differences in women's experience of later problems depending on who stitched them ($p < 0.05$). Twenty five per cent of those stitched by a doctor experienced postnatal problems as opposed to 13 per cent of those stitched by a midwife.

Women sutured by doctors (excluding medical students) were thus twice as likely to experience problems postnatally as those sutured by midwives. However, there is a debate about whether episiotomies or tears are more difficult to suture and which heal with least problems. To make sense of these figures it is therefore necessary to separate out the women who had episiotomies from those who had tears and re-examine the data.

Who sutured and with what result by episiotomies and tears

Once we controlled for the fact that doctors were more likely to suture episiotomies than tears, the differences disappeared. Women with episiotomies had an equal number of problems whether they were stitched by a midwife or a doctor. The women who had tears experienced, on the whole, fewer problems than those who had episiotomies. They were, however, slightly more likely to have problems with soreness and 'gaping' stitches if sutured by a doctor than if sutured by a midwife. This might be accounted for by the fact that doctors suture the more severe tears.

To further compare episiotomies and tears, analysis could be carried out comparing the problems experienced by women who had second degree tears because second degree tears involve the same tissue damage as episiotomies – skin and muscle.

Unit differences

Women at Willowford were much more likely to be sutured by a midwife and, consequently, were more likely to be sutured by the same person who delivered them. Women in any of the Exington units, on the other hand, were nearly always sutured by a doctor and therefore were seldom sutured by the same person who delivered them.

	Doctor		Midwife		Number of women who had stitches in each unit
	n	%	n	%	
Willowford	16	(15)	81	(77)	105
Exington consultant	62	(89)	4	(6)	70
Exington GP unit	24	(86)	4	(14)	28
Little Exington	29	(97)	1	(3)	30
Wychester	94	(78)	26	(21)	121
Zedbury	80	(80)	15	(15)	100

Percentages are of women in a given unit. Percentages do not always add up to 100 due to the exclusion of medical students from analysis.

Table 7.5: Person who sutured by unit

	Stitched by same person who delivered them		Number of women had stitches in each unit
	n	%	
Willowford	71	(68)	105
Exington consultant	16	(23)	70
Exington GP unit	4	(14)	28
Little Exington	5	(17)	30
Wychester	47	(39)	121
Zedbury	28	(28)	100

Table 7.6: Continuity of care for suturing by unit

Continuity of care for suturing thus varies widely between units ranging from just 14 per cent of women at Exington GP unit being sutured by the same person who delivered them to 68 per cent of those at Willowford where midwives routinely suture. There were no significant differences between units in the discomfort experienced; whether a local anaesthetic was used or whether there were any problems with the stitches.

Suturing and continuity of care

Does continuity of care for suturing make a difference to the pain?

It may be hypothesized that the continuity of care resulting from being stitched by the same person as delivered you (and the greater likelihood of no delay) makes it a less painful process. We did not, however, find a significant difference between the pain experienced at the time or in problems postnatally, although women who were stitched by the same person as delivered them were less likely to be given a local anaesthetic and more likely to be already anaesthetized.

	Local anaesthetic		No pain relief		Already anaesthetized (e.g. epidural)		Other	
	n	%	n	%	n	%	n	%
Women sutured by same person who delivered	109	(62)	35	(20)	21	(12)	11	(6)
Women sutured by different person	242	(86)	20	(7)	9	(3)	12	(4)

Percentages are of women in a given row.

$p < 0.05$

Table 7.7: Type of pain relief for suturing by who sutured

Types of suturing material

A variety of suturing materials were used in the units such as Decon, various types of catgut and black silk. In Exington women are sutured with a different type of material depending on which consultant they are booked with. However, most of the women in our sample were sutured with catgut – either soluble catgut or chromic catgut. There was too much variation within the Exington GP unit (depending on which GP is involved) to be able to determine which material was used and too few women sutured with Decon to include these in the analysis. However this still leaves us with a group of 174 women who were sutured with plain catgut and 226 who were sutured with chromic catgut.

Material	Where the material is used
Plain catgut	Wychester, Little Exington Women booked with Consultant No. 1 at Exington
Chromic catgut	Zedbury, Willowford Women booked with Consultant No. 2 at Exington
Decon	Women booked with Consultant No. 3 at Exington
Variety of materials	Exington GP unit

Table 7.8: Type of suturing material by unit

There was no difference between the two groups of women regarding whether they had a tear or episiotomy, what type of tear they had, or whether they had a local anaesthetic. Inevitably there were some differences in who sutured. Plain catgut was used in the units where doctors did the majority of suturing; chromic catgut was used in a group of units where, overall, the midwife was almost equally likely to suture as the doctor (because this group included Willowford). Similarly, women who were sutured with plain catgut were less likely to be sutured by the person who delivered them (because most of them were delivered by a midwife but then sutured by a doctor). Fifty four per cent of those sutured with chromic catgut were sutured by the same person as delivered them whereas 68 per cent of those sutured with plain catgut experienced continuity of care. There were no other differences in the suturing of the two groups or in the pain they experienced at the time or whether they experienced problems later. There were no differences in the type of problems they experienced except that women sutured with plain catgut had a slightly higher risk of infection ($p < 0.01$). This difference in infection rate is *not* accounted for by the fact that there was more continuity of care or midwife suturing of the women stitched with chromic catgut. Nor, as we showed earlier, does being sutured by a doctor increase the risk of infection. However, to really be able to say anything meaningful about these different suturing materials one would need larger numbers and a randomized controlled trial.

Summary

There was a wide variation in suturing practice in different units, both in which staff group performed the operation and what materials were used. Suturing is often seen as a routine 'tidying up' operation by staff ('a petty interruption to sleep' to quote an SHO from our phase I study; Green et al., 1986). However, it was clearly a major, and sometimes traumatic, event for women themselves. It is important that suturing be carried out quickly and skilfully with proper pain relief and staff also need training to ensure that there is minimum long term discomfort for women postnatally.

CHAPTER EIGHT

Women's Experiences of Care during Labour

Antenatally, the most common comment about previous experience of labour related to treatment by staff and this also emerged as central to women's experience of their current birth. Women had the opportunity to tell us about their experience of care during their recent labour in response to an open-ended question at the end of the postnatal questionnaire. In addition, they were also offered a list of adjectives to circle.

The questions and how women answered them

We noted in the pilot phase that women were very reluctant to circle any negative words to describe any of the staff. We therefore carefully phrased the question as follows:

> Finally, we'd like to know how you feel you were looked after while you were having your baby. Please circle whichever of the words below describe *any* of the staff who you saw during labour (circle as many as you wish). Please tell us about the negative as well as the positive things even if it was only one member of staff.
>
> | | | |
> |---|---|---|
> | rushed | humorous | insensitive |
> | unhelpful | sensitive | considerate |
> | supportive | off-hand | polite |
> | rude | warm | inconsiderate |
> | informative | bossy | condescending |

However, women were still reluctant to circle any negative words. Even where women wrote very negative responses to open-ended questions, many of them did not seem prepared to actually circle negative adjectives. One woman, for instance, circled 'supportive', 'informative', 'humorous', 'warm', 'considerate' and 'polite', but then added the comment:

> 'The only faults were the night staff, one in particular, she was very bossy and could be quite upsetting! Some of the night staff thought they were little Hitlers!'

Similarly, another woman only circled positive adjectives but added that:

> 'Unfortunately there were two rotten eggs who let the side down. One, a young sister I found very condescending and very insensitive, how on earth she ever qualified I will never know... when you are on a low you can do without staff such as these as this brings you down even more, hence postnatal blues!'

Even one encounter with an inconsiderate member of staff could destroy the occasion. One woman, for instance, who had established a very good relationship with her midwife said that the worst thing about her very straightforward birth was the actual moment of pushing the baby out because 'of a very rude, bossy auxiliary whose scolding distracted me from both midwife and baby. The actual moment of his birth was marred for me'.

	n	% of total sample who circled this adjective.
supportive	598	(84)
considerate	544	(77)
warm	492	(69)
polite	443	(62)
informative	432	(61)
humorous	395	(56)
sensitive	343	(48)
bossy	113	(16)
rushed	98	(14)
insensitive	83	(12)
off-hand	61	(9)
condescending	40	(6)
inconsiderate	38	(5)
unhelpful	34	(5)
n = 710		

Table 8.1: Description of staff

Often women explained that they selected the positive adjectives for one set of staff and the negative ones for another – midwives versus doctors, day staff versus night staff (or vice versa):

> 'All the good was for the midwife – smashing girl. The rest are for the doctor – Rude man!'

> 'Midwife – very nice. Doctor – really nasty, shame she had to spoil my day.'

> 'The day staff who delivered my son couldn't have been better. They were all super even the doctor made us laugh. But the night staff were unfriendly, cold and made me feel like a time wasting pest.'

Adjectives describing staff: parity, education and social class differences

For the individual adjectives, the only parity differences were that primips were significantly more likely to describe staff as 'supportive' on the one hand (88% compared to 82%) and 'inconsiderate' on the other (8% compared to 4%). There were also some education differences. The most educated women were most likely to describe staff as 'sensitive', whilst those who had left full-time education between 17 and 18 were most likely to describe them as 'informative'. The least educated women were most likely to describe staff as 'rude' on the one hand and 'polite' on the other.

	Education						
Adjective	16 and under		17–18		19 and over		p <
	n	%	n	%	n	%	
sensitive	145	(43)	97	(47)	99	(63)	0.001
polite	233	(68)	122	(59)	84	(54)	0.01
rude	23	(7)	10	(5)	2	(1)	0.05
informative	187	(55)	143	(69)	99	(63)	0.01

Percentages are of women of a given educational level

Table 8.2: Description of staff by education

Relationship between unit and description of staff

To obtain a general idea of how women felt about the staff in different units, we divided the adjectives into 'positive' and 'negative' ones and counted how many of each kind were circled by women in each unit. The greatest difference in the proportion of negative words circled was between women from Exington consultant unit (19% of the adjectives they circled were negative) and those from Little Exington (only 9% of the adjectives they circled were negative).

	Negative adjectives		Positive adjectives		Total number of adjectives circled by women in unit
	n	%	n	%	
Willowford	123	(14)	787	(86)	910
Exington Consultant	96	(19)	399	(80)	495
Exington GP	25	(10)	223	(90)	248
Little Exington	19	(9)	192	(91)	211
Wychester	94	(10)	825	(90)	919
Zedbury	117	(14)	733	(86)	850

(Percentages are of all comments made by women in each unit)

Table 8.3: Description of staff by unit

The importance of staff attitude

The attitude of the individual midwife was vital to women's experience of labour. A positive, supportive midwife greatly enhanced the occasion:

> 'I enjoyed the labour and had a very nice midwife deliver me – I think that it was because she was young and smiling that I did enjoy it. I feel that if it had been someone not so concerned it would have not been as happy an experience.'

Many women compared their much praised midwife who 'made it all worthwhile' with other midwives they had seen during this, or a previous labour:

> 'The midwife who delivered me was wonderful and I could not have imagined anyone else making it a better experience for me. I know from previous births how important her attitude is to the whole experience. My second birth was dreadful – I had a 'sour' midwife who never gave me any encouragement at all – in fact she probably never spoke more than three words to me during the whole ordeal.'

Women appreciated midwives keeping them informed, in control and praising them and they wanted their midwife to be friendly and involved, not just efficient:

> 'The midwife who "dealt with me" was very capable and experienced but had a brusque manner and was rather unenlightened in her attitude. I felt as if she was removing this baby from me, rather than assisting me to give birth. I found her rough and rather insensitive.'

Women were pleased when the staff made them feel 'special':

> 'It was obvious they loved their job and they made me feel very special (as I'm sure they do everyone).'

> 'The care I received could not have been better. I felt as though I was the only person that had ever given birth.'

They were pleased when the staff were on first name terms with them and respected their wishes:

> 'I feel very privileged to have had my baby at Willowford as the staff were great. It was all first names, even the doctor who delivered me, which made it much more comfortable. The doctor also thanked me for letting him take part.'

Women who had been treated like 'a lump of meat' felt humiliated and depressed about it:

> 'I felt I was another "body" not a person. They never once addressed me as a person. Discussed situation among themselves. I felt almost superfluous.'

(The 'lump of meat' issue and the importance of control is further discussed in Volume 1, Chapters 7 and 9).

When the staff were busy it was hard for them to give women individualized attention:

> 'I got the feeling I was just a number to be delivered as quickly as possible and wheeled back to the ward to be replaced by the next one. The staff however were very rushed that night and this probably accounted for it.'

Some staff, though, just seemed uninterested and uninvolved:

> 'When in labour staff were not very helpful and were talking about their shopping sprees and not interested in helping me cope with the pain at all.'

One woman who gave her birth experience an overall satisfaction score of just one out of ten simply wrote about the staff:

> 'They don't care.'

If the midwife appeared caring and also calm and confident this gave women confidence and helped them cope with labour pains:

> 'I felt as if I could have had triplets without batting an eyelid if she had said I could do it. It helped me keep my pain under control. If your midwife gives you confidence the pain seems to diminish.'
>
> 'I felt very pleased at not having drugs and think this is due to the fantastic midwife who helped so much, obviously very experienced and made me feel very calm and in control. I think the way you and your husband are treated makes a lot of difference.'

Some women seemed to feel that they probably would not have managed to give birth without their midwife:

> 'She was absolutely wonderful. She gave me encouragement and made me feel that there was no doubt in her mind that I could do it. And quite simply, if she wasn't on duty that particular morning I wouldn't have been able to do it all on my own.'

The individual midwife's support could be particularly important during a difficult labour:

> 'If it wasn't for the midwives I had I wouldn't have come through it. Sounds dramatic I know. But this baby will be my one and only child. Even my husband doesn't want me to go through that again.'

The staff support and involvement and the special support of one midwife in particular were also important for the woman whose baby died in utero:

> 'I believe I received the best care. The last midwife is inextricably linked with my positive feelings. I felt she was totally involved, totally on my side, that she was feeling it all with me.'

An unsupportive midwife on the other hand could really spoil the most straightforward birth:

> 'The midwife was awful. She made the whole of the birth seem like a nightmare. She wasn't encouraging me at all. She sat on the bed as I sat on a chair and just watched.'

Talking things through

Many women expressed gratitude to labour attendants who came to visit them postnatally, to see how things went:

> 'She came and visited me a few days later in the postnatal ward and made me feel really proud of myself. I feel very lucky to have had her as my midwife.'

Having the chance to talk things through postnatally was especially appreciated when problems had arisen. As one woman who had had a difficult birth wrote:

> 'They shared the experience with you and afterwards the midwife who delivered me came and talked about the delivery which I found invaluable. She discussed the problems they had had and how I coped.'

But another woman was less fortunate:

> 'I would have liked a member of the staff to sit with me and explain what happened and why things went wrong. I had to wait until I got home and saw my community midwife. I think that if I had had someone to talk to at the hospital, I would not have felt as though I had failed so miserably.'

The staff are, as we also discussed in Volume 1, very important participants in the experience of childbirth. They can, in some cases, make or mar a woman's memories irrespective of the actual events of the labour itself. They can also help a woman to come to terms with a difficult birth.

Interactions between staff

Interactions between staff were also important to women. Comments made about the woman which she could not hear, or which she was not meant to hear, were a source of worry:

> 'I was worried about the amount of whispering and worried looks they were giving each other.'

> 'Once I heard the midwife tell a nurse to get a paediatrician as baby may have swallowed meconium also she mentioned that there was *no resuscitation unit* available, I panicked, I thought they thought the baby was lost (dead) so I then pushed with all my might, and I found I panicked for nothing, baby was fine.'

Women were also annoyed by staff communicating with each other but ignoring them:

> 'All three stood at the bottom of the bed and discussed me like I wasn't there.'

> 'The midwife... must have thought that I was blind and/or stupid because she kept pulling faces to the medical student who was with us.'

Defining the start of labour: problems with staff

Unfortunately, for some women, problems between them and the staff started right at the beginning over the definition of the start of labour:

> 'When I first went into hospital after my waters broke the doctor and the sister examined me, but because I was not in any pain they did not believe me when I said that my waters had broken... After that I was left in a room with no-one coming in at intervals to check up on me.'

A few women mentioned such disputes in response to the question 'What was the worst thing about the birth?'

> 'The fact that the midwives on the ward refused to believe that I was in labour and left me in a room on my own, giving me two Panadol for the pain. I thought I would give birth on my own and was very frightened.'

For some, these arguments meant the whole event started off 'on the wrong foot':

> 'When my contractions were coming every five minutes I went into the labour ward. I was seen by a very rude sister who examined me internally with all the gentleness of an elephant (but that's probably cruel to elephants). She then informed me that I was not in labour and was not getting pains every five minutes. When I insisted that although they weren't very strong but I was still getting contractions she practically called me a liar and promptly told me that I should get somebody to fetch me home, and come back when I was in labour. The sister left my room with me nearly in tears. If it wasn't for the nice midwives that attended to me on my return to the labour ward I would have reported her without hesitation. As it is I feel that I never wanted to go back to Willowford to have another baby and if and when I become pregnant again I will insist on a home birth.'

On a few occasions women who came in thinking they were in labour were told by staff that they were not and were then given sleeping pills – sometimes with very sad consequences:

> 'I feel that the birth of my baby was completely spoiled. It was an experience I was so looking forward to, as the birth of my first son was so fulfilling. On arrival at the labour ward I was told that the pains I was having were only due to the enema and castor oil I was given. The midwife advised me to take two sleeping tablets and she would review the situation in the morning. My boyfriend

> was sent home and I was left alone. The next thing I remember, I was getting strong pains and my baby was born shortly after my boyfriend arrived. Everything was very fuzzy, but I remember my baby was taken away to another room and I had to send my boyfriend to find him... I felt utterly drunk and exhausted.'

Although we did not ask about the administration of sleeping pills, we were surprised by how many women volunteered that they had been given such drugs and then delivered their baby while still feeling only half-awake. It is clear that sleeping pills should not be given lightly and that, in some cases, staff need to listen with more sensitivity to women's own assessments of whether or not they are in labour.

CHAPTER NINE

Feeding The Baby

Twenty four per cent of the postnatal respondents (166 women) did not breastfeed their babies at all. Twenty three per cent (163 women) had started off breastfeeding but given up by the time they completed the questionnaire (about six weeks postnatally) and 53 per cent (377 women) were still breastfeeding.

Breastfeeding and education, social class and parity

The less educated women were less likely to breastfeed as were women in the lower social classes (defined both by woman's best ever occupation and partner's occupation).

Educational level	Did not breastfeed		Breastfed but stopped		Still breastfeeding	
	n	%	n	%	n	%
16 and under	119	(35)	88	(26)	133	(39)
17–18	39	(19)	54	(26)	112	(55)
19 and over	6	(4)	19	(12)	131	(84)

Percentages are of women in a given row.

$p < 0.0001$

Table 9.1: Breastfeeding by education

Multips and primips were equally likely to be breastfeeding at six weeks but multips were less likely to have tried to breastfeed and then given up than primips.

Parity	Did not breastfeed		Breastfed but stopped		Still breastfeeding	
	n	%	n	%	n	%
Primips	40	(15)	76	(32)	148	(54)
Multips	126	(29)	76	(18)	229	(53)

Percentages are of primips and multips.

$p < 0.0001$.

Table 9.2: Breastfeeding by parity

Reasons for giving up breastfeeding

The women who had given up breastfeeding were asked when they gave up and why. Thirty two (5% of the sample) had stopped before leaving hospital, 40 (6%) within a week of leaving hospital and the remaining 90 (13%) subsequently.

Over half of the women who gave up breastfeeding said that they did so because of 'insufficient milk' or problems getting the baby to feed. Women described being unable to get the baby to latch on to the breast and some gave up at a very early stage i.e. within hours of delivery. Thus one woman, who defined herself as having started but then given up breastfeeding, wrote:

> 'The midwife tried two to three times to get her to latch on. Eventually it seemed a lot less hassle just to bottlefeed.'

These women also talked about being 'unable to satisfy their baby', their milk 'drying up' and the baby 'needing' supplementary milk:

> 'My milk started drying up and the baby was very upset and hungry so I put her onto SMA milk.'
> 'The baby always seemed hungry and required a bottle to satisfy her.'

> 'He was a very hungry baby – so I was never sure he was getting enough to eat. Sister on the ward suggested I top him up with SMA Milk – which I did.'

It is unlikely that this many women (23%) were, in fact, incapable of satisfying their babies. Women's perceptions of having 'insufficient milk' depend on how they interpret their babies' behaviour. Babies will suck on almost anything but when a woman sees her baby continuing to suck she may interpret this as hunger and worry that her own milk supply is not adequate (Flint, 1986). Similarly, if a baby demands to be fed more frequently than every four hours, the mother may interpret that as meaning her milk is not good enough. Alternatively, if there are nipple problems the woman's anticipation of pain works against the milk ejection reflex (Greasley, 1986). The introduction of supplementary bottlefeeds can also lead to a reduction in the milk supply. However, supplementary bottlefeeds can be attractive to women who are anxious that their baby is not getting enough milk because they provide visible reassurance by allowing them to see how much their baby is drinking.

Once breastfeeding was interrupted for one reason or another, some women found it very hard to re-establish:

> 'I had fish food poisoning, unable to eat or drink anything for 36 hours. Although I tried both drinking and feeding baby during this time I had to supplement feeding with the bottle. When I fully recovered I tried to feed by the breast but I couldn't make up enough milk. I had help and advice from a Breast Counsellor during all this time, but found I was getting nowhere fast. All this and a 4 year old running around. I gave in gracefully!'

Reason for giving up breastfeeding	n	% of those women who gave up breastfeeding
Insufficient milk and latching on problems	87	(53)
Breast problems	46	(28)
Too tired/no time	33	(20)
Did not enjoy it	16	(10)
Lack of support from staff	3	(2)
Use of and 'top ups' of powdered milk	3	(2)
Other	18	(11)

n = 163

A maximum of two reasons were coded for each woman. A total number of 206 reasons were given.

Table 9.3: Reasons for giving up breastfeeding

Twenty eight per cent of the women who gave up breastfeeding wrote that breast problems had influenced their decision e.g. painful engorgement, cracked and sore nipples etc. Other studies have found that sore or cracked nipples are the major reason for women abandoning breastfeeding (Martin and Monk, 1980) and up to 40 per cent of mothers may suffer from this problem (Herd and Feeney, 1986). Descriptions of breast problems such as soreness were often given in conjunction with problems of getting the baby to suck or of having 'insufficient' milk:

> 'I could not satisfy my baby and I was getting very bad pains where he was draining my breasts.'

The two may of course be intertwined: sore nipples, for instance, can result from incorrect positioning of the baby on the breast (Inch, 1985). Sore nipples are thus, in many cases, an avoidable problem (Gunther, 1970).

Problems of exhaustion or lack of time were also mentioned by 20 per cent of the women – bottlefeeding was seen as more convenient:

> 'Breastfed for three weeks but was taking over an hour a time and with one child already it didn't work out. Now trying to get into a routine with bottles so we can plan things better.'

> 'Baby was not satisfied with feeds, fed every two hours night and day, and I got very tired (with two other children to cope with as well).'

> 'I found it a bind, being a single parent and living on my own, I just didn't have the time.'

Several women pointed out that breastfeeding meant less sharing of childcare:

> 'I think breastfeeding does isolate you from your husband in these early weeks when he can't really help out with the disturbed nights.'

Richards and Bernal (1971), for example, found that other people are more likely to be present when the baby is bottlefed than when it is breastfed.

Other problems arose for women who were feeling fatigued by the birth or debilitated by infection:

> 'I got an infection through having a swab left in my vagina for a couple of days until the midwife discovered it when I got home. This made me feel under the weather as I was losing blood for four weeks until the infection cleared up.'

All these reasons discussed above were not, of course, mutually exclusive. We coded up to two reasons for each woman, but several women gave a whole catalogue of reasons – everything seemed to conspire against their attempts to breastfeed:

> 'The first problem was that my right breast was constantly blocked, and I had to use a breast pump before each feed. The second problem was that he was constantly hungry and would sometimes want feeding every half an hour, plus he was not putting on very much weight, so I was told by the Health Visitor to supplement every feed with a bottle. The last and final problem was that my two year old daughter became unwell and needed more of my attention.'

Ten per cent of the women who gave up breastfeeding said they did not like it, often suggesting they found it distasteful:

> 'I found that most of the time I felt mucky, if she was late waking for her feed I used to become very wet very quickly and it used to make me feel dirty.'

A few said they were 'fed up with feeling like a cow', or, as one woman put it, 'I want my body back!'. One woman described her decision to give up breastfeeding in the following terms:

> '... too exhausted, too nervy, hated exposing myself and had problems regaining my dignity. I felt everyone was pawing me all the time.'

Other reasons ranged from the feeling that bottlefeeding was easier on the older sibling:

> 'My older child seemed to understand more, when I gave the baby a bottle, what was happening and could also see when the feed would end.'

To a lack of privacy on the postnatal ward:

> 'I was very unhappy being in a ward with seven other women and babies and could only tackle getting the baby to breastfeed when I was able to concentrate on it in peace.'

Only three women explicitly referred to lack of staff support as a factor in their decision to give up breastfeeding. However, as we shall see (and as some of the earlier quotations have implied), the skill and support of staff was much more important than this figure suggests.

Breastfeeding and information

The importance of staff attitude was made clear by the responses to the open-ended question: 'Is there anything in particular you wish you had known more about before you had your baby?'. Twenty per cent of the 141 women who answered 'yes' to this question specified breastfeeding as a topic they would have liked to have known more about (whether or not they would have absorbed such information antenatally is, however, another question (Flint, 1986)). The issue came up again in response to the question about misleading, contradictory or confusing information. Nineteen per cent of the 121 women who said that they had been given 'bad' information specified that this information had been about feeding their baby.

One woman gave a vivid account of how she was deluged by contradictory advice from different staff:

> 'The staff treated me as though my brain had been removed, with regard to breastfeeding. I was told 1) feed as long as you like, 2) 15 mins one side then change for next feed, 3) 8 mins each side, 4) 5 mins each side, 5) not to feed more than once every five hours, 6) feed whenever you like. This 'information' was all on the day of the birth and from different staff. The nearest approach to sensitivity and caring I received was a 'hockey-stick type' who stuck her head round the curtain when I had visitors and said "Titties all right, then?".'

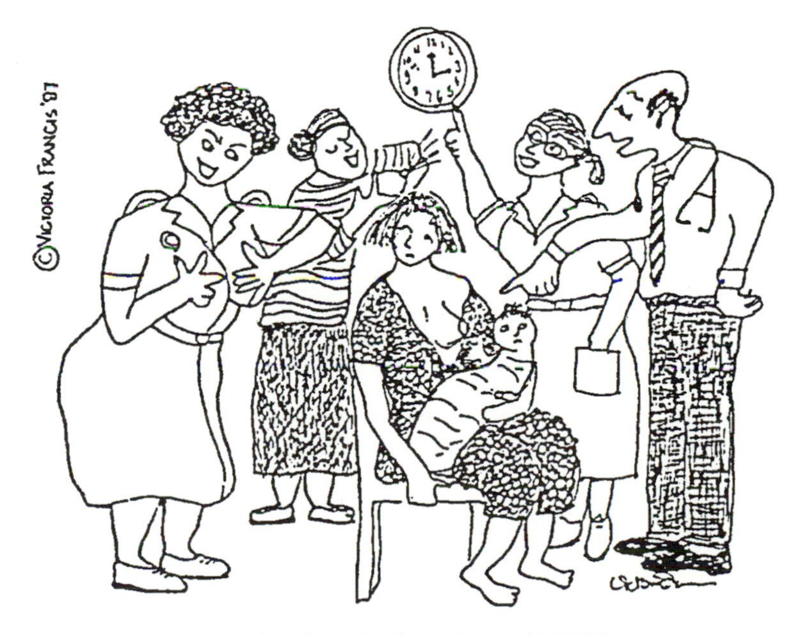

Reproduced with kind permission of MIDIRS

Conflicting advice about breastfeeding was a very common complaint, as other studies have also found (e.g. Hewat and Ellis, 1984). Some women were in no doubt that contradictory and condescending information was enough to make women give up breastfeeding:

> 'One sister said to feed when the baby wanted it i.e. every two hours whilst one of the nurses said to make him wait as he'd keep on going every two hours. Another case was one said to keep him alert whilst feeding making him suck continually whilst another said let him suck in his own time. No wonder so many give up breastfeeding in the first few days.'

Other women felt that the information they had been given was simply incorrect:

> 'The only thing I really didn't like about the nurses was they showed me how to breastfeed my baby wrong. That's why she messed me about in hospital because as soon as I got home and my mum showed me she took straight away.'

Staff attitudes to breastfeeding, even when there was a consensus, were not always constructive. Some women wrote about feeling generally unsupported in their efforts to breastfeed:

> 'I realize that it is difficult for the staff, dealing with all the personalities of the mums – however, it is also difficult the other way around if you have any ideas that are different from standard procedure. I had problems with cracked nipples that I think could have been prevented with more guidance. My baby was not latching on properly, but I didn't realize it until it was too late. This gave a few midwives more ammunition to make me feel I was being ridiculous with breastfeeding. I also have inverted nipples, but have done quite a lot to prepare them, and in my opinion they work just fine. However, I feel this was also a factor in their lack of support, which is very insensitive (if anything, I needed more support).'

Several women said that although some staff were supportive they had to face what amounted to harassment from others when they had problems breastfeeding:

> 'There were four midwives who were very supportive, especially after they realized how unsupportive others were being regarding my breastfeeding. Unfortunately they were not always there and I was left to deal with the rest, especially the night staff, whom I felt just wanted to keep the place quiet. Some comments:
>
> – 'If your baby does not gain by morning he will get a bottle' (he had only lost 9 per cent of his birth weight at that time and my milk had not come in yet).
>
> – 'You have a big boy – he needs to eat – you should be topping him up with a bottle.'
>
> – (said to another midwife in front of me): 'If it were your baby wouldn't you top up with a bottle?' (Reply was affirmative).'

Staff 'support' for breastfeeding was not always welcome when it came in the form of mauling and 'manhandling'. Some staff seemed to see a lactating breast as public property detached from the woman herself:

> 'A very insensitive silly nurse kept wiggling my nipple in front of the baby's mouth when we were doing fine – I was too exhausted to protest – but looking back that really did irritate. It seems that they can't keep their hands off you, and all your dignity goes out the window. Yes, I was furious at that.'

Other women felt they were put under undue pressure to breastfeed and were relieved to give up and turn to bottles:

> 'I did feel very pressurized to breastfeed. I understand that this is obviously best but I found it distasteful and difficult and felt guilty about this. I had three sleepless, tearful and fretful nights before I felt able to change over to bottlefeeding. One or two members of staff obviously thought I had given up too soon and I was very conscious that I was somehow a failure.'

> 'I felt under a lot of pressure in the after care to breastfeed even as it turned out I was unable to because I had no milk but I felt at the time baby got very upset by being pushed on to me, at the same time I felt myself being very upset. I even asked twice if I could have a bottle for baby but was told no, to carry on and that I had a lazy baby.'

A theme running through many women's comments is that staff support for women's choices about, or ability to, feed their babies was crucial to their feelings about their adequacy as mothers. One women wrote at length about the guilt and anxiety induced by insensitive treatment by some staff:

> 'I kept telling one midwife that I did not think the baby was getting any milk from me as I had lumps in my breast and even when I massaged and squeezed them nothing came out. The next thing I knew this nurse is shouting at me and telling me that I should feed my baby as she was very hungry. I was really upset I felt that she was trying to tell me I was neglecting my baby. One of the other midwives came to help me put her to the breast but where my baby had not been getting anything she had given up sucking. They tried the milk machine on me and it flowed for a few minutes then stopped as soon as my daughter had a few sucks. This went on all afternoon into the evening. I got really distressed, I ended up in tears. They kept telling me to persevere.'

This woman was finally rescued from the situation when the night staff came on:

> 'One of the nursery nurses came and talked to me and asked me what I wanted to do. I decided I could not bear my baby crying any more because she was hungry. This was not an easy decision. I felt I had failed my baby. I so wanted to breastfeed. But this nurse sat and talked to me. I felt better after she had talked to me. My little girl was given a bottle of milk. The nurse said she drank the whole bottle and had looked up at her as if to say thank you. She was taken to the nursery that night and fed by the nurses. She drank the whole bottle for about 24 hours so she must have been desperately hungry.'

When the day staff came back on duty however they were still very unsupportive:

> 'They made me feel really guilty because I had not kept on trying to breastfeed... I did not need their attitude, I needed reassurance that she would be alright breastfed or bottlefed and that I hadn't failed. I did not get that.'

Conflict with staff about, for instance, the baby's weight gain could be very distressing and, women suggested, could have repercussions for the woman's relationship with her baby. Another woman who wrote at length about the lack of support for breastfeeding commented:

> 'I have to say that on the whole the midwives were marvellous, and they agreed with me that I would be under less stress at home and so the feeding would improve. They also pointed out that the paediatrician's ideal weight gain chart was based on bottlefed babies, who tended to gain weight more quickly than breastfed babies.
>
> However, the paediatricians were very unsympathetic to the whole situation, and while I pointed out that the weight gain problem was due to my being under stress, and the exhaustion resulting from my previous experience, both of which would improve if I went home, their answer was that they 'weren't interested in the causes, only the effects'!
>
> I do think that as a result of these "upsets" in hospital I was left feeling quite depressed for some time, and initially even began to resent my baby for not gaining weight and for putting me in such a stressful situation. Since we have been at home my baby has put on more than the average amount of weight each week, and I have succeeded in breastfeeding her.'

Breastfeeding was not, of course, a central focus of our study. Had it been we would have asked all women directly what they had found supportive or unsupportive, instead of just asking women who had given up breastfeeding why they had done so. As it was, breastfeeding was clearly an important issue for the women who answered our questionnaire and many took every opportunity they could to write about it. This was the issue most often mentioned when women were asked about conflicting information and it would seem that there is still a long way to go if women are to be successfully helped to establish breastfeeding or supported in their decision to bottlefeed. We would suggest that, as Inch (1985) has pointed out, the hospital institutions may not be conducive to the establishment of breastfeeding. Separation from the baby, loss of social support and lack of control over the postnatal period may make it difficult for some women in hospital:

> 'Two things marred my stay in hospital and my memories of what could, and should have been a very happy occasion. One was the handling of the phototherapy given to my baby and the other was their handling of subsequent feeding problems. I was left in a separate room to look after my jaundiced baby whilst she received phototherapy, and had little help in spite of her constant diarrhoea and reluctance to feed. At one stage I had no sleep for 36 hours.

> Exhausted, my milk supply dwindled to nothing and I was pressurized into giving her a bottlefeed. I asked for soya milk and was given only cows milk, in spite of a strong history of allergy to cows milk in the family. Of course I complained to the nursing officer who was very apologetic about the events, but by then the damage was done.'

There are also issues to be explored around the fact that so many women felt that their own milk was not sufficient. Some researchers have suggested this may reflect the kind of messages that women are receiving from the baby milk companies (Eliot, 1984; Flint, 1986).

Breastfeeding also has important associations with the way women perceive their babies and the importance of what happens in the first few weeks cannot be underestimated (see Volume 1, Chapter 8).

References

Affonso, D., Domino, G. (1984). 'Postpartum depression: a review'. *Birth*, 11, pp. 231–235.

Affonso, D., Stichler, J.F. (1978). 'Exploratory study of women's reactions to having a caesarean birth'. *Birth and the Family Journal*, 5, pp. 88–94.

Allen, I., Dowling, B.S., Williams, S.A. (1997). *A Leading Role for Midwives? Evaluation of Midwifery Group Practice Development Projects.* Policy Studies Institute. Report No. 832.

Arizmendi, T., Affonso, D. (1984). 'Research on psychosocial factors and postpartum depression: a critique'. *Birth*, 11, pp. 237–240.

Arms, S. (1975). *Immaculate Deception.* Boston: Houghton Mifflin.

Arney, W.R., Neill, J. (1982). 'The location of pain in childbirth: natural childbirth and the transformation of obstetrics'. *Sociology of Health and Illness*, 4, pp. 1–24.

Astbury, J. (1980). 'The crisis of childbirth: can information and childbirth education help?'. *J. Psychosomatic Research*, 24, pp. 9–13.

Baker, R.A. (1978). 'Technological intervention in obstetrics. Has the pendulum swung too far?'. *Obstetrics and Gynecology*, 51, pp. 241–244.

Ball, J.A. (1987). *Reactions to Motherhood: The Role of Postnatal Care.* Cambridge: Cambridge University Press.

Bardon, D. (1972). 'Puerperal depression'. In: Morris, N. (Ed). *Psychosomatic Medicine in Obstetrics and Gynaecology.* 3rd International Congress. 1971. London: Basel, Karger.

Beaton, J., Gupton, A. (1990). 'Childbirth expectations: a qualitative analysis'. *Midwifery*, 6, pp. 133–139.

Beck, N.C., Hall, D. (1978). 'Natural childbirth. A review and analysis'. *Obstetrics and Gynecology*, 52, pp. 371–379.

Bennett, A., Hewson, D., Booker, E., Holliday, S. (1985). 'Antenatal preparation and labor support in relation to birth outcomes'. *Birth*, 12, pp. 9–16.

Bing, E., Karmel, M., Tanz, A. (1961). *A Practical Training Course for the Psychoprophylactic Method of Childbirth.* New York: ASPO.

Bluff, R., Holloway, I. (1994). '"They know best": women's perceptions of midwifery care during labour and childbirth'. *Midwifery*, 10, pp. 157–164.

Booth, C., Meltzoff, A. (1984). 'Expected and actual experience in labour and delivery and their relationship to maternal attachment'. *J. Reproductive and Infant Psychology*, 2, pp. 79–91.

Bourne, G. (1975). *Pregnancy.* London: Pan Books.

Boyd, C., Sellers, L. (1982). *The British Way of Birth.* London: Pan Books.

Brackbill, Y., Rice, J., Young, D. (1984). *Birth Trap.* St. Louis, Missouri: Mosby Press.

Bradley, C., Brewin, C.R., Duncan, S.L.B. (1983). 'Perceptions of labour: discrepancies between midwives' and patients' ratings'. *British J. Obstetrics and Gynaecology*, 90, pp. 1176–1179.

Bradley, C.F., Ross, S.E., Warnyca, J. (1983). 'A prospective study of mothers' attitudes and feelings following cesarean and vaginal births'. *Birth*, 10, pp. 79–83.

Bramadat, I.J., Driedger, M. (1993). 'Satisfaction with childbirth: Theories and methods of measurement'. *Birth*, 20, pp. 22–29.

Breen, D. (1975). *The Birth of a First Child.* London: Tavistock.

Brewin, C., Bradley, C. (1982). 'Perceived control and the experience of childbirth'. *British J. Clinical Psychology*, 21, pp. 262–269.

Brockington, I.F., Kumar, R. (1982). *Motherhood and Mental Illness.* London: Academic Press.

Brown, G., Harris, T. (1978). *Social Origins of Depression: A Study of Psychiatric Disorder in Women.* London: Tavistock.

Brown, S., Lumley, J. (1994). 'Satisfaction with care in labor and birth: a survey of 790 Australian women'. *Birth*, 21, pp. 4–13.

Brown, S., Lumley, J., Small, R., Astbury, J. (1994). *Missing Voices: The Experience of Motherhood.* Melbourne: Oxford University Press.

Cartwright, A. (1977). 'Mothers' experience of induction'. *British Medical Journal,* 2, pp. 745–749.

Cartwright, A. (1979). *The Dignity of Labour.* London: Tavistock.

Cartwright, A. (1987). 'Monitoring maternity services by postal questionnaires to mothers'. *Health Trends,* 19, pp. 19–20.

Chapman, M.G., Jones, M., Springs, J.E., de Swiet, M., Chamberlain, G.V.P. (1986). 'The use of a birthroom: a randomised controlled trial comparing delivery with that in the labour ward'. *British J. Obstetrics and Gynaecology,* 93, pp. 182–187.

Charles, A.G., Norr, K.L., Block, C.R., Meyering, S., Myers, E. (1978). 'Obstetric and psychological effects of psychoprophylactic preparation for childbirth'. *American J. Obstetrics and Gynecology,* 131, pp. 44–51.

Clark, N. (1986). 'Expectations about childbirth: the relationship between expectations, childbirth education and birth satisfaction'. Unpublished Ph.D. Thesis, Monash University, Victoria, Australia.

Clayton, S.G., Fraser, D., Lewis, T.L.T. (1975). *Obstetrics by Ten Teachers.* London: Edward Arnold.

Clinch, J. (1985). 'The third stage'. In: Studd, J. (Ed). *The Management of Labour.* Oxford: Blackwell Scientific Publications.

Cooper, P.J., Campbell, E.A., Day, A., Kennerley, M., Bond, A. (1988). 'Non-psychotic psychiatric disorder after childbirth: a prospective study of prevalence, incidence, course and nature'. *British J. Psychiatry,* 152, pp. 799–806.

Cox, J.L., Connor, Y., Kendell, R.C. (1982). 'Prospective study of the psychiatric disorders of childbirth'. *British J. Psychiatry,* 140, pp. 111–117.

Cox, J.L., Holden, J.M., Sagovsky, R. (1987). 'Detection of postnatal depression. Development of the 10-item Edinburgh Postnatal Depression Scale'. *British J. Psychiatry,* 150, pp. 782–786.

Crowe, K., Von Baeyer, C. (1989). 'Predictors of a positive childbirth experience'. *Birth,* 16(2), pp. 59–63.

Davenport-Slack, B., Boylan, C. (1974). 'Psychological correlates of childbirth and pain'. *Psychosom. Med.,* 36, pp. 215–223.

Department of Health (1993). *Changing Childbirth. Part 1. Report of the Expert Maternity Group.* London: HMSO.

Deutsch, H. (1945). *The Psychology of Women: A Psychoanalytic Interpretation.* Vol. II. New York: Grune and Stratton.

DHSS (1987). *Women's Experience of Maternity Services. DHSS Circular, DA(87)6.* London.

Dick Read, G. (1933). *Natural Childbirth.* London: Heinemann.

Dick Read, G. (1944). *Childbirth Without Fear: The Principles and Practices of Natural Childbirth.* New York: Harper.

Doering, S.G., Entwisle, D.R. (1975). 'Preparation during pregnancy and ability to cope with labor and delivery'. *Amer.J. Orthopsychiatry,* 45, pp. 825–837.

Elbourne, D., Prendiville, W., Chalmers, I. (1988). 'Choice of oxytocic preparation for routine use in the management of the third stage of labour: an overview of the evidence from controlled trials'. *British J. of Obstetrics and Gynaecology,* 95, pp. 17–30.

Eliot, E. (1984). 'Are we really free to choose?'. *New Generation,* March 23.

Elliott, S.A., Anderson, M., Brough, D.I., Watson J.P., Rugg, A.J. (1984). 'Relationship between obstetric outcome and psychological measures in pregnancy and the postnatal year'. *J. Reproductive and Infant Psychology,* 2, pp. 18–32.

Enkin, M.W. (1984). 'Smoking and pregnancy – a new look'. *Birth,* 11, pp. 225–228.

Enkin, M.W., Smith, S.L., Dermer, S.W., Emmett, J.D. (1972). 'An adequately controlled study of the effectiveness of PPM training'. In: Morris, N. (Ed). *Psychosomatic Medicine in Obstetrics and Gynecology.* New York: Karger.

Erb, L., Hill, G., Houston, D. (1983). 'A study of parents' attitudes toward their Cesarean births in Manitoba hospitals'. *Birth,* 10, pp. 85–91.

Evans, R., Durward, L. (1984). *Maternity Rights Handbook.* Harmondsworth: Penguin.

Felton, G.S., Segelman, F.B. (1978). 'Lamaze childbirth training and changes in belief about personal control'. *Birth and the Family Journal*, 5, pp. 141–150.

Festinger, L. (1957). *A Theory of Cognitive Dissonance.* Evanston, Illinois: Row, Peterson.

Flint, C. (1986a). 'Maternity services today: do they help women to become confident mothers?'. Seminar given to the Child Care and Development Group, University of Cambridge, 21st October.

Flint, C. (1986b). *Sensitive Midwifery.* London: Heinemann.

Fox, J.S. (1979). 'Episiotomy'. *Midwives Chronicle*, October.

Francis, H.H. (1985). 'Obstetrics: a consumer orientated service? The case against'. *Maternal and Child Health*, 10, pp. 69–72.

Fridh, G., Gaston-Johansson, F. (1990). 'Do primiparas and multiparas have realistic expectations of labor'. *Acta Obstetrics Gynecology Scand.*, 69, pp. 103–109.

Garcia, J. et al. (1985). 'Views of women and their medical and midwifery attendants about instrumental deliveries using vacuum extraction and forceps'. *J. Psychosomatic Obstetrics and Gynaecology*, 4, pp. 1–9.

Garcia, J., Corry, M., MacDonald, D., Elbourne, D., Grant, A. (1985). 'Mothers' views of continuous electronic fetal heart monitoring and intermittent auscultation in a randomized controlled trial'. *Birth*, 12, pp. 79–85.

Garcia, J., Garforth, S., Ayers, S. (1987). 'The policy and practice in midwifery study: introduction and methods'. *Midwifery*, 3, pp. 2–9.

Garel, M., Lelong, N., Kaminski, M. (1987). 'Consequences de l'analgesie peridurale sur l'experience de la cesarienne et les premieres reactions mere–enfant'. In progress on *Journal d'Obstetrique et de Biologie de la Reproduction.*

Garforth, S., Garcia, J. (1987). 'Admitting – a weakness or a strength. Routine admission of a woman in labour'. *Midwifery*, 3, pp. 10–24.

Graham, H. (1977). 'Women's attitudes to conception and pregnancy'. In: Chester, R., Peel, J. (Eds). *Equalities and Inequalities in Family Life.* New York: Academic Press.

Graham, H. (1984). *Women, Health and the Family.* Brighton: Wheatsheaf Books.

Greasley, V. (1986). 'Breastfeeding'. *Nursing*, 3, pp. 63–70.

Green, J M. (1998). 'Postnatal depression or perinatal dysphoria? Findings from a longitudinal community-based study using the Edinburgh Postnatal Depression Scale'. *Journal of Reproductive & Infant Psychology* (in press).

Green, J., Kitzinger, J., Coupland, V. (1986). *The Division of Labour: Implications of Medical Staffing Structure for Doctors and Midwives on the Labour Ward.* Child Care and Development Group, University of Cambridge.

Green, J., Kitzinger, J., Coupland, V. (1994). 'Midwives responsibilities, medical staffing structures and women's choice in childbirth'. In: Robinson, S., Thomson, A. (Eds). *Midwives, Research and Childbirth.* Vol. III. London: Routledge, Chapman and Hall.

Green, J.M. (1990). 'Who is unhappy after childbirth?: Antenatal and intrapartum correlates from a prospective study'. *J. of Reproductive & Infant Psychology* , 8, pp. 175–83.

Green, J.M. (1993). 'Expectations and experiences of pain in labor: Findings from a large prospective study'. *Birth*, 20(2), pp. 65–72.

Green, J.M., Curtis, P., Price, H., Renfrew, M.J. (1998). *Continuing to Care: The Organisation of Midwifery Services in the UK: A Structured Review of the Evidence.* Hale, Cheshire: Books for Midwives Press (in press).

Green, J.M., Kafetsios, K. (1997). 'Positive experiences of early motherhood: predictive variables from a longitudinal study'. *J. of Reproductive & Infant Psychology* ,15, pp. 141–157.

Green, J.M., Murray, D. (1994). 'The use of the EPDS in research to explore the relationship between antenatal and postnatal dysphoria'. In: Cox, J.L., Holden, J. (Eds). *Perinatal Psychiatry: use and misuse of the Edinburgh Postnatal Depression Scale.* London: Gaskell Press.

Green, J.M., Shearn, D.C.S., Bolton, N. (1983). 'A numeracy course for arts undergraduates'. *Studies in Higher Education*, 8, pp. 57–65.

Greenshield, W. (1987). 'Postnatal infection survey'. *New Generation*, 6, pp. 6–7.

Gunther, M. (1970). *Infant feeding.* London: Methuen.

Haire, D. (1978). 'The cultural warping of childbirth'. In: Ehrenreich, J. (Ed). *The Cultural Crisis of Modern Medicine.* New York: The Monthly Review Press.

Harmond, K. (1994). 'Midwives must be directive as well as supportive'. *British J. of Midwifery,* 2(11), pp. 543–544.

Herd, B., Feeney, J. (1986). 'Two aerosol sprays in nipple trauma'. *The Practitioner,* 230, pp. 31–34.

Hewat, R., Ellis, D. (1984). 'Breastfeeding as a maternal–child team effort: women's perceptions'. *Health Care Women Int.,* 5, pp. 437–452.

Hodnett, E. (1989). 'Personal control and the birth environment: comparisons between home and hospital settings'. *Journal of Environmental Psychology,* 9, pp. 207–216.

Hodnett, E.D., Osborn, R.W. (1989). 'Effects of continuous intrapartum professional support on childbirth outcomes'. *Research in Nursing and Health,*12, pp. 289–297.

Hodnett, E.D., Simmons-Tropea, D. (1987). 'The Labor Agentry Scale: psychometric properties of an instrument measuring control during childbirth'. *Research in Nursing & Health,* 10, pp. 301–10.

Hoult, I.J., MacLennan, A.H., Carrie, L.E. (1977). 'Lumbar epidural analgesia in labour: relation to fetal malposition and instrumental delivery'. *British Medical Journal,* 1, pp. 14–16.

Hubert, J. (1974). 'Beliefs and reality: social factors in pregnancy and childbirth'. In Richards, M. (Ed). *The Integration of a Child Into a Social World.* New York: Cambridge University Press.

Humenick, S. (1981). 'Mastery: the key to childbirth satisfaction? A review'. *Birth and the Family Journal,* 8, pp. 79–83.

Humenick, S.S., Bugen, L.A. (1981). 'Mastery: the key to childbirth satisfaction? A study'. *Birth and the Family Journal,* 8, pp. 84–90.

Huntingford, P. (1985). *Birth Right: The Parent's Choice.* London: British Broadcasting Corporation.

Huttel, F.A., Mitchell, I., Fischer, W.M., Meyer, A.E. (1972). 'A quantitative evaluation of psychoprophylaxis in childbirth'. *J. Psychosomatic Research,* 16, pp. 81–92.

Inch, S. (1982). *Birthrights – A Parents Guide to Modern Childbirth.* London: Hutchinson.

Jackson, J.E., Vaughan, M., Black, P., D'Souza, S.W. (1983). 'Psychological aspects of fetal monitoring: maternal reaction to the position of the monitor and staff behaviour'. *J. Psychosomatic Obstetrics and Gynaecology,* 2, p. 97.

Jacoby, A. (1987). 'Women's preference for and satisfaction with current procedures in childbirth – findings from a national study'. *Midwifery,* 3, pp. 117–124.

Jones, A.D., Dougherty, C.R.S. (1984). 'Attendance at ante–natal classes and clinics, medical intervention during birth and implications for "Natural Childbirth"'. *J. Reproductive and Infant Psychology,* 2, pp. 49–60.

Kendell, R.E. (1985). 'Emotional and physical factors in the genesis of puerperal mental disorders'. *J. Psychosomatic Research,* 29, pp. 3–11.

Kirkham, M.H. (1987). 'Basic supportive care in labour. Interaction with and around labouring women'. Unpublished PhD thesis, University of Manchester, Faculty of Medicine.

Kitzinger, J., Green, J., Coupland V. (1990). 'Labour relations: doctors and midwives on the labour ward'. In: Garcia, J., Kilpatrick, R., Richards, M.P.M. (Eds). *The Politics of Maternity Care.* Oxford University Press.

Kitzinger, S. (1978). *Some Mothers' Experiences of Induced Labour.* London: National Childbirth Trust.

Kitzinger, S. (1979). *The Good Birth Guide.* London: Fontana.

Kitzinger, S. (1983). *The New Good Birth Guide.* Harmondsworth: Penguin.

Kitzinger, S. (1987a). *Freedom and Choice in Childbirth.* Harmondsworth: Penguin.

Kitzinger, S. (1987b). *Some Women's Experiences of Epidurals – A Descriptive Study.* London: National Childbirth Trust.

Kitzinger, S., Walters, R. (1981). *Some Women's Experiences of Episiotomy.* London: National Childbirth Trust.

Knight, R.G., Thirkettle J.A. (1987). 'The relationship between expectations of pregnancy and birth, and transient depression in the immediate post-partum period'. *J. Psychosomatic Research,* 31(3), pp. 351–357.

Kumar, R., Robson, K.M., Smith, A.M.R. (1984). 'Development of a self-administered questionnaire to measure maternal adjustment and maternal attitudes during pregnancy and after delivery'. *J. Psychosomatic Research*, 28, pp. 43–51.

Lamaze, F. (1958). *Painless Childbirth.* London: Burke.

Leverton, T. (1987). 'Psychological problems in the longer term following childbirth'. *Maternal and Child Health Journal of Family Medicine*, 12, pp. 60–65.

Lewis, B.V., Rana, S., Crook, E. (1975). 'Patient response to induction of labour'. *Lancet*, May 24th.

Lindsay, A. (1987). 'Italian women's experience of childbirth in two English towns'. Unpublished paper, Child Care and Development Group, University of Cambridge.

Lomas, J., Dore, S., Enkin, M., Mitchell, A. (1987). 'The labour and delivery satisfaction index: the development and evaluation of a soft outcome measure'. *Birth*, 14, pp. 125–129.

Lumley, J. (1985). 'Assessing satisfaction with childbirth'. *Birth*, 12, pp. 141–145.

Lumley, J. (1987). 'Stopping smoking'. *Br. J. Obstetrics and Gynaecology*, 94, pp. 289–294.

Lumley, J., Astbury, J. (1980). *Birth Rites, Birth Rights: Childbirth Alternatives for Australian Parents.* Melbourne: Thomas Nelson.

Macarthur, C., Newton, J.R., Knox, E.G. (1987). 'Effects of anti-smoking health education on infant size at birth: a randomized controlled trial'. *Br. J. Obstetrics and Gynaecology*, 94, pp. 295–300.

MacDonald, R.R. (1987). 'In defence of the obstetrician'. *Br. J. Obstetrics and Gynaecology*, 94, pp. 833–835.

MacFarlane, A., Mugford, M. (1984). *Birth Counts: Statistics of Pregnancy and Childbirth.* London: HMSO.

MacIntyre, S. (1981). 'Expectations and experiences of first pregnancy'. Institute of Medical Sociology, Occasional Paper No. 5, University of Aberdeen.

Martin, C.J. (1984). 'Monitoring maternity services by postal questionnaire: congruity between mothers' reports and their obstetric records'. *Statistics in Medicine*, 6, pp. 613–627.

Martin, J., Monk, J. (1982). *Report on Infant Feeding.* London: HMSO.

May, I. and the Farm Midwives (1975). *Spiritual Midwifery.* Summertown, Tennessee: The Book Publishing Company.

McClain, C.S. (1983). 'Perceived risk and choice of childbirth service'. *Soc. Sci. Med.* 17, pp. 1857–66.

McCleary, E. (1974). *New Miracles of Childbirth. How Modern Miracles are Making Childbearing Safer and Easier.* New York.

McIntosh, J. (1986). 'Expectations and experiences of childbirth in a sample of working class primigravidae'. *Research and the Midwife Conference Proceedings*, pp. 40–57.

Melzack, R., Tanzer, P., Feldman, P., Kinch, R.H. (1981). 'Labour is still painful after prepared childbirth training'. *Canadian Medical Association Journal*, 125, pp. 357–363.

Milner, I. (1988). 'Water baths for pain relief in labour'. *Nursing Times*, 84, pp. 38–40.

Molfese, V., Sunshine, P., Bennett, A. (1982). 'Reactions of women to intrapartum fetal monitoring'. *Obstetrics and Gynecology*, 59, p. 705.

Morcos, F.H., Snart, F.D., Harley, D.D. (1989). 'Comparison of parents' expectations and importance ratings for specific aspects of childbirth'. *Canadian Medical Association Journal*, 141, pp. 909–914.

Morgan, B., Bulpitt, C.J., Clifton, P., Lewis, P.J. (1982a). 'Effectiveness of pain relief in labour: survey of 1000 mothers'. *British Medical Journal*, 285, pp. 689–90.

Morgan, B., Bulpitt, C.J., Clifton, P., Lewis, P.J. (1982b). 'Analgesia and satisfaction in childbirth'. *Lancet*, ii, pp. 808–810.

Morgan, B.M. (1982). 'Pain relief in labour'. *Maternal and Child Health*, April, pp. 152–155.

Morgan, B.M. et al. (1983). 'Anaesthesia for caesarian section; a medical audit of junior anaesthesia staff practice'. *Br. J. Anaesth.*, 55, pp. 885–889.

Morgan, B.M., Bulpitt, C.J., Clifton, P., Lewis, P.J. (1984). 'The consumer attitude to obstetric care'. *British J. Obstetrics and Gynaecology*, 90, pp. 624–628.

Moss, N. (1984). 'Hospital units as social contexts: effects on maternal behaviour'. *Soc. Sci. Med.*, 19, pp. 515–522.

Mother and Baby Survey (1988). 'Having a baby in 1988'. *Mother and Baby*, October, pp. 8–11.

Munns, J., Galsworthy, E. (1995). 'Expectations of pregnancy and birth in first-time mothers'. *British Journal of Midwifery*, 3(4), pp. 231–236.

Nelson, M.K. (1982). 'The effect of childbirth preparation on women of different social classes'. *J. Health and Social Behaviour*, 23, pp. 339–352.

Nelson, M. (1983). 'Working class women, middle class women and models of childbirth'. *Social Problems*, 30, pp. 785–796.

Nettlebladt, P., Fagerstrom, C.F., Uddenberg, N. (1976). 'The significance of reported childbirth pain'. *J. Psychosomatic Research*, 20, pp. 215–221.

Niven, C., Gijsbers, K. (1984). 'Obstetric and non–obstetric factors related to labour pain'. *J. Reproductive and Infant Psychology*, 2, pp. 61–78.

Nordholm, L.A., Muhlen L. (1982). 'Experiences of childbirth: how effective is childbirth education?'. *Australian J. Physiotherapy*, 28, pp. 3–6.

Norr, K.L., Block, C.R., Charles, A., Meyering, S., Meyers, S. (1977). 'Explaining pain and enjoyment in childbirth'. *J. Health and Social Behaviour*, 18, pp. 260–273.

Oakley, A. (1980). *Women Confined: Towards a Sociology of Childbirth.* Oxford: Martin Robertson.

Oakley, A. (1983). 'Social consequences of obstetric technology: the importance of measuring "soft" outcomes'. *Birth*, 10, pp. 99–108.

Oakley, A., MacFarlane, A., Chalmers, I. (1982). 'Social class, stress and reproduction'. In: Rees, A.R, Purcell, H. (Eds). *Disease and the Environment.* Chichester: John Wiley.

Oakley, A., Richards, M.P.M. (1990). 'Women's experience of caesarean delivery'. In: Garcia, J., Kilpatrick, R., Richards, M.P.M. (Eds). *The Politics of Maternity Care.* Oxford: Oxford University Press.

Office of Population Censuses and Surveys (1988). *Birth Statistics 1986. England and Wales. Series FM1 No. 15.* London: HMSO.

Office of Population Censuses and Surveys (1988). *Hospital in–patient enquiry (England). Maternity Statistics 1985. OPCS Monitor MB4 88/1.* London: OPCS.

Office of Population Censuses and Surveys (1988). *OPCS Monitor MB4 88/1: Hospital in-patient enquiry (England). Maternity Statistics 1985.* London: OPCS.

Open University with the Health Education Council and the Scottish Health Education Group (1985). *Understanding Pregnancy and Birth.* Milton Keynes: The Open University.

Oppenheim, A.N. (1966). *Questionnaire Design and Attitude Measurement.* London: Heinemann.

Ounstead, M., Simons, C. (1979). 'Maternal attitudes to obstetric care'. *Early Human Development*, 3, pp. 201–204.

Paykel, E.S., Emms, E.M., Fletcher, J., Rassaby, E.S. (1980). 'Life events and social support in puerperal depression'. *British J. Psychiatry*, 136, pp. 339–346.

Peterson, G., Mehl, L. (1978). 'Some determinants of maternal attachment'. *American J. Psychiatry*, 135, pp. 1168–1173.

Philipp, E. (1986). 'Personal view'. *British Medical Journal*, 292, p. 1011.

Pitt, B. (1968). 'Atypical depression following childbirth'. *British J. Psychiatry*, 114, p. 1325.

Prendiville, W., Elbourne, D., Chalmers, I. (1988). 'The effects of routine oxytocic administration in the management of the third stage of labour; an overview of the evidence from controlled trials'. *British J. Obstetrics and Gynaecology*, 95, pp. 3–16.

Raphael-Leff, J. (1985). 'Facilitators and regulators: vulnerability to postnatal disturbance'. *J. Psychosomatic Obstetrics and Gynaecology*, 4, pp. 151–168.

Reid, M.E., Gutteridge, S., McIlwaine, G.M. (1982). *A Comparison of the Delivery of Antenatal Care between a Hospital and a Peripheral Clinic.* Glasgow: University of Glasgow.

Richards, M.P.M. (1982). 'The trouble with "choice" in childbirth'. *Birth*, 9, pp. 253–260.

Richards, M.P.M., Bernal, J.F. (1971). 'Social interaction in the first days of life'. In: Schaffer, M.R. (Ed). *The Origins of Human Social Relations.* London: Academic Press.

Riley, E.M.D. (1977). 'What do women want? The question of choice in the conduct of labour'. In: Chard, T., Richards, M. (Eds). *Benefits and Hazards of the New Obstetrics.* London: Spastics International Medical Publications.

Robson, K.M., Kumar, R. (1980). 'Delayed onset of maternal affection after childbirth: association with a routine obstetric procedure'. *British J. Psychiatry*, 136, pp. 347–353.

Romito, P. (1988). 'Post-partum depression or the medicalization of unhappiness'. Unpublished paper. Istituto Scientifico Burlo Garofalo, Trieste, Italy.
Savage, W. (1986). *A Savage Enquiry: Who Controls Childbirth?* London: Virago.
Shaw, N.S. (1974). *Forced Labour: Maternity Care in the United States.* New York: Pergamon Press.
Shearer, E.C. (1983). 'How do parents really feel after cesarean birth?'. *Birth*, 10, pp. 91–92.
Shearer, M.H. (1983). 'The difficulty of defining and measuring satisfaction with perinatal care'. *Birth*, 10, p. 77.
Shearer, M.H. (1987). 'Commentary: How well does the LADSI measure satisfaction with labor and delivery?'. *Birth*, 14, pp. 130–131.
Sikorski, J., Wilson, J., Clement, S., Das, S., Smeeton, N. (1996). 'A randomized controlled trial comparing two schedules of antenatal care visits: the antenatal care project'. *British Medical Journal*; 312, pp. 546–553.
Simkin, P. (1980). *The Birth Plan.* Seattle: Pennypress.
Slade, P., MacPherson, S.A., Hume, A, Maresh, M. (1993). 'Expectations, experiences and satisfaction with labour'. *British Journal of Clinical Psychology*, 32, pp. 469–483.
Sleep, J., Grant, A., Garcia, J., Elbourne, D., Spencer, J., Chalmers, I. (1984). 'West Berkshire perineal management trial'. *British Medical Journal*, 289, pp. 587–590.
Snell, M. (1983). 'A plan for birth'. *Nursing Times*, 79, pp. 62–63.
Society for Reproductive and Infant Psychology (1983). 'Painful satisfaction'. Editorial Bulletin, No. 4, *Society for Reproductive and Infant Psychology.*
Sosa, R., Kennell, J., Klaus, M., Robertson, S., Urrutia, J. (1980). 'The effect of a supportive companion on perinatal problems, length of labor and mother-infant interaction'. *New England J. Medicine*, 303, pp. 597–600.
Spielberger, C.D., Gorsuch, R.L., Lushene, R.E. (1970) *The State-Trait Anxiety Inventory.* Palo Alto: Consulting Psychologists Press.
Stein, A., Campbell, E.A., Day, A., McPherson, K., Cooper, P.J. (1987). 'Social adversity, low birth weight and pre-term delivery'. *British Medical Journal*, 295, pp. 291–293.
Stewart, A., Prandy, K., Blackburn, R.M. (1980). *Social Stratification and Occupations (Cambridge Studies in Sociology).* London: Macmillan.
Stewart, N. (1982). 'Natural third stage of labour – a personal account'. *AIMS Quarterly J.*, Autumn.
Stolte, K. (1987). 'A comparison of women's expectations of labor with the actual event'. *Birth*, 14, pp. 99–10.
Stone, M.L. (1979). 'Presidential address'. *American College of Obstetricians and Gynaecologists Newsletter*, 23, pp. 4–6.
Tanzer, D. (1968). 'Natural childbirth: pain or peak experience'. *Psychology Today*, 2, p. 17.
Tanzer, D. (1972). *Why Natural Childbirth?* New York: Schocken.
Timm, M.M. (1979). 'Prenatal education evaluation'. *Nursing Research*, 28, pp. 338–342.
Waldenström, U., Borg, I-M., Olsson, B., Sköld, M., Wall, S. (1996). 'The childbirth experience: A study of 295 new mothers'. *Birth*, 23, pp. 144–153.
Walker, B., Erdman, A. (1984). 'Childbirth education programs: the relation between confidence and knowledge'. *Birth*, 11, pp. 103–108.
Walker, J.M., Hall, S., Thomas, M. (1995). 'The experience of labour: a perspective from those receiving care in a midwife-led unit'. *Midwifery*, 11, pp. 120–129.
Ward, A. (1983). 'Syntometrine – a midwife's view'. *Association of Radical Midwives Newsletters*, No. 19, Summer.
Willmuth, L.R. (1975). 'Prepared childbirth and the concept of control'. *JOGNN*, 4, p. 38.
Woollett, A., Lyon, L., White, D. (1983). 'The reactions of East London women to medical intervention in childbirth'. *J. Reproductive and Infant Psychology*, 1, pp. 37–46.
World Health Organization (1985). *Having a Baby in Europe.* Report on a Study. Public Health in Europe, 26. Copenhagen, WHO.
Wright, J.T., Toplis, P.J. (1986). 'Alcohol in pregnancy'. *British J. Obstetrics and Gynaecology*, 93, pp. 201–202.
Zastowny, T.R., Roghmann, K.J., Hengst, A. (1983). 'Satisfaction with medical care: replications and theoretic re-evaluation'. *Medical Care*, 21, pp. 294–322.

Publications from Great Expectations

Green, J., Coupland, V., Kitzinger, J. (1990). 'Expectations, experiences and psychological outcomes of childbirth: a prospective study of 825 women'. *Birth,* 17(1), pp. 15–24.

Green, J.M., Kitzinger, J.V., Coupland, V.A. (1990). 'Stereotypes of childbearing women: a look at some evidence'. *Midwifery,* 6, pp. 1–8.

Green, J.M. (1990). 'Who is unhappy after childbirth?: Antenatal and intrapartum correlates from a prospective study'. *J. of Reproductive & Infant Psychology,* 8, pp. 175–83.

Green, J., Richards, M., Kitzinger, J., Coupland, V. (1991). 'Mothers' perceptions of their 6-week-old babies: Relationship with antenatal, intrapartum and postnatal factors'. *Irish Journal of Psychology,* 12, pp. 133–144.

Green, J.M. (1993). 'Expectations and experiences of pain in labor: Findings from a large prospective study'. *Birth,* 20(2), pp. 65–72.

Green, J., Kitzinger, J., Coupland, V. (1994). 'Midwives responsibilities, medical staffing structures and women's choice in childbirth'. In: Robinson, S., Thomson, A. (Eds). *Midwives, Research and Childbirth* Vol. III. London: Routledge, Chapman and Hall.

Green, J.M. (1996). 'Do women want to be involved in decision making?'. Paper presented to the Changing Childbirth Workshop on 'Unbiased Information and Risk Assessment', July 1995, summary published in the workshop proceedings by the NHS Executive (DoH).

Publications based on data from the Cambridge Prenatal Screening Study

Green, J., Statham, H., Snowdon, C. (1991). 'EPDS by post'. (letter) *British Journal of Psychiatry,* 158, p. 865.

Statham, H., Green, J., Snowdon, C. (1991). 'When is a fetus a dead baby?'. (letter) *Lancet,* 6th April.

Green, J., Statham, H., Snowdon, C. (1992). 'Screening for fetal abnormality: attitudes and experiences'. In: Chard, T., Richards, M.P.M. (Eds). *Obstetrics in the 1990's: Current Controversies.* London: MacKeith.

Statham, H., Green, J., Snowdon, C. (1992). 'Psychological and social aspects of screening for fetal abnormality during routine antenatal care'. In: *Proceedings of Research and the Midwife.* November.

Statham, H., Green, J., Snowdon, C., France-Dawson, M. (1993). 'Choice of baby's sex'. (letter) *Lancet,* 341, pp. 564–65.

Green, J.M., Murray, D. (1994). 'The use of the EPDS in research to explore the relationship between antenatal and postnatal dysphoria'. In: Cox, J.L., Holden, J. (Eds). *Perinatal Psychiatry: Use and Misuse of the Edinburgh Postnatal Depression Scale.* London: Gaskell Press.

Statham, H., Green, J.M. (1994). 'The effects of miscarriage and other "unsuccessful" pregnancies on feelings early in a subsequent pregnancy'. *Journal of Reproductive and Infant Psychology,* 12, pp. 45–54.

Green, J.M., Snowdon, C., Statham, H. (1993). 'Pregnant women's attitudes to abortion and prenatal screening'. *Journal of Reproductive and Infant Psychology,* 11, pp. 31–39.

Green, J.M., Statham, H., Snowdon, C. (1993). 'Women's knowledge of prenatal screening tests. 1: Relationships with hospital screening policy and demographic factors'. *Journal of Reproductive and Infant Psychology*, 11, pp. 11–20.

Richards, M.P.M., Green, J.M. (1993). 'Attitudes toward prenatal screening for fetal abnormality and detection of carriers of genetic disease: a discussion paper'. *Journal of Reproductive and Infant Psychology*, 11, pp. 49–56.

Statham, H., Green, J., Snowdon, C. (1993). 'Mothers' consent to screening newborn babies for disease'. (letter) *British Medical Journal*, 306, pp. 858-59.

Green, J.M., France-Dawson, M. (1993). 'Women's experiences of routine screening during pregnancy: the sickle cell study'. Proceedings of a symposium entitled *Targeting Health Promotion: Reaching Those in Need.* Cambridge: Health Promotion Research Trust.

Green, J.M., France-Dawson, M. (1997). 'Women's experiences of screening in pregnancy: ethnic differences in the West Midlands'. In: Clarke, A., Parsons, E. (Eds). *Culture, Kinship and Genes.* Basingstoke: Macmillan Press.

Green, J.M., Kafetsios, K. (1997). 'Positive experiences of early motherhood: predictive variables from a longitudinal study'. *Journal of Reproductive & Infant Psychology*, 15, pp. 141–157.

Green, J.M. (1998). 'Postnatal depression or perinatal dysphoria? Findings from a longitudinal community-based study using the Edinburgh Postnatal Depression Scale'. *Journal of Reproductive & Infant Psychology* (in press).

Statham, H., Green, J. M., Kafetsios, K. (1997). 'Who worries that something might be wrong with the baby? A prospective study of 1062 pregnant women'. *Birth* (in press).

List of Appendices

Appendix A

Appendix B

Appendix C

Appendix D

A complete set of these appendices can be obtained from *Book for Midwives Press* at the address below.

Books for Midwives Press
174a Ashley Road
Hale
Cheshire
WA15 9SF

Tel: 0161 929 0929